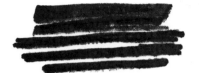

3/7/2000

FUNDAMENTALS OF HEALTHCARE FINANCIAL MANAGEMENT

A Practical Guide to Fiscal Issues and Activities

STEVEN BERGER, CHE, FHFMA, MS, CPA

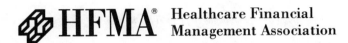 **HFMA**® Healthcare Financial Management Association

Educational Foundation

McGraw-Hill

New York   San Francisco   Washington, D.C.   Auckland   Bogotá
Caracas   Lisbon   London   Madrid   Mexico City   Milan
Montreal   New Delhi   San Juan   Singapore
Sydney   Tokyo   Toronto

Library of Congress Cataloging-in-Publication Data

Berger, Steven H.
    Fundamentals of healthcare financial management: a practical
guide to fiscal issues and activities / Steven Berger.
        p.   cm.
    Includes bibliographical references and index.
    ISBN 0-07-134671-6
    1. Health facilities—Business management.   2. Health facilities—
Finance.   I. Title.
RA971.3.B465   1999
362.1'068'1—dc21   99–23627
                                                              CIP

McGraw-Hill

*A Division of The **McGraw·Hill** Companies*

1 2 3 4 5 6 7 8 9 0 BKM/BKM 9 0 9 8 7

ISBN 007-134671-6

Printing and binding by Book-Mart Press, Inc.

Cover illustration by Steve Dininno.

This book was typeset using 10 point Times Roman.

This publication is designed to provide accurate and authoritative
information in regard to the subject matter covered. It is sold with the
understanding that neither the author nor the publisher is engaged in
rendering legal, accounting, or other professional service. If legal
advice or other expert assistance is required, the services of a
competent professional person should be sought.

> *—From a Declaration of Principles jointly adopted by a Committee
> of the American Bar Association and a Committee of Publishers.*

*To the memory of my dad, Jack Berger, who always
inspired me to do more.*
May he rest in peace.

PREFACE

Starting now, we will embark on a journey into the interesting and compelling world of the healthcare financial manager. Because of the nature of the work, and though not on the front line of the patient's care, the healthcare financial manager needs to be involved in or apprised of all decisions related to the operations or planning of the facility. Because of this, the financial manager develops a unique understanding of the business of healthcare.

And whether the business is in hospitals, skilled nursing facilities, physician offices, home health agencies, psychiatric facilities, or any of the other operations doing business in this industry, the basic concepts are essentially the same. Healthcare and the way it is financed have several characteristics unique to this industry alone. Following are the most important.

1. The health insurance system separates the consumer from the buying decision. Because of this, the consumer seldom has had to make a rational choice in the amount or level of product consumption. This is the number one reason that the cost of healthcare is so high in America.

2. The healthcare system is pluralistic—a mixture of government and nongovernment providers and payors.

3. The payment system is very technical and complex. Every payor has a different set of benefits and often they are not spelled out clearly. The consumer (patient) may believe they have a certain set of benefits, but when they finally need care, they may find out that they, in fact, are not covered for that particular set of illnesses or therapies. This often puts the provider in the difficult situation of denying or postponing care until these coverage issues are settled.

4. Ultimately, though, healthcare is personal. And it affects everyone. No other industry provides the intensity of emotions engendered in healthcare. The patient, whose illness may lead to death, or in the case of maternity care, life, is always at personal risk. So, too, are the loved ones who congregate around the patient and the provider, often with great anxiety and trepidation.

This then is why healthcare, and the way it is financed, is so important. It helps to explain why the role of the finance manager takes on a great importance within the industry. The financial manager is responsible for the financial reporting and the budget, both of which summarize financial results of the organization, both actual and projected. These summaries are a direct reflection of the decisions made before the fiscal year begins and day to day as the year moves along. The astute financial manager, who needs to learn as much about every aspect of the organization's operation as possible, is often in a better position than any other manager to assess the operation in an objective and nonpartisan manner.

At the same time, the healthcare financial manager will need to learn, understand, and absorb a series of rules, regulations, policies, and procedures that reflect the highly unique world of American healthcare practices and its finances. This book is dedicated to the proposition that the reader can learn much about the unique financial underpinnings of this industry. There is so much to know and so little time. The challenge is how to make these complex ideas presentable in a basic text.

Imagine, if you will, an industry in which the billing rules for only one of its many payors, Medicare, is 45,000 pages long. Then imagine, that in 1997, Medicare's enforcement division claiming that billing mistakes constitute fraud, not honest errors.

Or, an industry in which the largest group of nongovernmental payors, known as health maintenance organizations (HMOs), or preferred provider organizations (PPOs), commonly referred to as managed care, create incentives to their contracted providers of care—the hospitals, doctors, and other caregivers—to limit the care given. This is done in the name of saving money for the premium payor, usually the employer. Yet, these same insurers generally do not provide coverage for screening tests that could either rule out or determine illness, which when caught early, would cost those self-same insurers less money through less intensive treatments.

Okay, so you get the idea. Crazy policies. Not always in the best interest of the patient. More than likely in the best interest of the insurer. But also ask yourself, when was the last time you reached into your own pocket to pay the full list price for your healthcare. Most probably never. Very few employed, elderly, or poor people in America have. And they seldom ask the question, which we will do, "Why does healthcare cost so much?" The biggest part of the answer is because when one of your loved ones get sick, you will spare no expense (primarily the insurance company's money) to make sure he or she gets well. The providers of care in America have therefore built their industry to respond to the needs and desires of the market.

The problem here is what the market desires is conflicted. Because very few patients (customers) pay out of pocket, the patient's desires are often at odds with the desires of the payors and employers who pay the premiums. Caught in the middle then are the providers, attempting to be cost-efficient, provide quality outcomes, and produce high levels of patient satisfaction while earning a positive financial return on their investment.

How it happened and how a particular provider contributes to the overall industry expenditures provides a case study for learning. This book will cover the basic healthcare financial management issues but from a distinct perspective. You, the reader, will get to act like a healthcare financial manager for the most common financial reporting period, a year. Starting on January 1, you will experience the highs and lows of a healthcare finance officer as he weaves his way through busy times and slow times (mostly busy!) and through the conflicting issues that populate the healthcare financing landscape.

This particular book is written from the perspective of a finance officer for a hospital. However, many of the other primary industry providers are also profiled because this case-studied organization also operates a hospital-based skilled nursing facility, home health agency, psychiatric unit, and it employs a dozen physicians in office practices.

Finally, this text is not intended as an academic treatise. Rather, it is intended as a practical guide to how an integrated healthcare finance division operates in this era, on a day-to-day basis. It is an attempt to meld practice with theory. As we go through the year, various concepts will be highlighted and re-highlighted, just as it often really happens. This will help to clarify those issues that are of overriding importance to sound financial management.

Steven Berger

A C K N O W L E D G E M E N T S

I would like to thank a number of people for bringing me to this point in my life where the opportunity to write this book coincided with the reality. On the professional side, I would like to thank two of the best bosses anyone could possibly be lucky enough to have had, Ken Knieser and Jack Gilbert, for never telling me to stop doing what I thought was right. Also, John Dalton, for encouraging me to become a writer and editor of healthcare finance material more than 10 years ago. Finally, my thanks to Jim Curcuruto, who, over 20 years ago, was the very first professional I worked with to take the time to stop what he was doing and give me my first taste of understanding healthcare finance concepts.

I would also like to thank those people with the experience and knowledge to help me improve this book. They took the time and effort to read the entire manuscript in draft and offer terrific suggestions for refinement and embellishment. They are my very good friends Mary Grace Wilkus, Bob Carlisle, and the aforementioned Jack Gilbert and Ken Knieser.

In addition, several people with expertise in some very specific healthcare financial management areas contributed their time and effort to review those sections and offer cogent comments that helped to improve this book. They are Catherine Kleinmuntz for capital decision analysis, Vincent Ciotti for information systems, Bruce Kite for corporate compliance, and Theresa Bebout for physician practice management.

I would also like to thank my staff at Highland Park Hospital for doing such a good job that I felt comfortable taking the time to write this book. My particular thanks to Keri Wulf, Guy Sanchez, and Diana Wright without whom I would not be as effective, and my secretary Patty Holland who always keeps me heading in the direction I need to be going.

On the personal side, I am indebted to my family who made the biggest sacrifice in the creation of this book. The nights and weekends I labored on the book often took me away from them. My wife Barbara kept the household together, holding a menagerie of very active children in a relative state of equilibrium. I am blessed to have four kids who keep me younger in spirit than in body. Ben, Arlie, and Emmalee make me smile all the time. But how would I have ever been able to finish this book without Sam who looked over my shoulder every day to check my progress and whisper encouragement in my ear, like, "Come on, Dad, what do you mean you did only one page since yesterday. Let's move it, move it, move it."

C O N T E N T S

Chapter 3

March   53

Chapter 4

April   80

Chapter 5

May   108

Chapter 6

June   133

Chapter 7

July 159

Chapter 8

August 190

1
C H A P T E R

January

"Daddy, what do you do all day at work?" the seven year old asked plaintively.

"What do you mean?" blinked Samuel Barnes, the daddy.

"You know, like when you go out so early in the morning and then don't come back until after other daddies are already home. What are you doing, and why does it take so long?" asked the curly haired tot.

Sam had to think for a moment. "Well, honey, that's a good question. I guess I'm out there trying to make the hospital I work for as successful as it can be."

"But what do you do?" she asked again.

"Susie, I am in charge of all the money that comes into the hospital. I'm also responsible for all the money that is paid out to the people who work there and all the other people who send us stuff that we have to use to make the sick people better, like food and medicine," said Sam.

"Daddy, do you ever have any money left over after you pay these people?"

"Well, Susie, that's the whole point. To be successful, you want to have as much left over as you can."

"But, Daddy, what do you do with all that leftover money? Do you put it in the bank like I do with my allowance?"

"Well, sort of. But instead of putting it into the bank, we put it into a kind of bank that lends it out to other people who need money in their businesses. They then pay us back with a little extra money to thank us for letting them use our money for a while. It's called interest."

"So, Daddy, the hospital has all this leftover money and then you have even more money from these other people or companies paying you interest. I'm glad that you work at a company that is doing well because I heard on the news the other night that some people were losing their jobs. I guess you or any of the people who you work with won't lose their jobs."

"Actually, Susie, I wish I could tell you it was that clear-cut, but it is not. Part of my job is to make sure that the hospital makes as much money as we decided we wanted to make before the year starts. Sometimes that means that we believe we will need less people working for us if we think less people will come to the hospital to be taken care of."

"But, Daddy," Susie asked quizzically, "how can you know about all these things?"

"Ah, honey," he said, "that's a long story."

It is one minute past midnight on January 1.

Outside, the New Year's revelers are just beginning their celebrations. Inside the bowels of the powerful computers of Ridgeland Heights Medical Center (RHMC), a different kind of ritual is taking place. At this time, the automated pricing mechanism is executing its programming, effectively increasing the 10,000 or so charges related to individual services or supplies provided to patients. These increases, so carefully planned, are meant to help the organization improve its bottom line.

How these charges came to be, and why they are important, is only a small part to the story that constitutes the *art* of healthcare financial management. Financial management in most any industry will have its own policies, procedures, and practices. In most cases, generally accepted accounting principles (GAAP) and financial procedures will require estimates and approximations based on the company's and the estimator's previous experiences within the industry. These experiences are often time-worn. Financial statements are produced month after month, year after year. Over time, most companies doing business within any industry will report financial results in conformance with industry standards.

Standards are "something considered by an authority or by general consent to be an approved or acceptable model."[1] In the healthcare industry, these standards represent the ability to properly report the operating results for any particular period of time requested as well as the net assets of any organization.

For RHMC, the price increase, although not entirely desired by the organization's administration because of its possible negative public relations, is vital to its continued financial success. The size of the price increase is a function of volume, severity, and expense changes that have been forecast and budgeted by the medical center. These changes are the result of strategic planning initiatives, newly planned services, payor mix shifts, and demographic fluctuations. They are also related to expense increases and/or decreases projected as a result of the volume changes.

---

[1] Random House Unabridged Dictionary, 2nd ed. 1993.

This book examines these issues and many more. To begin to get an understanding of healthcare financial management and many of its key components it is necessary to build a framework from which to operate. This framework takes the form of a diary and a primer. It is a year in the life of one healthcare institution and one healthcare financial administrator. It explores how this organization, its board of directors, and its clinical and financial executives go about making decisions and how these decisions are then implemented. It further explores it through the natural life cycle of the institution, day by day and month by month, just as a real institution operates.

This book offers practical and informative points on healthcare decision making, usually from the financial point of view. In the end, the book's objective is to create a greater understanding of how the industry operates on a detailed financial level. Our fictional medical center, Ridgeland Heights, was chosen because its bed complement of 256 falls in the range of a great deal of hospitals in the United States today. According to Health, United States, 1996/1997 Edition, an annual compilation of healthcare statistics across the United States, of the 33 million admissions to all hospitals in 1994, 6.5 million admission were made to hospitals in the 200–299 bed range. When you add up the admissions of hospitals in the 100–399 bed range, the result is 17.3 million, just over 50% of all admissions.[2] Thus, this book is representative of more than half of the typical hospitals in the country.

Before we begin to explore healthcare financial management systems and techniques, it is necessary to first define some terms.

WHAT IS HEALTHCARE?

What is healthcare? Healthcare is "the field concerned with the maintenance or restoration of the health of the body or mind."[3] This may seem obvious. Maybe not! The healthcare industry at the current time encompasses much more than just hospitals and doctors. And although together they make up the majority of industry expenditures, there are considerable numbers of other reputable healthcare providers that make up the remainder. Table 1–1 shows the current breakdown of expenditures within the healthcare industry.

Remarkably, the largest growing segment of the industry is in the "other" category. "Alternative" or "complementary" medicine currently dominates this category. This is generally categorized as non-Western therapies, which are not currently accepted as a standard of care by most U.S. doctors. Some therapies included in this grouping are chiropractic, massage therapy, acupuncture, Chinese herbal medicine, aromatherapy, meditation, and yoga. According to a study published in the *New England Journal of Medicine* (NEJM) in 1993, consumers spent about $13.7 billion on alternative care in 1990.[4] Of that amount, $10.3 billion was out-of-pocket expenditures,

---

[2] National Center for Health Statistics. (1997). *Health, United States, 1996/1997*. With Socioeconomic Status and Health Chartbook, Hyattsville, Md.

[3] Random House Unabridged Dictionary, 2nd ed., 1993.

[4] Eisenberg, D.M., et al. (1993). Unconventional Medicine in the United States. *New England Journal of Medicine* 328(4):246.

TABLE 1-1

Current Breakdown of Expenditures within the Healthcare Industry

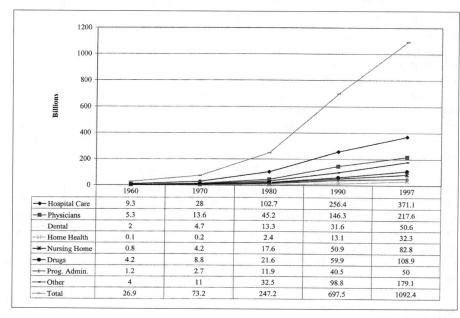

	1960	1970	1980	1990	1997
Hospital Care	9.3	28	102.7	256.4	371.1
Physicians	5.3	13.6	45.2	146.3	217.6
Dental	2	4.7	13.3	31.6	50.6
Home Health	0.1	0.2	2.4	13.1	32.3
Nursing Home	0.8	4.2	17.6	50.9	82.8
Drugs	4.2	8.8	21.6	59.9	108.9
Prog. Admin.	1.2	2.7	11.9	40.5	50
Other	4	11	32.5	98.8	179.1
Total	26.9	73.2	247.2	697.5	1092.4

not paid for by any insurance. The NEJM study further indicated that 34% of the respondents in the national survey said they had used at least one alternative therapy in the past year. The important principle here is the recognition of the industry's breadth. It would be foolhardy to jump to any particular conclusions on its size or scope.

Still, the industry is huge and has grown that way in the most dramatic fashion over the past 30 years, really starting its climb in 1966 with the advent of the Medicare and Medicaid programs. These programs are explored in greater detail in Chapter 4. However, suffice it to say that these programs opened the floodgates of money to the industry. At the time the programs began, the industry absorbed 5.7% of the gross domestic product (GDP) in the country.[5] The GDP is the market value of goods and services produced by labor and property located in the United States. In the intervening 32 years, the percentage of GDP has grown to 13.4%, a 235% increase.[6] This means that, as a country, we have decided, either by intent or accident, to expend a considerable amount of additional national resources and wealth in the pursuit of our health.

It is important to note that the 13.4% of the GDP absorbed for healthcare by the United States leads the industrialized world—by a large margin. The next five

[5] National Center for Health Statistics. (1997). *Health, United States, 1996*, Hyattsville, Md., p. 250.
[6] Ibid.

highest GDPs by country are Canada at 9.8%, Austria and France at 9.7%, Switzerland at 9.6%, and Germany at 9.5%.[7] So, the United States spends significantly more on healthcare than anyplace else in the world. And there are many reasons for this. First, Americans have more discretionary income than anyone else and have chosen to spend some of it on healthcare. Second, Americans have been trained over the past 50 years (since World War II) to expect unlimited treatments for illnesses. This training has come from organized medicine—defined as the American Medical Association, the American Hospital Association, the American College of Surgeons, and many more groups. Healthcare is big business and major administrative services have sprung up to handle the load.

Table 1–1 highlights the financial scope of the healthcare industry. It is over one trillion dollars. $1,000,000,000,000. That's a lot of zeros. It is also the total amount of money spent on healthcare services in 1996. This means that there are tremendous resources available to the companies that service patients. Tremendous resources and tremendous opportunities! Healthcare is now one of the largest industries in the country. This money should be consumed in the pursuit of the best possible outcomes, provided in the most consumer friendly way, and at the least possible cost. That is the role and objective of healthcare. And the financial manager plays a large role in trying to achieve these outcomes through his or her involvement and leadership in budget planning and reporting, charge setting, contract negotiations, and general financial consulting to the organization's department managers.

WHAT IS MANAGEMENT?

Before looking for a definition of financial management, it is first important to define general management. In most for-profit firms, management's overarching objective is to maximize the owners' or shareholders' wealth. In order to accomplish this goal, management has been assigned roles and responsibilities that are generally defined as the following.

- Leading
- Planning
- Organizing
- Coordinating
- Motivating
- Controlling

In the case of the healthcare industry, an overwhelming majority of hospitals and skilled nursing facilities are classified as not-for-profit through section 501(c)(3) of the Internal Revenue Code. Still, although not-for-profit, healthcare industry managers are required to produce the best possible bottom line. They simply need to do so in the context of providing optimal patient care in the most efficient manner.

---

[7] Ibid.

In the for-profit world, "management must administer the assets of the enterprise in order to obtain the greatest wealth for the owner."[8] Therefore, management's goal is to find the combination of earnings, and the associated risk involved in producing those earnings, that will yield the highest possible value.

In the not-for-profit world, earnings or profits are called margins. In the case of both for-profit and not-for profit healthcare firms, the profits or margins are what remains after expenses, or costs, are subtracted from revenues. So, to reiterate, the role of management is to produce the best possible financial outcomes while minimizing risk to the organization. The healthcare industry places a somewhat greater emphasis on social goals as well, but in the end, management's success or failure as defined by each organization's board of directors is primarily related to the quality of its bottom line.

WHAT IS FINANCIAL MANAGEMENT?

Financial management can be defined as the strategizing of the organization's financial direction as well as the performance of its day-to-day financial operation.

Therefore, financial management has a twofold purpose. The first one is to provide the strategic financial direction of the organization. This function is usually performed at the executive level of the financial ladder by the chief financial officer (CFO). The primary job is to prepare and present the organization's strategic financial plan to the board for endorsement and approval. In many organizations this job may also include the treasury function, which is charged with investing the organization's financial assets in the most prudent manner as set down in the board-approved investment policies.

The second purpose is management of the day-to-day financial operations of an organization. The organization's second in command finance officer, often called a controller, usually carries this out. The function means making sure that the payroll and suppliers are paid and the revenues generated by the operation are billed out in an accurate and timely manner and collected efficiently with a minimum of write-offs.

Financial management has a role within the overall context of general management. Sound financial management will aid the general managers in the six management concepts expressed previously. According to Berman, Weeks, and Kukla, "financial management tools and techniques can aid management in providing the community with quality services at least cost by furnishing the data that are necessary for making intelligent capital investment decisions, by guiding the operations of certain hospital subsystems, and by providing the systems and data needed to monitor and control operations."[9]

So, providing data and helping to analyze the financial implications of the data across the healthcare organization's setting is a primary role of financial management.

---

[8] Berman, H.J., Weeks, L.E., Kukla, S.F. (1986). *The Financial Management of Hospitals*, 6th ed., Health Administration Press, Ann Arbor, Mich., p. 4.

[9] Ibid, p. 6.

Financial management involves the finance staff in a number of highly visible and important matters, such as the following.

- The setting of prices for the services provided (often called gross charges)
- The production and analysis of the discounts (often called contractual allowances) taken by a third-party payor—defined as anyone other than the patient who pays for the patient's services (The large third-party payors are Medicare, Medicaid, and hundreds of different managed care organizations [MCOs and often called HMOs or PPOs] across the country.)
- The recording and analyzing of cost information across the organization and at the department level (This involves comparing actual costs to budgeted costs and determining variance analysis. It may also involve a more detailed cost accounting program.)
- The preparing and reporting of financial projections to help successfully guide the organization in its future endeavors (Short-term projections [up to a year into the future] are called budgets and long-term projections [one to five years into the future] are called strategic financial plans.)

There is much more to financial management. The above is merely an opening view of some of the issues involved in financial management.

WHY IS FINANCIAL MANAGEMENT IMPORTANT?

Financial management has both a primary and a secondary role in the financial health of the healthcare organization. Its secondary role constitutes the reporting of financial results on a periodic basis, usually monthly. Its primary role, however, is as a broker of information. Those who control the information usually have quite a bit of power in any organization. The finance division of most organizations, and in most industries, have generally been the storers and reporters of information.

Remember there is very little success that an organization can have without the proper financial information with which to base its decisions. The whole purpose of having and using information is to make the most appropriate decisions. Making decisions is any manager's number one priority. Making the proper decision is a function of experience and appropriate information.

Keep in mind that there is a significant difference between information and raw data. Data streams inundate most managers all day long. Raw data are often useless, sometimes harmful in the process of making the best decision. The value of information is that it brings *context* to the data, presenting them in a format that enhances a manager's ability to understand what is happening and to make good decisions.

In the section above, management was described as the art of making decisions, usually under uncertain conditions. Thus, financial management can be said to be important because, if applied properly, it maximizes the operating manager's ability to make good decisions, under uncertainty, by presenting information in the best possible format. In addition, it allows the finance division to maximize reimbursement (net revenues) for the healthcare organization. (This is covered in Chapter 4.)

TABLE 1-2

Ridgeland Heights Medical Center
1998 Actual and 1999 Budgeted Inpatient Volumes

		Admissions			Patient Days			Length of Stay		
	No. of of Beds	1998 Actual	1999 Budget	Percent Variance	1998 Actual	1999 Budget	Percent Variance	1998 Actual	1999 Budget	Percent Variance
Medical/ surgical	120	2,700	2,800	3.7	13,000	14,000	7.7	4.81	5.00	3.8
Intensive care	24	1,800	1,900	5.6	6,500	7,220	11.1	3.61	3.80	5.2
Pediatrics	10	600	660	10.0	1,500	1,716	14.4	2.50	2.60	4.0
Maternity	24	2,000	2,200	10.0	4,000	4,400	10.0	2.00	2.00	0.0
Births	26	1,950	2,145	10.0	3,900	4,290	10.0	2.00	2.00	0.0
Psychiatric	20	1,000	1,200	20.0	6,500	8,160	25.5	6.50	6.80	4.6
Skilled nursing facility	30	800	840	5.0	8,800	8,400	−4.5	11.0	10.0	−9.1
Totals	254	10,850	11,745	8.2	44,200	48,186	9.0	4.07	4.10	0.7

RIDGELAND HEIGHTS MEDICAL CENTER

The Primary Statistics

Ridgeland Heights Medical Center is a medium-sized medical center in a northern Chicago suburb. For Internal Revenue Code purposes, it was classified as a community, not-for-profit hospital under Internal Revenue Code Section 501(c)(3) because of its charitable mission dating back to 1925. In addition to its current complement of 180 acute care medical and surgical beds, it also has a 20-bed maternity unit, a 22-bed Medicare PPS-exempt psychiatric unit, a Medicare-certified home health agency (HHA) and hospice, and a 30-bed hospital based skilled nursing facility (SNF).

Ridgeland Heights also owns 10 primary care physician practice sites, which employ 13 full time physicians. This practice is managed through a corporate affiliated management service organization (MSO), which also manages 6 nonowned primary care physician practices.

In addition, RHMC is half owner of a physician hospital organization (PHO), the other half owned by an independent practice association (IPA), a group of physicians legally organized to negotiate contracts with managed care organizations (MCOs). The PHO negotiates contracts on behalf of both the medical center and the IPA. In many instances, this is well received by the managed care companies because of its time-saving and cost-reducing principles.

Volume indicators are critical to understanding any institution. It generally defines the level of financial viability. RHMC provides both inpatient and outpatient services. Table 1–2 highlights the *inpatient* volumes for the year just ended as well as the current budgeted year.

T A B L E   1–3

Ridgeland Heights Medical Center
1998 Actual and 1999 Budgeted Outpatient Visits

	Visits		
	1998 Actual	**1999 Budget**	**Percentage Variance**
Emergency department	19,000	20,000	5.3
Outpatient surgery	4,500	5,000	11.1
Same day surgery	3,700	4,000	8.1
Observation patients	1,950	2,000	2.6
Home health services	26,000	30,000	15.4
Other outpatients	112,000	120,000	7.1
Total	167,150	181,000	8.29

While the medical center had always received a majority of its gross revenues from its inpatient services the 11,000 or so inpatient admissions are now dwarfed by over 180,000 outpatient services each year. (See Table 1–3 for the analysis.) This brought a series of unexpected consequences to the medical center. Although the administration had, for several years talked about redefining its service lines to be somewhat more aligned with the outpatient business, it had not yet done so. The continuing decline in the inpatient census coupled with the outpatient increases drove the powers-that-be to complete plans for a renovation and expansion, primarily for improved and updated outpatient and physician services. At the same time, the medical center has decided to take some dramatic action with regards to its dwindling inpatient census.

Managed Care Inroads

Over the past few years, managed care companies have made significant inroads into RHMC's primary and secondary service areas. In doing so, these companies have brought with them a utilization review philosophy that generally reduces access to care to those beneficiaries covered by these insurances. This was not by accident. The employers, who usually foot the bills for employee medical insurance, had grown tired of the seemingly never-ending round of double digit premium increases each year throughout the 1980s. When the old-style indemnity insurance, which generally paid the healthcare providers (hospitals, physicians, SNFs, home health agencies, etc.) failed to reign in these increases, the employers turned to the managed care companies.

Managed care companies claimed that they could control the rate of premium increases using a series of strategies that would reduce both the number of healthcare

BOX 1–1

COST CONTROL STRATEGIES USED BY MANAGED CARE ORGANIZATIONS

UTILIZATION CONTROLS

- Preauthorization of necessity (before approval for service)
- Second opinions to determine need for service or alternatives
- Concurrent review and case management of continuing service necessity during hospital stays
- Quality management programs, monitoring treatment type, and duration for outpatient services
- Patient outcomes research to determine efficacy of new clinical services

REIMBURSEMENT AND PAYMENT CONTROLS

- Minimizing level of payments to service providers through tough negotiations
- Approval of payment methodologies that minimize provider incentives to continue treatments
- Imposition of patient copayments to discourage utilization of services

provider contacts as well as the intensity of the services received. Box 1–1 summarizes the cost control strategies used by managed care companies.

RHMC's Actions to Counter Dwindling Inpatient Census

The rate of decline in the inpatient census was alarming to the RHMC administration. They recognized that the decline in the inpatient census was partially causing the increase in the lower-paying outpatient services. Still, to maintain viability as a full service medical center, the administration knew they needed to increase the admissions. They determined that there were only a few ways to do this.

1. Steal market share from other service providers (always an option in any business in any industry. The secret was not in the trying but in the succeeding). This could be attempted in the following ways.

   - Improved and/or more consumer marketing—historically not the most effective means. Healthcare is an industry that has historically resisted consumer marketing because referrals have generally been through physicians and more recently through managed care contractual coverages.
   - Improved and/or more physician marketing.

- A better mix of clinical services—this would be a much more effective strategy given the reasons that previous marketing strategies have not worked. A healthcare organization that can meet the demands of the physicians and the payors is more likely to survive and thrive in the current climate of downsized institutions.
2. Grow the market share by providing services that are not being provided in the service area. This could mean being on the leading edge of technology (a potentially very expensive place to be) or assessing the local market through focus groups and surveys to determine the current needs, wants, and desires of the community. An example of this could be alternative or complementary care services, as mentioned earlier in this chapter.
3. Grow market share by recruiting additional physicians at RHMC and encouraging physicians who practice at more than one hospital to practice exclusively at RHMC.

RHMC Decision Time

RHMC, through its administration, decided to try a mix of solutions. It would perform more targeted marketing and advertising to highlight those services where it already had a substantial clinical advantage as well as those services that it wanted to build on.[10] In addition, it plans to build new services, particularly outpatient surgeries and services, that appear to be where the heaviest industry growth is headed. Finally, it will put some of its limited financial and intellectual resources into developing more advanced clinical services (often called tertiary services) to differentiate itself from some of its other community-based, nonacademic teaching facility competitors.

Financial Management Implications

Almost every decision made by the healthcare organization's administration has financial management implications. There should be intended consequences that were expected and in fact desired when the decision was made. There are also *unintended consequences,* those results that were unforeseen. (There is a 100% likelihood of it happening!) In any event, the finance division will be counted on (no pun intended) to provide the most appropriate and conservative estimate of the likely projected financial results. This usually means producing what are called pro formas, which are projected income statements, incorporating all known assumptions. This should be done using assumptions that represent best case, worst case, and most likely scenarios.

---

[10] The concept of target marketing and advertising in healthcare is complex because it is difficult to identify the decision makers who ultimately purchase the service. For instance, is it the patient, patient's family, physician, insurer, or someone else? The answer is, it depends on the particular healthcare service.

PRO FORMA DEVELOPMENT

The development of pro formas is extremely important to the financial well being of the organization. Pro formas are usually performed when the organization is planning to develop a new service or acquire any type of equipment, the capitalized cost of which exceeds some internally generated amount of money. They are also usually performed in conjunction with the organization's strategic plan. While this book goes into some detail on the concept of strategic plans, strategic financial plans, capital goods and capital budgeting in Chapter 3, for now let us assume that RHMC always performs pro forma analysis for all capital acquisitions costing more than $500,000.

Net Present Values and Internal Rates of Return

The art of pro forma development is best described as the ability to assemble a series of assumptions that lead to *go/no go* decisions with respect to capital acquisition. This is generally accomplished by having the final result of the pro forma produce either a net present value (NPV) or internal rate of return (IRR) for the project.

NPV is defined as the present value of the future cash inflows of an investment less the investment's cash outflows. Whereas NPV measures a project's *dollar* profitability, IRR measures a project's *percentage* profitability, or its expected rate of return.[11] These computations summarize a sizable number of assumptions into a single percentage that has value to the decision maker. The organization may well have a "hurdle rate" established for its IRR for a new project. A hurdle rate is defined as the minimum percentage return that the organization expects to achieve through funding of the project. The hurdle rate reflects the percentage return on its investment that the organization wants to realize. It is a function of the amount of interest income it could earn if it were to invest in the stock or bond market and the additional risk associated with the volume and rate projections used in the pro forma. By concluding a pro forma with an IRR, it is easy, at a glance, to determine whether the hurdle rate has been exceeded, thus providing the decision maker with the appropriate information with which to make the go/no go decision.

The reason for establishing hurdle rates and internal rates of return involves money (i.e., the capital resources used to pay for all purchases, whether it be operating expenses or capital expenses). Money, or the organization's capital, is scarce. There is always a list of conflicting priorities to be funded. Therefore, it is imperative that any healthcare organization establish its own hurdle rate, know why they did so, and stick to it if they plan to stay financially viable into the future.

Volume Assumptions

The most important feature of pro forma development is the "validity" or best guess nature of the assumptions. And the most sensitive assumption in any pro forma is

[11] Gapenski, L.C. (1996). *Financial Analysis and Decision Making for Healthcare Organizations*. Irwin Professional Publishing: Chicago, p. 233.

that of *volumes*. Absolutely no other assumption, whether revenue or expense, will drive the bottom line result as much as the volumes. The age old question is always how to verify, validate, or just believe that the volumes being proposed will be achieved in the future for a service that has never been performed at the organization in the past.

There are various methods that can be used to construct a best guess for volumes, but again, because it will be in the future, the are no guarantees that it will be achieved.

A very good example of volume uncertainty and its potential validity can be seen in a pro forma that was developed at RHMC three years prior to this January. The medical center decided that it would make good clinical sense to install a magnetic resonance imaging (MRI) device, a highly sophisticated diagnostic radiology tool costing $1,750,000. Up to this time, when a physician ordered an MRI test for a patient, RHMC staff had to load the patient into an ambulance, at a cost of $60,000 a year, to be taken to a MRI provider 20 minutes away. An in-house unit would provide better patient satisfaction and better physician satisfaction as a result of faster turnaround time on results. But, it was the responsibility of the finance division to determine whether or not it would a good financial investment.

Working with the radiology department manager, RHMC's finance manager developed a series of assumptions (Table 1–4). The radiology manager provided the all-important verifiable volumes while the finance manager developed the information on the gross and net revenues. Volumes are the most important numbers on the page because both revenues and expenses are driven by it. In this case, the volumes were developed from two sources, one internal and one external.

The internal source was the number of MRI scans that RHMC was already sending to the outside provider on an annual basis. This number had great validity since it was historical. The external source was vendor generated (usually suspect because they are trying to sell their product). It consisted of the average number of MRI scans that should be needed at the medical center based on the number of current diagnostic radiology tests being performed. The vendor backed up their figures through a number of years of research. It is usually difficult to validate this type of claim, but it is important to try, particularly if the healthcare organization is considering spending almost $2,000,000. A survey of RHMC physicians most likely to order MRI scans can be used to validate the reasonableness of the vendor projection. In addition, external benchmarks of user rates per existing radiological procedures are available to help validate the projections.

Revenue and Expense Assumptions

Other aspects of the pro forma become almost as critical to the ultimate success or failure of the venture. In this case, the published price per scan (the gross charge) needed to be set at a prevailing market rate. So various individuals performed "secret shopper" phone calls to other MRI providers over a 30-mile radius. This helped the finance manager to set prices for the different types of scans able to be performed

TABLE 1–4

Ridgeland Heights Medical Center
Pro Forma of Proposed MRI Service
Financial and Volume Assumptions
January, 1999

		Capital Costs		Useful Life		
Equipment (MRI)		$1,750,000		5 years		
Construction/renovation		0				
Total		$1,750,000				
Volumes	**Year 1**	**Year 2**	**Year 3**	**Year 4**	**Year 5**	**Total**
Inpatient	350	371	393	417	442	1,973
Outpatient	1,610	1,710	1,809	1,918	2,033	9,076
Total volumes	1,960	2,078	2,202	2,335	2,475	11,049
Total per day	8	8.48	8.99	9.53	10.1	
Charge per test	$680	$680	$680	$680	$680	
Revenues	**Year 1**	**Year 2**	**Year 3**	**Year 4**	**Year 5**	**Total**
Inpatient	$238,000	$252,280	$267,417	$283,462	$300,470	$1,341,628
Outpatient	$1,094,800	$1,160,488	$1,230,117	$1,303,924	$1,382,160	$6,171,489
Total revenues	$1,332,800	$1,412,768	$1,497,534	$1,587,386	$1,682,629	$7,513,117
Payor Mix	**Year 1**	**Year 2**	**Year 3**	**Year 4**	**Year 5**	
Medicare	34.20%	35.00%	35.50%	36.00%	37.00%	
Medicaid	3.80%	4.00%	4.20%	4.40%	4.60%	
Managed care	26.80%	30.00%	33.00%	36.00%	39.00%	
All other	35.20%	31.00%	27.30%	23.60%	19.40%	
Total payor mix	100.00%	100.00%	100.00%	100.00%	100.00%	
Contractual Allowances	**Year 1**	**Year 2**	**Year 3**	**Year 4**	**Year 5**	
Inpatient						
Medicare	100.00%	100.00%	100.00%	100.00%	100.00%	
Medicaid	100.00%	100.00%	100.00%	100.00%	100.00%	
Managed care	20.00%	20.00%	20.00%	20.00%	20.00%	
All other	5.00%	5.00%	5.00%	5.00%	5.00%	
Outpatient						
Medicare	53.00%	53.00%	53.00%	53.00%	53.00%	
Medicaid	80.00%	80.00%	80.00%	80.00%	80.00%	
Managed care	15.00%	15.00%	15.00%	15.00%	15.00%	
All other	5.00%	5.00%	5.00%	5.00%	5.00%	
Free Care	**Year 1**	**Year 2**	**Year 3**	**Year 4**	**Year 5**	
All other						
Inpatient	0	0	0	0	0	
Outpatient	10.00%	10.00%	10.00%	10.00%	10.00%	

by the MRI machine that should maximize the return to RHMC and be acceptable to the community.

Maximization of net revenues is a function of the number of Medicare, Medicaid, and managed care patients that are expected and in what percentages to the total. This is important because none of these payors reimburses the organization by its set price. Instead, Medicare and Medicaid mandate what they will pay (no negotiations, thank you very much!) while each managed care payor attempts to negotiate the lowest price that the provider is willing to accept.

Direct variable expenses for this new service are purely a function of volume. The number of employees, often called full time equivalents (FTEs) that are needed to be hired will be a function of the number of scans expected to be performed and the amount of time it takes to perform the tests. Because staffing costs generally account for a majority of service costs, it is useful to project conservatively (i.e., lower volumes).

Fringe benefits are always a significant expense within any pro forma that has staffing expenses. There are two ways to reflect fringe benefits. One way is to determine the exact cost of fringe benefits. Fringe benefits are commonly represented by items such as the following.

- FICA (which is the Social Security and Medicare Part A Trust Fund taxes withheld)
- Medical, dental, and life insurance
- Short- and long-term disability
- Pension expense
- Tuition reimbursement
- The value of sick, vacation, and holiday time off

The only amount that is easily quantifiable is FICA, which the federal government has set at 7.65% of an employee's gross wages. All other fringe benefits are much harder to quantify if only because none of them are paid for as a percentage. Instead, they are all employee specific with criteria such as sex, age, family size and employment longevity as factors.

Therefore, a second method to reflect fringe benefit cost on a pro forma is generally preferred and used. This method is a percentage of gross salaries. Different healthcare organizations may use different percentages to represent their particular institution. RHMC has settled on a 30% rate, which is reflective of their experience over a several year period. Table 1–5 provides an analysis of the fringe benefit rate.

The results, as shown in Table 1–6, are presented in financial statement format with an IRR calculated over a five-year period. IRRs are easily calculated by the popular brands of electronic spreadsheets, a real time saver because the assumptions change constantly throughout the process. The 8.02% IRR is below RHMC's hurdle rate of 14%. But, this project was ultimately accepted because 1) it was going to improve customer satisfaction, 2) make the testing more efficient for the on-site clinical staff, and 3) it did show a positive IRR.

T A B L E   1–5

Ridgeland Heights Medical Center
Analysis of Fringe Benefit Percentage

1. FICA 7.65% of gross salary		
(up to a maximum of $65,400)		7.65%
2. Non-FICA fringe benefits		
Total non-FICA fringe benefit costs	$4,600,000	
Total gross salaries	÷ $36,000,000	
Non-FICA fringe benefit percentage	12.78%	12.78%
3. Staffing replacement fringe benefits		
Average allowable days off		
Sick	8	
Holiday	6	
Vacation	10	
Total allowable days off per year	24	
Total paid days per year	÷ 260	
Staffing replacement fringe benefit percentage	9.23%	9.23%
Total fringe benefits as a percentage		
of gross salaries		29.66%

Convinced that this was a worthwhile project, the medical center administration recommended this for approval to the finance committee of the board of directors, which approved it. But, as with all major projects, the finance committee wanted to track this investment over time. It requires that projects costing over $1,000,000 be brought back to the committee annually for review.

So, the finance manager, through finance staff, prepares an actual profit and loss statement for this program on an annual basis. The report was prepared in January 1999 so that at the February finance committee meeting, the CFO could present this second annual report on the MRI program that went "live" two years earlier in January 1997. The results are presented in Table 1–7. As can be seen, this new clinical program is performing acceptably on a financial return basis, coming up a little short in the first year, but doing better than budget on the bottom line in only its second year.

LIVING WITH THE FINANCE COMMITTEE'S AND BOARD OF DIRECTOR'S CALENDAR

An important aspect of proper healthcare financial management is an understanding of the information needs of the ultimate decision makers in any organization, the board of directors. This is true whether the organization is set up as a taxable or nontaxable entity. The board sets the policy direction for the organization, which is then carried out by the administration through its management team.

The board and its standing committees expect and require certain information, in a certain format, at specified intervals, which are committee meetings. It is essential

T A B L E 1–6

Ridgeland Heights Medical Center
Proposed MRI Service
Pro Forma Statement of Revenues and Expenses
January, 1999

	Year 1	Year 2	Year 3	Year 4	Year 5	Total
			Revenues			
Gross revenues	$1,332,800	$1,412,678	$1,497,534	$1,587,386	$1,682,629	$7,513,117
Less: contractual allowances	379,219	418,154	457,483	500,027	551,193	2,306,076
Less: free care allowances	27,615	25,808	24,092	22,076	19,236	118,827
Net revenues	925,966	968,806	1,015,959	1,065,283	1,112,200	5,088,214
			Expenses			
Variable expenses						
Salaries						
2.0 Technicians	70,000	73,500	77,175	81,034	85,085	386,794
1.0 Clerical	18,000	18,900	19,845	20,837	21,879	99,461
Total salaries	88,000	92,400	97,020	101,871	106,965	486,256
Fringes @30%	26,400	27,720	29,106	30,561	32,089	145,877
Medical supplies	82,320	91,622	101,975	113,499	126,324	515,740
Reduction of ambulance cost	(60,000)	(60,000)	(60,000)	(60,000)	(60,000)	(300,000)
Total variable expense	136,720	151,742	168,101	185,931	205,378	847,873
Fixed expenses						
Cryogens	23,000	35,000	36,750	38,588	40,517	173,854
Eqt. maintenance contracts	—	115,000	120,750	126,788	133,127	495,664
Utilities	40,000	42,000	44,100	46,305	48,620	221,025
Legal and acctg (incl. billing)	20,000	21,000	22,050	23,153	24,310	110,513
Insurance	30,000	31,500	33,075	34,729	36,465	165,769
Office supplies	5,000	5,250	5,513	5,788	6,078	27,628
Marketing	50,000	52,500	55,125	57,881	60,775	276,282
Facility lease	96,665	101,498	106,573	111,902	117,497	534,135
Interest	—	—	—	—	—	—
Miscellaneous	10,000	10,500	11,025	11,576	12,155	55,256
Total Fixed expense	274,665	414,248	434,961	456,709	479,544	2,060,127
Total cash outflows	411,385	565,990	603,062	642,640	684,922	2,907,999
Net cash inflows/(outflows)	514,581	402,816	412,897	422,643	427,278	2,180,215
Less: depreciation expense	350,000	350,000	350,000	350,000	350,000	1,750,000
Net operating profit/(loss)	164,581	52,816	62,897	72,643	77,278	430,215
Internal rate of return						8.02%

TABLE 1–7

Ridgeland Heights Medical Center
MRI Service
Annual Statement of Revenues and Expenses
January, 1999

	1997 Budget	1997 Actual	Percent Variance	1998 Budget	1998 Actual	Percent Variance
			Revenues			
Gross revenues	$1,332,800	$1,264,800	−5.1%	$1,413,040	$1,562,470	10.6%
Less: contractual allowances	379,219	379,440	0.1%	418,154	561,111	34.2%
Less: free care allowances	27,615	24,034	−13.0%	25,808	24,034	−6.9%
Net revenues	925,966	861,326	−7.0%	969,078	977,325	0.9%
			Expenses			
Variable expenses						
Salaries						
2.0 Technicians	70,000	72,000	−2.9%	73,500	76,000	−3.4%
1.0 Clerical	18,000	17,000	5.6%	18,900	18,500	2.1%
Total salaries	88,000	89,000	−1.1%	92,400	94,500	−2.3%
Fringes @30%	26,400	26,700	−1.1%	27,720	28,350	−2.3%
Medical supplies	82,320	74,500	9.5%	91,622	88,900	3.0%
Reduction of ambulance costs	(60,000)	(60,000)	0.0%	(60,000)	(60,000)	0.0%
Total variable expense	136,720	130,200	4.8%	151,742	151,750	0.0%
Fixed expenses						
Cryogens	23,000	20,000	13.0%	35,000	34,550	1.3%
Eqt. maintenance contracts	—	—	n/a	115,000	115,000	0.0%
Utilities	40,000	34,000	15.0%	42,000	45,000	−7.1%
Legal and acctg (incl. billing)	20,000	—	100.0%	21,000	—	100.0%
Insurance	30,000	—	100.0%	31,500	25,000	20.6%
Office supplies	5,000	4,500	10.0%	5,250	4,900	6.7%
Marketing	50,000	60,900	−21.8%	52,500	64,000	−21.9%
Facility lease	96,665	96,665	0.0%	101,498	101,498	0.0%
Interest	—	—	n/a	—	—	n/a
Miscellaneous	10,000	—	100.0%	10,500	—	100.0%
Total fixed expense	274,665	216,065	21.3%	414,248	389,948	5.9%
Total cash outflows	411,385	346,265	15.8%	565,990	541,698	4.3%
Net cash inflows/ (outflows)	514,581	515,061	0.1%	403,088	435,627	8.1%
Less: depreciation expense	350,000	350,000	0.0%	350,000	350,000	0.0%
Net operating profit/(loss)	164,581	165,061	0.3%	53,088	85,627	61.3%
Volumes (tests)	1,960	1,860	−5.1%	2,078	2,210	6.4%
Gross revenue per test	680	680	0.0%	680	707	4.0%

B O X 1–2

DUTIES AND RESPONSIBILITIES OF THE BOARD OF DIRECTOR'S FINANCE COMMITTEE

- Present an annual budget, consistent with the medical center's plan for providing care to meet patient needs, to the board for approval
- Present a long-term capital expenditure plan to the board for approval
- Review monthly and quarterly reports on financial matters
- Review and approve budgets of special projects or committees, when appropriate
- On an annual basis review the sources of funding for the corporation in conjunction with preparation of the budget
- Recommend the independent auditors for the medical center

that the information expected by the board be delivered in an accurate and timely manner. Many healthcare organizations have a calendar, published before the year begins, specifying which topics will be discussed throughout the year. The finance committee of the board of directors is one such committee. The finance committee has very specific authority and responsibility to the organization. These are enumerated in the bylaws to the organization. In the case of RHMC, these duties and responsibilities are shown in Box 1–2.

The finance committee of RHMC meets periodically to carry out its responsibilities. Table 1–8 is the finance committee calendar for Ridgeland Heights Medical Center. In addition to the routine matters that are brought forth at every meeting, the calendar clearly defines those topics that will be formally reviewed in defined time frames. As can be seen, the RHMC finance committee meets every other month except March, which is special with an additional meeting dedicated solely to the organization's strategic financial plan. Every organization determines its own preferred timing between meetings. Common intervals are monthly, bimonthly, and in some cases, quarterly.

Each of the items that the finance committee requires to be reviewed is important, if only because they are the governing board and this information aids in the conduct of their fiduciary responsibility.

Routine Matters

There are several items that the RHMC finance committee reviews each meeting. The most important of these are the monthly financial statements. Although the committee meets every other month, it still receives individual monthly financial statements for its review. At the meeting, the most recent financial statement will be reviewed, while the prior statement will only be mentioned if there was some

T A B L E   1–8

Ridgeland Heights Medical Center
Annual Finance Committee Agenda

	Routine Agenda Items—Every Meeting	
		Chapter #
	1. Approval of minutes	
	2. Financial statement review—including review of financial ratios	2
	3. Accounts receivable update	5
	Bimonthly Standing Agenda Items	
February	1. Bond debt status	2
	2. Health insurance annual review	2
March	3. Strategic financial plan	3
April	4. Results of annual audit and management letter review	4
June	5. Human resources report—salary budget decisions	6
	6. Pension status and actuaries report review	6
August	7. Review next year's budget assumptions	8
	8. Annual materials management/inventory level review	8
October	9. Finalize and approve operating and capital budgets	10
	10. Review progress towards management letter comment	10
December	11. Review insurance coverages	12
	12. Review and approve auditors and fees for next year	12
	As Needed Items	
	1. Information system plans	10
	2. Investment opportunities	

event that warranted discussion. The preparation and review of the financial statements by the finance division are discussed in Chapter 2.

The other routine item that will be presented at every meeting is an analysis of the organization's accounts receivable. Accounts receivable is often the largest current asset in a healthcare organization and has the most significant impact on the daily cash flow. A smaller accounts receivable balance is considered better because any organization would much rather have cash assets to invest instead of noninterest-bearing receivables. Accounts receivable practices are discussed in Chapter 5 while the all-important accounts receivable ratio, which is the number of days of revenue represented by the receivables, is discussed in Chapter 3.

The finance committee is primarily interested in *the number of days of receivable* calculation, how it compares to the recent months, and how it compares to the budget in order to judge the performance of the organization's management. The committee is also interested in the amount of bad debt write-offs and whether or not they judge it to be excessive. Finally, with respect to receivables, the committee is interested in the aging of the various open balances to judge whether management is allowing accounts to grow too old to collect.

Periodic Review Matters

As can be seen from Table 1–8, there are a number of areas under the periodic review of the finance committee. Each of these items, their importance, and implications to financial management are discussed at various lengths throughout the book. For the moment, though, the real importance to the financial managers is that they will be expected to produce reports and information that allow the governing board to pursue their duties. It allows the financial managers to set up their upcoming year, knowing the schedule they will be required to keep.

YEAR-END CLOSING

At the same time that the finance managers are preparing for the next finance committee meeting in February, they are engaged in one of the two most onerous tasks that they are required to perform each year, the year-end closing. (The other is the budget process.) While the regular monthly closing becomes a routine, the year-end closing always requires an extraordinary amount of extra effort. This is because an outside accounting firm will audit the financial books and records of these organizations and the year-end balances take on added importance.

Preparing for the auditors is an arduous time-consuming task, *particularly if the organization has not performed ongoing account analysis throughout the year.* The auditor's job is to validate the transactions that are reflected in the financial statements by its client, in this case, Ridgeland Heights Medical Center. Because it is the auditor's role to determine that the financial statements "present fairly, in all material respects, the financial position (balance sheet) of its client, as well as the results of the operations, changes in net assets and cash flows for the years then ended, in conformity with generally accepted accounting principles (GAAP)," the auditors need to examine the underlying transactions.[12]

---

[12] AICPA Audit and Accounting Guide, Health Care Organizations, Revised June 1, 1996.

T A B L E   1–9

Ridgeland Heights Medical Center
Year-End Accounting Procedure, December 31, 1998

Account Number and Person Responsible	Account Name	Procedure	Due Date
		Cash	
	Petty cash accounts	Verify balances are correct.	1/16/99
	Accounts payable—checking	Complete December and all prior month reconciliation. Adjust general ledger balance accordingly.	1/16/99
	Payroll	Complete December and all prior month reconciliation. Adjust general ledger balance accordingly.	1/16/99
		Investment	
	Money market sweep	Tie out to bank statement	1/16/99
	Unrestricted investments	Tie out to month-end investment schedule. Adjust valuation allowance so all investments are stated at market value. Verify balance in unrealized gain/loss account is proper	1/19/99
	Trusteed investments	Tie out to investment manager statement. Verify balance in unrealized gain/loss account is proper	1/16/99
	Endowment fund	Tie out balance to statement. Adjust for interest if necessary. Verify balance in unrealized gain/loss account is proper.	1/16/99
		Patient Accounts Receivable	
	Patient posted cash	Reconcile G/L balance to cash summary from patient accounts. Adjust if necessary.	1/20/99
	Accounts receivable	Complete December reconciliation of accounts receivable trial balance to the general ledger. Adjust if necessary.	1/12/99
	Refund clearing	Determine validity of balances. Verify refunds issued in January. Reclassify to liability section.	1/16/99
	Contra A/R—in-house and discharged—not final billed	Record adequate contra accounts receivable reserve to reflect accounts receivable at net realizable value.	1/16/99
	Allowance for doubtful accounts (bad debt reserve)	Test reserve by applying approved percentage allowances against the appropriate aging category of receivables. Recommend adjustment for excess/shortage of reserve requirement.	1/12/99

TABLE 1–9

Year-End Accounting Procedure, December 31, 1998 continued

Account Number and Person Responsible	Account Name	Procedure	Due Date
	Other Accounts Receivable		
	Credit card clearing	Verify that the G/L balance represents December charges not yet reimbursed.	1/16/99
	Collection agency clearing	Reconcile balances to collection agency statements. Follow-up on outstanding items.	1/16/99
	Inventory/Prepaid/Deferred Costs		
	Pharmacy inventory	Adjust balance to physical inventory.	1/16/99
	Dietary inventory	Verify G/L balance per inventory schedule.	1/16/99
	Central supply inventory	Verify G/L balance per inventory schedule.	1/16/99
	Prepaid insurance	Review schedule of all policies for completeness and accuracy. Determine prepaid amount remaining at year-end. Adjust G/L if necessary. Tie out amortized amount in 1997 per schedule to insurance expense on the income statement.	1/14/99
	Bond issues	Verify balances to amortized schedules. Analyze actual bond issue costs paid and compare to estimate of bond issue costs used for amortization schedule. Investigate differences. Adjust if necessary.	1/14/99
	Annual financing costs	Verify zero balances—all 1997 costs should be expensed. Balance only if amount prepaid for 1999.	1/14/99
	Fixed Assets/Depreciation		
	Fixed assets	Reconcile December plant ledger reports to G/L, both by fixed asset category and in total. Recommend adjustments and/or reclassifications, if necessary. Make all necessary adjustments for disposal of fixed assets. Tie out net of all disposal adjustments to gain/loss in disposal on the income statement.	1/26/99
	Construction in progress (CIP)	Verify that all completed projects have been included in fixed assets at year-end. Validate balances in CIP as ongoing projects that have not been completed at year-end.	1/20/99

T A B L E 1–9

Year-End Accounting Procedure, December 31, 1998 concluded

Account Number and Person Responsible	Account Name	Procedure	Due Date
	Depreciation reserve	Reconcile plant ledger reports to G/L, both by fixed asset category and in total. Recommend adjustments and/or reclassifications, if necessary.	1/26/99
	Accounts Payables/Accrued Expenses		
	Accounts payable	Reconcile subsidiary ledger to general ledger.	1/16/99
	Accrued accounts payable	Update schedule identifying balance in detail. Determine propriety of accruals at year-end. Recommend adjustment if necessary.	1/16/99
	Security deposits	Agree to schedule maintained by facilities.	1/16/99
	Accrued payroll	Determine if any adjustments are necessary due to voids or any other reason.	1/20/99
	Interest payable	Verify payable balances including current year expense for all bond issues not paid as of year-end. Tie out annual expense to debt schedules.	1/16/99
	Accrued pension	Verify balance against actuarial report. Adjust if necessary.	1/20/99
	Accrued malpractice	Test against 12/31/97 malpractice insurer report. Round balances due to estimate.	1/16/99
	Unemployment compensation	Adjust balance to estimated liability at year-end based on historical claims. Prepare schedule supporting calculation.	1/16/99
	Worker's compensation (WC)	Determine necessary accrual based on WC agent's estimate of future claims and estimate of future liability based on unreported claims.	1/16/99
	Third-party reserves	Determine adequacy of reserves/realizability of receivables. Adjust if necessary.	1/16/99
	Current retirement of long-term debt	Agree current portion for all bond issues to debt schedules. Adjust, if necessary.	1/16/99
	Long-Term Debt		
	Bonds payable	Agree amounts payable for all bond issues to debt schedules.	1/16/99
	Unamortized bond discount	Agree unamortized discount for all applicable bond issues to amortization schedules.	1/16/99

Therefore, the finance staff of RHMC needs to provide the auditors with a series of analyses for every balance sheet account, listing by category and dates the transactions made as well as the other side of each entry. If the staff performed this throughout the year, the task would be less onerous. However, many organizations have trouble maintaining and updating these analyses on a monthly basis and, thus, are required to recreate their annual transactions in a short time frame (say, one month). This is necessary because most administrators and boards require the audit to be complete and the auditor's report to be presented to the board within a very few months after the close of the fiscal year.

The staff and accounting director at RHMC do a better job than some of their peers, and thus, do not have as great an obstacle in finishing their tasks. Still, the accounting manager has created a list enumerating the tasks ahead of it during the months of January and part of February (Table 1–9). This will consume a majority of the staff time during these two months.

2
CHAPTER

February

"Honey, you sure have been working some late nights the last few weeks," said Becky Barnes to her nearly exhausted husband, Samuel.

"Yeah, you know how it is," said Sam, "we have the finance committee meeting in two weeks and we have some extra stuff to prepare for this month. In addition to the usual stuff, like the financial statements and accounts receivable report, we are in the middle of the year-end closing and audit that follows. So, it's been a tough month."

"But Sam, I'm confused," said Becky. "I know that you've been doing this healthcare financial management thing for a long time, but how can you, with only your finance background, know enough to deal with and understand all the things that are required in a clinical program like an MRI?"

"Well, Becky, you know that's a question that I have been asked before," Sam said to his long-suffering wife. "You've heard me say that I believe no finance person, no matter what level of responsibility they have, can be truly effective unless they intimately know the operations of the business they are in. This is true whether the industry is manufacturing, banking, industrials, or airlines. The only way to be sure the financial statements accurately reflect the results of operations is to know those operations. It's imperative that the finance person learn how those operations work, whether it be through formal study, continuing education, or on the job training."

"Yeah, Sam, I've heard you say that before," said Becky, "but MRIs are just one clinical program. Being an ICU (intensive care unit) nurse, I'm deeply involved in some complicated clinical programs and I know you have been involved in preparing the financial analyses for these. How can you be sure that you are being given enough or all the information you need to put together the proper analysis?"

"Actually, Becky, the truth of the matter is that there is never enough information. That's because we're dealing with the future and no one can accurately predict the future. So we get as much information as we can about an entire program by asking questions developed over years of asking the same kinds of questions and hope that we haven't missed anything big," said Sam emphatically.

"Sam, I know you haven't missed much over the past few years, but it seems like its getting tougher and tougher lately, with you working on shorter and shorter time frames with fewer and fewer staff people to help with the analysis," said Becky empathetically.

"Yeah," said Sam, "it's the nature of this beast."

———

It was a cold, clear and crisp day in northern Illinois in early February. While the ice and snow of the previous week were clinging to the narrow branches of dormant trees creating a beautiful frozen tableau, the accountants of Ridgeland Heights Medical Center were busy at work. Their priority assignment was to finish preparing analyses required to be presented to the auditors by the third week of February. The auditors, from one of the Big Five international accounting and auditing firms, scheduled their usual three week audit in order to be ready to present their findings at the April finance committee meeting.

Preparation and attestation of the year-end financial statement is one of the critical aspects of healthcare financial management. These statements are the backbone of the financial reporting and analysis of this $1 trillion industry. Because healthcare as an industry does not stand in isolation in this country, it is important that the reporting be accurate and timely so that industry statistics can be combined for aggregate national data.

ACCOUNTING PRINCIPLE AND PRACTICES

Just like other industries, healthcare has a set of principles and practices established through authoritative pronouncements, regulation, and historical precedents. All books and records of organizations that are audited, whether for-profit or not-for-profit, are required to follow Generally Accepted Accounting Principles (GAAP). For the healthcare industry, GAAP is formally presented in the American Institute of Certified Public Accounting (AICPA) Audit and Accounting Guide for Health Care Organizations (AAG-HCO).[1]

---

[1] AICPA Audit and Accounting Guide, Health Care Organizations, Revised June 1, 1996.

The hierarchy of GAAP for not-for-profit organizations starts at paragraph 1.23 of the AAG-HCO. It states that "not-for-profit organizations should follow the guidance in effective provisions of ARBs (Accounting Research Board), APB Opinions (Accounting Principles Board) and FASB Statements and Interpretations (Financial Accounting Standards Board), unless the specific pronouncement explicitly exempts not-for-profit organizations or their subject matter precludes such applicability."[2] The AAG-HCO also defines the GAAP hierarchy for government organizations as well as all other healthcare organizations that do not qualify as not-for-profit or government entities (generally for-profit organizations).

The general definitions of the three major types of healthcare organizations, as listed in the AAG-HCO on page 1, are as follows.

- *Not-for-profit, business-oriented organizations,* which are characterized by no ownership interests and essentially are self-sustaining from fees charged for goods and services. The fees charged by such organizations generally are intended to help the organization maintain its self-sustaining status rather than to maximize profits for the owner's benefit. Such organizations are exempt from federal and state income taxes and may receive tax deductible contributions from corporations or individuals that support their mission.
- *Investor-owned healthcare enterprises,* which are owned by investors or others with a private equity interest and provide goods or services with the objective of making a profit.
- *Government health care organization,* which are public corporations and bodies corporate and politic. Also organizations are presumed to be governmental if they have the ability to issue directly (rather than through a state or municipal authority) debt that pays interest exempt from federal taxation.

All of the accountants at RHMC have formal accounting training, and thus, understand the background of these pronouncements. In addition, they are aware that the interpretation of accounting rules for their industry are often covered in the AAG-HCO, and as such, each accountant keeps one within reach at all times.

As we saw in Chapter 1, RHMC is a not-for-profit corporation and therefore it will follow the rules for such organizations. These rules, for not-for-profit organizations, will be essentially the same whether the organization is a hospital, skilled nursing facility, psychiatric facility, or home health agency. Physician office practices are generally some form of for-profit partnership or corporation and, as such, will follow for-profit accounting rules.

OBJECTIVES OF FINANCIAL REPORTING

Because RHMC has a hospital-based skilled nursing facility, home health agency, and psychiatric unit, it will employ these basic not-for-profit accounting rules across

---

[2] Ibid, p. 7.

the various financial statements. It will also follow the objectives of financial reporting that were set down and are summarized in the Financial Accounting Standards Board Statement of Financial Accounting Concepts Number 1, which stated that financial reporting should provide information:

- Useful to present and potential investors, creditors, and other users in making rational investment, credit, and similar decisions
- About the economic resources of an enterprise, the claims to those resources, and the effects of transactions, events, and circumstances that change resources
- Regarding an enterprise's financial performance during a period
- Describing how an enterprise obtains and spends cash, about its borrowing and its repayment of borrowing, about its capital transactions, and about other factors that may affect its liquidity or solvency
- Describing how management of an enterprise has discharged its stewardship responsibility for the use of enterprise resources
- Useful to managers and directors in making decisions in the interest of owners

Ultimately, the whole point of preparing, auditing, and disseminating enterprise financial reports is *to allow the stakeholders to determine the financial performance of the organization.* This is true whether these stakeholders are any of the following.

- For-profit equity shareholders
- Not-for profit community board members and the community members themselves
- The politicians, who charged the governmental agencies with spending the budgeted dollars

BASIC ACCOUNTING CONCEPTS

At RHMC, the accountants are well aware of the importance of their work. They are in fact extremely diligent in the care they give to preparing the financial statements. In addition, because of their accounting training, they are aware of the basic accounting concepts that have been developed over the years that they follow along with their peers. There are six basic accounting concepts with which they are particularly aware.[3]

1. Entity concept—the concept that expresses that the corporate structure, or entity, is capable of taking economic actions apart from the individuals running the entity. Accounts are kept for the business entity and reflect events that affect the business. This concept is further expanded by the "going concern" theory, which suggests that the entity will live on

---

[3] Adapted from Berman, H.J., Weeks, L.E., Kukla, S.F. (1986). *The Financial Management of Hospitals,* 6th ed., Health Administration Press: Ann Arbor, Mich., p. 39.

indefinitely, regardless of the individuals who control. This is important because it allows the accountants to use a continuity assumption in valuing assets, rather than "fire sale" liquidation value at the end of each accounting period.

2. Transactions concept—a simple concept that requires all financial transactions that affect an organization to be included in the accounting records and reports. This is necessary in order to ensure that accounting data and reports are dependable and valid. If all transactions are not included, then the financial records could be inaccurate, creating the possibility that the accounting numbers could be massaged or finessed in an undesirable and inappropriate way.

3. Cost valuation concept—a corollary to the transaction concept, this concept requires that all financial transactions be recorded at "cost," that is, the price paid to acquire any item or good. Cost is preferable to any other valuation because it is determinable, definite, objective, and verifiable. Other valuation methods such as sale price and replacement cost are not always definite and may be a matter of conjecture or opinion. While the cost method of valuation is not perfect, primarily because it does not properly value inflationary or deflationary trends in times of highly fluctuating prices, its merits outweigh its demerits.

4. Double entry concept—the granddaddy of all accounting concepts. Developed in 1492, it requires that accounting records be constructed in such a manner as to reflect the two aspects of each transaction, that is, the change in assets, and the change in the source of financing—liabilities. Thus, for the accounting records to reflect fully the effect of any transaction, *two* entries must be made.

5. Accrual concept—a concept that acts as a guide in accounting for revenues and expenses. The accrual concept requires that revenues be recorded in the accounts when they are realized and that expenses be recorded in the period when they contribute to operations. In practice this means, for example, that supplies purchased and used at the end of a month should be recorded as expenses for that month. But, if the supply distributor has not sent out the invoice for those goods, the accrual concept requires the organization's accountants to estimate the value of the supplies and record it in that month's financial records. This concept allows for the proper allocation of income and expenses to the appropriate fiscal period.

6. Matching concept—this concept requires that all *associated* revenues and expenses must be matched in the financial records in any given month to properly determine net income. If it were not necessary to match related items, revenues, and expenses, then it would be possible to manipulate income from different types of activities to produce whatever type of operating picture is desired.

TABLE 2–1

Basic Financial Statements of a Healthcare Organization

Financial Statement	Primary Purpose
Balance sheet	Presents a snapshot of the financial condition of the healthcare organization at a single point in time
Statement of operations	Presents summarized revenues and expenses of an organization, resulting in a profit or loss, for a given period of time
Statement of changes in net assets (or equity, if for-profit)	Presents a summary of the financial elements that caused a change in net assets, or equity, during a given period of time
Statement of cash flows	Presents a summary of the assets and liabilities that caused a change in the main cash balances during a given period of time
Notes to the financial statement	Presents disclosure and discussion of the information underlying the numbers reported on the financial statements

As the accountants prepare their entries, the above concepts are second nature, being used in all their work. They know it is critical that their work be accurate and timely. Accuracy is a function of properly applying the basic concepts. Timeliness is a function of management's will and persistence. As the accountants prepare their automated and manual journal entries, they are repeatedly reminded of the lessons learned along the way.

BASIC FINANCIAL STATEMENTS OF A HEALTHCARE ORGANIZATION[4]

What the RHMC accountants are preparing are financial statements. The basic financial statements of a healthcare organization consist of a balance sheet, a statement of operations, a statement of changes in net assets, a statement of cash flows and footnotes (notes) to the financial statement (Table 2–1). It is important to note that when presented with a financial statement, every one of these five items must be present, or else it is not complete. Each one of these items is only a part of the whole, a whole that can tell the knowledgeable reader a great deal about the organization whose financial statement he or she is reviewing.

---

[4] Part of the analysis for this section is derived from the Healthcare Financial Management Association's (HFMA) Certification Examination Preparation—CORE manual, 1998, Chapter 11, as authored by Phyllis Cowling, Chief Financial Officer at Baptist St. Anthony's Health System in Amarillo, Texas.

USES OF FINANCIAL INFORMATION

As we said earlier in this chapter, the reason for preparing, auditing, and disseminating enterprise financial reports is to allow the stakeholders to determine the financial performance of the organization. Additionally, financial reporting is important because it enhances the ability of many different stakeholders to make decisions about the organization. According to Dr. William Cleverly, a professor of healthcare financial management, there are five uses of financial information that may be important in decision making.

1. Evaluating the *financial condition* of an entity
2. Evaluating *stewardship* within an entity
3. Assessing the *efficiency* of operations
4. Assessing the *effectiveness* of operations
5. Determining the *compliance* of operations with directives[5]

Some of these stakeholders that would want to be able to make appropriate decisions about the organization using financial information would include the following.

- Governing board—to review the financial performance (the bottom line results and the asset and liabilities levels—financial condition) as well as the organization's actual financial ratios compared to budget and industry benchmarks. The governing board will also be interested in the auditor's review of the organization's internal financial controls during its attestation process, sometimes called the "management letter" (stewardship).
- Senior management—same criteria as the governing board. In addition, senior management would want to review operating ratios such as departmental productivity (efficiency) and departmental budget variances (effectiveness).
- Department management—to review the results during the period to determine their efficiency (did they make their budget numbers?) and to prepare analysis for any budget variances.
- Investment bankers, rating agencies, and bondholders—to determine whether the value of any outstanding bonds has deteriorated or increased during the reviewed period (financial condition). Millions of dollars could be at stake in the secondary market for individuals or mutual fund holders.
- Community—to determine if their community resource is functioning in an appropriate manner. This may mean different things to different communities. For example, the standard in one community may mean that the not-for-profit board of directors prescribes that the organization should not earn a "profit" greater than 2%, because if it does, the community may

---

[5] Cleverly, W.O. (1997). *Essentials of Healthcare Finance*, 4th ed., Aspen Publishers: Gaithersburg, Md., p. 4.

think it is "gouging" its community members. Another community's standard, however, may lead the not-for-profit organization to be able to budget and achieve a much higher net margin.

- Benefactors—a subset of community, inasmuch as most organizations or individuals who give charitable donations reside in or around the community. These donors want to know whether or not their donations are being used appropriately for an organization that will remain self-sustaining (financial condition).
- Equity investors—those individuals and investment fund managers who are concerned with their investment and may require either stock price appreciation and/or dividends to maintain their participation with the stock.

THE FINANCIAL STATEMENTS

So, we have theories, concepts, and practices of accounting that both the preparers and the users of the financial statement information have been trained to analyze and understand. It is time to review these financial statements and the value that they bring to the users in providing an understanding of the financial health of the organization.

Balance Sheet

The order of financial statement presentation is always the same, as was indicated in Table 2–1. This has been established over time. The balance sheet has always been first because of the age-old concept that has placed the organization's assets, liabilities, and net assets or equity balances in a primary position ahead of periodic profits or losses (the income statement). The rationale is that an organization with a strong balance sheet can withstand a short run of losses or reduced profits while those organization's with a weak balance sheet will not be able to as easily. So, an investor's eye quite naturally looks first to the balance sheet and then the income statement.

Table 2–2 is the balance sheet of Ridgeland Heights Medical Center at December 31, 1998. A significant amount of financial information can be extracted from the balance sheet alone. Yet, it will also be used in conjunction with the other parts of the financial statements as well as additional financial and volume related information to form a complete picture of the medical center's financial resources.

Although just one part of a complete financial statement, the balance sheet by itself, can yield some very interesting information applicable to internal or external users, a quick perusal of RHMC's balance sheet highlights several matters of import. First, it can be noted that RHMC has $213,900,000 in total assets, a considerable amount.

Next, it can be noted that RHMC has three very large grouping of assets, cash (in several forms), accounts receivable, and fixed assets. The large percentage of assets tied up in fixed assets (characterized as property, plant, and equipment [PP&E]) indicates that RHMC, illustrative of the industry as a whole, is capital intensive. We

TABLE 2–2

Ridgeland Heights Medical Center
Balance Sheet (in thousands)

	December 1998	December 1997
Assets		
Current assets		
Cash	$1,200	2,000
Investments — short term	6,500	5,400
Total cash and cash equivalents	7,700	7,400
Accounts receivable	22,000	22,800
Less: allowance for doubtful accts	(5,800)	(5,600)
Net patient receivables	16,200	17,200
Inventory	500	400
Prepaid expenses	400	300
Other current assets	900	700
Total current assets	24,800	25,300
Long-term investments — unrestricted	95,500	87,000
Trusteed investments	22,000	30,000
Endowment fund investments	300	300
Deferred financing costs	3,300	3,400
Other noncurrent assets	121,100	120,700
Property, plant & equipment (PP&E)		
Land and land improvements	8,000	7,600
Buildings	70,000	66,000
Leasehold improvements	3,000	2,800
Equipment and fixtures	56,000	54,000
Construction in progress	3,000	4,000
Total PP&E	140,000	134,000
Less: accumulated depreciation	(72,000)	(70,000)
Net PP&E	68,000	64,400
Total Assets	213,900	210,400
Liabilities		
Current liabilities		
Accounts payable and accrued liabilities	12,000	10,000
Third-party liabilities	4,000	4,500
Current retirement on long-term debt	3,500	3,400
Total current liabilities	19,500	17,900
Long-term debt	120,000	123,400
Other long-term liabilities	4,000	4,100
Total long-term liabilities	124,000	127,500
Long-term liabilities	143,500	145,400
Net Assets		
Unrealized gain/(loss) on investments	2,000	3,000
Other unrestricted	67,900	61,500
Temporarily restricted	200	200
Permanently restricted	300	300
Total Net Assets	70,400	65,000
Total Liabilities and Net Assets	$213,900	210,400

will see later when we review the income statement (or statement of operations) that it is also labor intensive.

Third, it is reported that there is $125,200,000 in cash and investments on the asset side of the balance sheet (which is made up of the cash of $1,200,000, short-term investments of $6,500,000, plus the unrestricted long-term investments of $95,500,000 and trusteed investments of $22,000,000). There is also $120,000,000 of debt on the liability side, which may indicate a highly leveraged financial position. The organization will be able to determine its leverage position during ratio analysis (see Chapter 3).

Finally, it can be seen that RHMC has net assets of $70,400,000. Net assets in a not-for-profit organization are the equivalent of equity in a for-profit organization. There are some very technical aspects of net assets, particularly the concepts surrounding the classification of unrestricted, temporarily restricted, and permanently restricted. In general though, the unrestricted net assets in most organizations constitute a large majority of the total net assets. At first glance RHMC looks to be financially stable.

A word of interest is in order here. You can see that RHMC has only $400,000 in inventory on its balance sheet, a very low amount of dollars compared to the $216,000,000 in total assets. This is one area where the healthcare industry as a service industry differs considerably from most manufacturing and industrial industries, which have a considerably larger percentage of their total assets tied up in inventory.

Statement of Operations

The Statement of Operations (previously known as the Income Statement before the 1992 publication of the new Healthcare Audit Guide) can provide a knowledgeable reader with both summary and some detailed information as to the periodic financial results of an organization. Depending on the amount of line items provided in the statement of operations and the amount of trending information conveyed a reader could glean a wealth of intelligence.

For example, the initial review of the RHMC income statement, appearing in Table 2–3, would indicate that for the year ending December 31, 1998, the organization had an operating margin of $5,200,000 and a net margin of $6,400,000. Without additional trending information or ratio analysis, this appears to be a good set of bottom lines for the organization. These margins were the result of $145,000,000 in gross patient revenues less discounts, and charity care provided of $51,600,000. The gross patient revenues are a manifestation of charging list prices for all services rendered by the healthcare facility. The majority of the discounts were the consequence of contracting with managed care companies and accepting a variety of discounts through negotiations.

It should be noted that the AAG-HCO mentioned earlier in this chapter has taken a position that gross patient revenues and contractual adjustments and charity care should no longer be reported on audited financial statements. While the

T A B L E 2–3

Ridgeland Heights Medical Center
Statement of Operations
For the Year-to-Date Ending December 31, 1997 and 1998 (in thousands)

	1998	1997	Percentage Change
Revenues	73,000	74,000	−1.35
Inpatient revenue	72,00	69,000	4.35
Outpatient revenue			
Total patient revenue	145,000	143,000	1.40
Less			
Contractual and other adjustments	(49,000)	(48,000)	2.08
Charity care	(2,600)	(2,200)	18.18
Net patient service revenue	93,400	92,800	0.65
Add			
Premium revenue	2,100	1,300	61.45
Investment revenue	6,400	5,500	16.36
Other operating income	1,200	1,200	0.00
Total revenue	103,100	100,800	2.28
Expenses			
Salaries	36,000	34,000	5.88
Contract labor	1,000	1,500	−33.33
Fringe benefits	7,000	6,800	2.94
Total salaries and benefits	44,000	42,300	4.02
Bad debts	4,600	4,400	4.55
Patient care supplies	15,500	15,000	3.33
Professional and management fees	3,600	3,600	0.00
Purchased services	5,400	5,600	−3.57
Operation of plant (including utilities)	2,600	2,500	4.00
Depreciation	11,000	10,500	4.76
Interest & financing expenses	7,400	7,600	−2.63
Other	3,800	4,600	−17.39
Total expenses	97,900	96,100	1.87
Operation margin	5,200	4,700	10.64
Nonoperating income			
Gain/(loss) on investments	1,200	600	100.00
Total nonoperating income	1,200	600	100.00
Net income	6,400	5,300	20.75

industry has had to adopt this for annual external reporting (e.g., the audited financial statement), in practice the monthly financial statements prepared for the administrators and the board continues to include this information. Healthcare facilities know that reported patient service revenue is an indicator of business growth or decline and is important in relation to its variances between both this year's budgeted and prior year's revenues. The increase or decrease in contractual adjustments is likewise important to budgeted and prior year's results. Large variances cause the reviewers to raise pertinent questions, such as what caused the changes, are they part of a trend, and what can be done to improve them?

Premium revenues indicate that the healthcare facility has contracted with insurance type organizations (usually managed care companies) to accept *capitation* payments for treating members of the managed care companies. This concept of capitation is reviewed in Chapter 3. For purposes of the financial statement, however, suffice it to say that premium revenue on the statement of operations means that the healthcare organization has decided to take the *risk* of a financial gain or loss for the provision of healthcare services. They do this by agreeing to provide all contracted healthcare for insurance members, with no additional payments beyond the insurance premiums. In other words, healthcare organizations that take capitation have effectively, for at least part of their services, turned themselves into insurance companies.

Interest income is the revenue earned on investments of excess funds made by the organization. RHMC has over $120,000,000 in excess funds and its investment policies will determine the most appropriate mix of equities (stocks), bonds, and other financial instruments. As you can see, RHMC earned $6,400,000 on the investment of its money. That is a return of 5.33%. By itself, this return does not look substantial. But this represents only the interest paid out by its holdings in bonds and other fixed instruments and the dividends paid out by its holdings in stocks. It does not include the unrealized appreciation (or depreciation) in the price of its stocks and bonds. The cumulative amount of these unrealized gains and/or losses is available on the balance sheet in the net assets section. For purposes of analysis, total investment returns, which are reported internally, include the appreciation or depreciation amount as a percentage.

The placement of interest income in the other operating section of the statement of operations is somewhat controversial. GAAP appears to allow the placement in this section, which is "above the line" and therefore included in the operating margin. The more common and traditional treatment is "below the line" in the nonoperating income section of the statement of operations and therefore not part of the operating margin. A review of financial statements around the country will reveal that one or the other methods are used and certified to by the CPA firms that issue audit opinions. In fact, an article that appeared in *Modern Healthcare* states that, "Much like medicine, auditing is not an exact science. One set of numbers can be interpreted many ways, each of which may be correct. Finance experts say healthcare accounting rules allow a great deal of leeway in accounting for investment income, for example. Some systems may classify those earnings as 'nonoperating income.' Other systems lump investment income with 'other revenue.'"[6] Interestingly, because of this lack of consistency, operating margins are no longer considered a good benchmark. Many investment managers and consultants only use the net margin ratio as a consistent indicator for comparison.

---

[6] Pallarito, K. (1998). Auditing the Auditors. *Modern Healthcare*, September 21, p. 2.

Other operating income is an aggregation of many disparate types of miscellaneous incomes not directly related to patient care. The most common type of other operating income would be cafeteria revenue, revenues from drugs sold to patients, sale of the silver in old x-ray film, and rebates for volume discounts from vendors. It should be noted that some of these items of other operating income are subject to income taxes even though the healthcare organization is tax-exempt. A tax-exempt organization needs to file an IRS 990-T form along with its IRS 990 form for all appropriate items of other operating income that qualify as taxable.

Salaries are the most significant expenses on the statement of operations. This line includes only wages paid to its employees by the organization that are subject to employment taxes.

Any work being carried out in the organization by individuals who are not subject to employment taxes are reported on the statement of operations as either contract labor or purchased services. Contract labor represents laborers employed by an outside organization. The healthcare organization has contracted with this outside organization to have its employees perform work within the organization. Contract labor often mounts when there is a shortage of certain types of skilled labor within the industry. For example, RHMC spent $1,000,000 in 1998 on contract labor. The majority of these funds where spent on physical therapists because there is a shortage in the region. Their budget had assumed that they could hire more of their own therapists, but they were not successful in doing so and hence they needed to resort to these outside agencies at twice the price.

Purchased services often represent the engagement of outside help in a larger context. The organization's administration may decide that it wants to outsource management of a department or departments to companies that specialize in certain skilled or unskilled areas rather than recruit and retain their own management staff. They therefore purchase the services for these areas. For example, RHMC purchases management services for environmental services (previously called housekeeping), laundry, operation of plant, dietary, and information systems.

Fringe benefits are an aggregation of several types of expenses paid for by the organization to enhance the quality of life for its employees or to comply with federal, state, and local laws. The development and magnitude of fringe benefit expenses was previously explored in Chapter 1.

Bad debts represent the amount of gross charges that the provider of healthcare services will not collect from the financial guarantor of the individual who receives the health services. The financial guarantor could be the patient, the patient's relative, or the third-party payor (an insurance company). Usually, it is not the insurance company, but the patient or family member who has to pay out of pocket, either for the entire scope of services or just a deductible or coinsurance amount. Following is a useful definition that distinguishes a bad debt expense from a charity care write-off.

- Charity care—patients are *unable* to pay for their healthcare services received
- Bad debts—patients are *unwilling* to pay for their healthcare services received

Patient care and other supplies, professional and management fees, operation of plant and other expenses represent the normal costs of doing business in healthcare. For example, the patient care supplies line includes medical supplies and drugs used in the patient's care as well as mundane office supplies needed to run the operation. Professional and management fees include the costs of external auditors, attorneys, and consultants. Operations of plant costs represent the expenses of running the physical facility, such as the nuts, bolts, and screws used in minor repairs as well as the heat, light, and power bills needed to keep the facility operating.

Depreciation is the periodic portion of the cost of building the physical plant and the purchase of all the capital equipment used within it. Depreciation expense is determined by dividing the original cost of a building project or capital equipment purchase by the estimated useful life of the asset. A review of RHMC's statement of operation's reveals that depreciation is the second largest expense. This is in keeping with the capital-intensive nature of the healthcare industry. Depreciation therefore has a large impact on the organization's bottom line. Because of its size and the nature of the calculation, depreciation expenses are subject to being finessed. There are three major ways that an organization could attempt to manipulate its bottom line through the use of depreciation expense. They are use of the following.

1. Nonstandard estimated useful lives
2. Accelerated methods of depreciation rather than a straight-line method
3. Capitalization policy inconsistent with reasonable industry standards

Nonstandard Estimated Useful Lives

In theory, an organization could pick any useful life, which allowed it to alter the bottom line of its statement of operations to suit its needs. In practice however, the industry has adopted a generally accepted source for establishing asset lives—a pamphlet called Estimated Useful Lives of Depreciable Hospital Assets.[7] The Guide was developed for two reasons.

1. GAAP would not permit a wide range of options for useful lives. If allowed, there would be no "general acceptance." So the external auditors wanted to be sure that an authoritative source was available.

2. Medicare was established in 1966 as a third-party payor that reimbursed providers for service based on cost. They did not want to pay more than reasonable cost and so they also needed an authoritative source for the denominator of the calculation. Medicare has stated that using the lives in the AHA book will be deemed acceptable for cost reporting purposes.

---

[7] Estimated Useful Lives of Depreciable Hospital Assets, American Hospital Association.

Accelerated Methods of Depreciation

The second major way for any organization to manage depreciation expense is through the use of any method that accelerates it. The most common method of depreciation is called straight line. This method is simple to use. To determine the depreciation expense, you simply divide the cost of the asset by the number of years of estimated useful life. Table 2–4 shows a comparison of the straight line method of depreciation with two different accelerated methods, double declining balance and sum of the years digits. The main point is that the method used can have a big impact on the total depreciation expense recorded each accounting period. As you can see, the straight line method literally smoothes the depreciation expense of each asset for each year of its estimated useful life. Yet, the two accelerated methods place a greater proportion of the expense in the early years and smaller portions in the later years.

One reason to use an accelerated depreciation methodology is when a financial advantage can be gained from doing so. It needs to be done thoughtfully because, as

TABLE 2–4

Comparison of Straight Line and Accelerated Depreciation Methods

		Accelerated Depreciation Method				
	Straight Line	Double Declining Balance with optimum switch*	Actual Declining Balance	Optimum Switch double declining balance	Sum of the Years Digits	SYD Years
Cost of asset (Radiology fluoroscope)	$300,000	$300,000			$300,000	
Estimated useful life	5	5			5	
Annual depreciation						15
Year 1	60,000	120,000	180,000		100,000	5
Year 2	60,000	72,000	108,000		80,000	4
Year 3	60,000	43,200	64,800		60,000	3
Year 4	60,000	32,400	38,800	25,920	40,000	2
Year 5	60,000	32,400	23,328	15,552	20,000	1
Total depreciation	$300,000	$300,000		$41,472	$300,000	15

*Optimum switch method allows the organization to switch to straight line depreciation after the straight line method exceeds the double declining balance method. On a five year life, the switch would occur in the fourth year. On a ten year life, the switch would occur in the seventh year. Without optimum switch, the declining balance will extend many years past the original useful life determination.

we have seen, the acceleration of depreciation puts extra expense on the statement of operation, which will make the bottom line worse than it really is. But, it is an established practice in the for-profit world because the income tax code provides favorable treatment. Specifically, because the tax code allows accelerated depreciation to be used for tax reporting purposes, the extra expense that decreases the bottom line means that the for profit organization will pay *less* taxes. Further, the organization is not harmed financially for doing so because depreciation is a noncash expense. The organizations are, in fact, helped financially.

As stated earlier, most healthcare organizations in this country are not-for-profit. So therefore there is no tax advantage to using accelerated depreciation. However, while there is no tax advantage, there may be an advantage because of the cost reimbursement nature of the Medicare program. Although we explore the Medicare program in greater detail in Chapter 4, it is important to note that at least through 1998, all Medicare costs except those for acute inpatient services are reimbursed at cost. All outpatient costs are reimbursed at cost. However, because Medicare was aware of this potential advantage, it specifically forbid the use of any type of accelerated depreciation for cost reporting purposes. Therefore, with no tax advantage and no Medicare advantage, most not-for-profit organization chose to stick with the easy and familiar straight-line method.

So it turns out that the only real advantage to using accelerated depreciation is operational. It makes sense to charge the new capital acquisition a higher depreciation in the early years when it needs little maintenance. Then in later years, it is financially responsible to charge the asset a lower level of depreciation when it will need and receive service and maintenance charges.

Capitalization Policies Inconsistent with Industry Standards

Once again, Medicare has had a large impact in this area. The question is "at what dollar level should a purchase be capitalized?" When Medicare came into existence in 1966, they established a rule that defined a capital asset as having a useful life greater than one year and a cost over $500. Therefore anything bought under $500 was, by definition, an operating expense. At that time it was important to the Medicare program to use as small a dollar figure as possible because it wanted to limit its cost reimbursement. Although a Medicare provider could conceivably set its capital policy at a higher level, there was no incentive to do so because it still had to report to Medicare at the $500 level.

Although Medicare changed its method of reimbursing for the capital related to acute inpatient care in 1990, thereby rendering some of the rationale no longer applicable, it was not until 1998 that Medicare revised its 1966 practice. Since 1998 Medicare has allowed providers to consider purchases with useful lives of more than one year and costs at $5,000 and above to be considered capital. This allows providers to more properly classify many purchases as operating expenses, bringing more reality to the operations, and hence, decreasing depreciation expense in the future.

Over the course of the last 30 years RHMC has always followed the prescribed guideline, recognizing that was is in their best interest to use the American Hospital

Association Estimated Useful Lives of Depreciable Hospital Assets along with the straight-line method and the $500 capitalization policy. However, it is pleased that the $500 level has been revised—a long overdue need. RHMC has in fact decided to revise its capitalization to $2,500 next year. It further recognizes that in doing so, it needs to provide additional operational budget dollars for those purchases that in prior years would have fallen into the $500–$2,499 range.

Interest and financing expenses are a result of the $123,400,000 of prior-year tax-exempt bond debt on the liability side of the balance sheet. In fact, at $7,400,000 per year, it is evident that at the time the bonds were issued, the tax-exempt interest rate that RHMC was able to obtain for 1998 was 5.5% (0.055 x $123,400,000 = $6,787,000 + $600,000 in bond insurance fees). This rate was 85 basis points less than the 30-year taxable rate at the time the bond was issued. This amounted to savings of several million dollars that RHMC will not have to pay over the life of the bonds. The entire topic of interest and financing for each organization falls under the heading of "Treasury Management" and is the subject of several books. (We touch on some of the topic briefly in Chapter 3 when we review strategic financial planning.)

Finally, the next to last line on the RHMC statement of operations is *realized gains or losses on investments.* This is the profit or loss made when the organization or its investment managers sell any financial instrument that it had been holding for investment. These instruments are usually bonds or stocks and the difference between the purchase price and the selling price is always reported in the nonoperating section.

Statement of Changes in Net Assets (or Equity)—Table 2–5

This is the least used part of the financial statement. Its primary purpose is to roll-forward the net assets from the end of the prior period to the current period. In many cases the most common changes in the unrestricted net assets from one period to the next will be the change in the following.

T A B L E 2–5

Ridgeland Heights Medical Center
Statement of Changes in Unrestricted Net Assets
For the Year-to-Date Ended December 31, 1997 and 1998

	1998	1997
Unrestricted net assets		
Excess of revenues over expenses	$ 6,400	$ 5,300
Change in net unrealized gains and losses on other than trading securities	(1,000)	500
Increase (decrease) in net assets	5,400	5,800
Net assets, beginning of year	65,000	59,200
Net assets, end of year	$70,400	$65,000

- The excess of revenues over expenses
- Any unrealized gains or losses on other than trading securities
- Net assets released from restrictions used for the purchase of property and equipment

All positive results in any of these areas will increase the organization's "equity" while negative results will decrease the "equity."

More complex organizations, such as RHMC, may require separate statements of changes in net assets, segregating the net assets into the three categories of unrestricted, temporarily restricted, and permanently restricted.

Statement of Cash Flows—Table 2–6

The statement of cash flows is generally the most useful section of a typical financial statement. While many financial statement readers turn first to the income statement and then to the balance sheet in an attempt to understand an organization's financial results and financial position, they often overlook the cash flow statement. At a glance, this statement provides the knowledgeable reader with an interesting set of information regarding the organization's sources and uses of cash.

The statement begins by recording the organization's change in net assets, (which primarily consists of the bottom line). After that, all noncash items included in the bottom line, such as depreciation and amortization, are added back because the purpose of this statement is to recognize cash transactions only. Finally, the statement is then designed to show the balance sheet items that increase and decrease an organization's cash balances. In the not-for-profit industry, the statement of cash flows is divided into cash flows from operations, investing activities, and financing activities. These designations represent cash flows from the organization's principal activity (operations), investments and capital expenditures (investing) and proceeds of debt activities (financing). Although for-profit organizations do not use the same categorizations, the end result is the same, that is to describe the net increases or decreases in cash and cash equivalents.

Some interesting and useful line items on the statement of cash flows are the following.

- Capital expenditures—this line shows the total change in the capital expenditures during the reporting period. The changes involve the acquisition of any new capital as well as any capital items that are discarded.
- Proceeds from the issuance of long-term debt—this line exhibits any long-term debt issued by the organization during the reporting period. At a glance the reader can determine the amount of debt taken on by the organization.
- Payments on long-term debts—this line represents all principle payments made during the reporting period. It quickly isolates the amounts in question.

TABLE 2–6

Ridgeland Heights Medical Center
Statement of Cash Flows
For the Year-to-Date Ended December 31, 1997 and 1998

	1998	1997
Cash Flows from Operating Activities		
Increase (decrease) in net assets	6,400	4,700
Change in net unrealized gains and losses		
on investments other than trading securities	(1,000)	(2,000)
Changes in net assets		
Adjustments to reconcile changes in net assets		
Depreciation and amortization	11,000	10,500
Net accounts receivable (increase) decrease	1,000	(700)
Other current assets (increase) decrease	(200)	(1,500)
A/P & accrued liabilities (decrease) increase	2,000	(1,000)
Other long-term liabilities (decrease) increase	(100)	200
Third-party settlement (decrease) increase	(500)	1,200
Current portion of long-term debt (decrease)	100	100
Net cash provided by (used in) operating activities	18,700	11,500
Cash Flows from Investing Activities (increase) decrease		
Net investments	(9,500)	—
Other noncurrent assets	100	(200)
Capital expenditures — net	(5,600)	(6,200)
Net cash provided by (used in) investing activities	(15,000)	(6,400)
Cash Flows from Financing Activities		
Proceeds from the issuance of long-term debt	—	—
Payments on long-term debts	(3,400)	(2,500)
Net cash provided by (used in) financing activities	(3,400)	(2,500)
Net increase (decrease) in cash and cash equivalents	300	2,600
Cash and cash equivalents, beginning of year	7,400	4,800
Cash and cash equivalents, end of year	7,700	7,400

Supplement disclosure of cash flow information — cash paid for interest. Cash paid for interest (net of amount capitalized) in 1998 and 1997 was $7,7000,000 and $7,500,0000, respectively.

Notes to the Financial Statements

The financial statement notes have considerable importance to the overall quality of a full-scope financial statement. Generally accepted accounting principals require notes to be included in an audited statement. They add a level of understanding to the other four statements by describing various accounting concepts used by the reporting organization. In addition, the notes allow the organization to present any message they want to illustrate to the readers of the statements. The notes provide supporting detail that cannot easily be placed on the face of the financial statements themselves. Internal monthly financial statements often exclude a formal set of notes because it is assumes that the readers of these internal statements are already familiar with the information that may be included in the notes.

PREPARING FOR THE AUDITORS

As stated earlier in this chapter, the RHMC accounting director and her accountants have spent several weeks just prior to the end of the fiscal year as well as several weeks into the new calendar year employing once-a-year actions getting ready for the arrival of the auditors. They are paying special attention to the preparation of analysis to be given to the auditors for both balance sheet and income statement accounts. That is, in fact the biggest difference between regular month-end and end-of-year closing.

During regular month-end closings, the accountants are generally more concerned with getting the books closed, publishing the financial statement, and getting ready for the next month's close. There is usually not enough time during a regular month-end closing to be concerned with the type of accuracy involved in a year-end closing. That is because the senior administration and the board want to know the results of operations as soon as possible after the close of the month.

For the year-end closing, extra time is allotted for the close of the month and hence the year end. This is allowed because finance administration is aware that there will be the extra scrutiny of the audit and, from a *political* viewpoint, it is much better to make sure that the accounting staff makes all required accounting entries and none are proposed by the auditors. This extra time is always used for additional analysis which, due to time constraints, is not always performed during the rest of the year.

In the previous chapter, the tasks involved in a year-end closing were enumerated in Table 1–9. This is the baseline for the workpaper analysis that will be prepared by the RHMC accounting staff and given to the external auditors. This workpaper preparation is referred to as prepared by client (PBC), and allows the auditors to begin their audit already armed with the details behind the financial statement accounts. The extra closing time, coupled with the PBCs permits a clean year-end financial statement, and almost assures that the auditors will not find any financial transactions that should have been recorded but were not, were recorded in error and need to be eliminated, or were recorded in error and need to be changed.

Following are a couple items of note.

1. A healthcare facility would be better served if they maintained good account analysis on a month-by-month basis. This simply follows good management practices. Not maintaining monthly account analysis means that the administration and the accounting staff are absolutely sure that the published financial statements may not be as accurate as possible. Because of this, they are not sure if a major adjustment will be required which can make the already published statements misleading and get the

accountants, the accounting director, and/or the chief financial officer *fired*.

2. Following are the six most sensitive accounts (i.e., those most likely to receive audit adjustments in the financial statements).
   a. Contractual adjustments (income statement)
   b. Accounts receivable (balance sheet)
   c. Allowance for doubtful accounts (ADA) (balance sheet)
   d. Bad debt expenses (income statement)
   e. Allowance for contractual adjustments (ACA) (balance sheet)
   f. Due to/from third-party settlements (balance sheet)

Their sensitivity involves greater analytical difficulty because each account involves a great deal of *estimation*. There are, of course, accounting rules that set down proper estimation techniques. These are, in fact, the rules that the auditors use when they do their analysis. But, amazingly, many healthcare organizations either want to follow these techniques but have trouble because of time or talent, or they decide they have a better way and thus choose to follow their own methodology. This often causes significant audit adjustments after the healthcare facility has closed its books for the year.

There is some very good advice to follow in this regard. Always ask your auditors to share the exact methodology they use to analyze these accounts. Ask them to explain their methodology. Then, after it becomes understandable, adopt it. When the healthcare organization is using the same methodology as the auditors, then as long as there is no problem with the numerical input, there is no potential for audit adjustment. In other words, unless the facility has some reason (often a long-standing tradition) not to adopt the auditor's method, just do it! It significantly minimizes the risk of adjustments, and that is the name of the game in year-end preparation for the auditors.

Analysis of Sensitive Accounts

Because Chapter 2 is being used to explain the financial statements and its elements, this is a good opportunity to provide further discussion of the six sensitive accounts identified above.

1. Contractual adjustments—Contractual adjustments have become the second largest line item on the income statement of many healthcare organizations after gross revenues. This has happened because many organizations have chosen not to limit increases to their gross charges (price list) while at the same time they have had to absorb extraordinary increases to the discounts (contractual adjustments) they agreed to provide to the third parties. Because of its size on the income statement, even a small discrepancy can have big consequences on earnings. The timing of the contractual adjustment on the patient's account as well as

the accuracy of the adjustment are crucial items that could have impacts on potential audit adjustments. The development of contractual adjustments is further reviewed, along with the concept of net revenue generation in additional detail in Chapter 4.

2. Accounts receivable—The concept of accounts receivable management is discussed in further detail in Chapter 5. It is a detailed analysis of methods to minimize the dollar levels and aging of the amounts owed to the healthcare facility for the services it provided to its patients (customers). The reason for its importance and its sensitivity lies in its size and the percentage of assets that it represents. In most other industries, accounts receivable is usually the third largest current asset behind inventories and cash. In healthcare however, accounts receivable are often the largest asset. In addition, accounts receivable involves a high degree of detailed analysis to verify that the amount of gross and net receivables on the books are, in fact, valid.

3. ADA—One of the oldest, time honored concepts in accounting, it has its own special rules in the healthcare industry. ADA represents the amount of dollars that are subtracted from the gross accounts receivable to help arrive at net amounts expected to be collected from all patients. It is always an estimate, because it is impossible to know, with certainty, how many accounts receivable dollars will not be collected. Because of the high dollar value of ADA (which is often between 12% to 30% of the gross accounts receivable depending on each organization's payor mix), there are significant implications for bottom line adjustments if not done appropriately. We review, in detail and with examples, how to prepare a monthly ADA analysis in Chapter 5.

4. Bad debt expense—sometimes called the provision for bad debts, the finance committee keeps a close eye on this income statement line. This expense is also called a provision because, like the ADA, it is also an estimate. It is, in fact specifically related to the ADA. The higher the ADA, the higher the bad debt expense and visa versa. Bad debt expenses have a direct effect on the bottom line. The ability to minimize this expense is dependent on the kind of accounts receivable management practiced and in many cases the socioeconomic neighborhood in which the organization is located. Still, in those aspects that are controllable, the finance committee will require that these expenses not vary greatly from year to year without very good reason. In addition, it is important that the bad debt expenses be properly estimated throughout the year so that no large negative entry is made to the income statement in December or as an audit adjustment.

5. ACA— Like ADA, the ACA is used to reduce the gross accounts receivable down to its net collectible value. ACA is an estimate of contractual adjustments that should be taken when the healthcare

organization receives payment for services from the many third-party payors with which it has contracted. These third-party payors are usually categorized into groups such as Medicare, Medicaid, or managed care. Also like ADA, this allowance, or estimate, can have a meaningful impact on earnings. If the organization does not properly prepare its estimate, the audit adjustment can cause havoc with the year-end closing numbers. Detailed explanations of ACA are also discussed in Chapter 5.

6. Due to/from third parties— An accounting concept that has been used in most healthcare organizations since 1966, with the inception of Medicare. This balance sheet account represents the amount of monies either owed back to the third-party payor by the provider (liability) or additional reimbursement owed by the payor back to the provider (asset). This is necessary only when the type of reimbursement agreed to between provider and payor is cost-based and retrospective, which means that all payments throughout the year were only interim (temporary) and would be finalized (or final settled) after a year-end cost report was filed. This was how Medicare originally reimbursed providers (mostly hospitals). Since 1983, inpatient hospital reimbursement was changed, is no longer retrospective, and all such rates are set before the year begins (called prospective). However, all but inpatient care is still retrospective (at least through federal fiscal year end 1998). This means that the dollar amount used by the provider to estimate the due to/from third party each month, before the cost report is filed, is critical to both the income statement and balance sheet.

FEBRUARY FINANCE COMMITTEE SPECIAL REPORTS

As we have reported earlier, Ridgeland Heights Medical Center's finance committee of the board meets bimonthly to review routine matters, such as the operating results of the organization, as represented by the statement of operations (income statement) as well as the balance sheet and statement of cash flows. Other routine items of interest are a review of the accounts receivable balances and capital expenditures, both budgeted and unbudgeted.

In addition, at every meeting, there are items that are formally reviewed on a specific periodic schedule. This is done so that these items, which have been deemed important but not necessary to review at every meeting, are not forgotten. In February, two of these items are on the agenda.

Bond Debt Status

RHMC has issued $150,000,000 of bond debt over the last several years. This is a substantial amount of money, particularly to the individuals and corporations that have bought the debt. In fact, both the purchasers of the debt and the issuers of the debt (as represented by the RHMC board) have the same concerns. Namely, is the value of the organization that issued the bond still financially viable and able to continue to repay both the principal and interest of the outstanding bond issue?

One of the best ways to determine financial viability and the ability to repay principal and interest on a bond issue is through the use of financial statement ratios,[8] particularly the following three ratios.

1. Long-term debt to capitalization ratio—This ratio is defined as the proportion of long-term debt divided by long-term debt plus unrestricted net assets or equity. Higher values for this ratio imply a greater reliance on debt financing and may imply a reduced ability to carry additional debt.

2. Debt service coverage ratio—This ratio measures total debt service coverage (interest plus principal) from the organization's cash flow. Higher values for this ratio indicate better debt repayment ability.

3. Cash flow to total debt—This ratio is defined as the proportion of cash flow to total liabilities, current and long-term. It has been found to be an important indicator of future financial problems or insolvency.

These ratios are the most commonly used throughout the healthcare industry to measure bond repayments capability. The actual calculations for these ratios are presented in Box 2–1.

B O X 2–1

SELECTED BOND REPAYMENT RATIOS

1. Long-term debt to capitalization ratio

$$\frac{\text{Long-term liabilities}}{\text{Long-term liabilities} + \text{unrestricted net assets}}$$

2. Debt service coverage ratio

$$\frac{\text{Cash flow (total margin} + \text{depreciation expense)} + \text{interest expense}}{\text{Principal payment} + \text{interest expense}}$$

3. Cash flow to total debt ratio

$$\frac{\text{Revenues and gains in excess of expenses and losses} + \text{depreciation}}{\text{Current liabilities} + \text{long-term debt}}$$

---

[8] The following analysis of these capital structure ratios were adapted from Cleverly, W.O. (1998). *The Almanac of Hospital Financial and Operating Indicators*, 1998–1999 edition, The Center for Healthcare Industry Performance Studies: Columbus, Ohio, pp. 77–109.

We further explore ratios in Chapter 3.

Because of its importance, these ratios are computed and presented on the financial statement each month for review and any discussion by the finance committee. Still, once a year, the administration has deemed it important to prepare an in-depth review of the organization's debt status for the finance committee.

The review includes the following.

1. A summary of the bond debt expenses for the past 10 years
2. A discussion of any changes in the organization's bond debt rating by either of the two major rating agencies, Moody's and Standard and Poor's

Table 2–7 shows the analysis and review.

T A B L E 2–7

Ridgeland Heights Medical Center
Analysis of 30-Year Bond Debt (1986–1998)

				Bond Analysis		
	Interest Rate (%)	**Principal**	**Interest Expense**	**Total Annual Payments**	**Debt Balance**	**Additional Expenses***
1986					$150,000,000	
1987	4.4	$1,740,000	$6,600,000	$8,340,000	148,260,000	$600,000
1988	4.7	1,900,000	6,968,220	8,868,220	146,360,000	600,000
1989	4.9	2,000,000	7,171,640	9,171,640	144,360,000	600,000
1990	5.0	2,100,000	7,218,000	9,318,000	142,260,000	600,000
1991	5.2	2,220,000	7,397,520	9,617,520	140,040,000	600,000
1992	5.3	2,320,000	7,422,120	9,742,120	137,720,000	600,000
1993	5.3	2,440,000	7,299,160	9,739,160	135,280,000	600,000
1994	5.3	2,660,000	7,169,840	9,829,840	132,620,000	600,000
1995	5.4	2,820,000	7,161,480	9,981,480	129,800,000	600,000
1996	5.4	3,100,000	7,009,200	10,109,200	126,700,000	600,000
1997	5.5	3,300,000	6,968,500	10,268,500	123,400,000	600,000
1998	5.5	3,400,000	6,787,000	10,187,000	120,000,000	600,000

*Additional expenses include the following.
- The cost of bond insurance at 40 basis points, or 0.4% (in order to receive a AAA rating from the bond rating agencies)
- Related consulting fees
- Related legal fees, all of which are being amortized over the life of the bond

Based on the ratio analysis of RHMC's current financial statement, there have been no upgrades or downgrades of RHMC's bond ratings by Moody's or Standard and Poor's.

B O X 2–2

RIDGELAND HEIGHTS MEDICAL CENTER, 1997 HEALTH INSURANCE INFORMATION

During 1998, RHMC offered a single health insurance plan through ABC Healthcare—a Midwest regional-based health maintenance organization. We offered a point-of-service (POS) plan that offered managed care benefits for the employees staying in the ABC network antindemnity-type benefits for going outside of the ABC network.

The budget for health insurance for 1998 was $2,400,000. Actual premiums paid during 1998 were $2,000,000. The savings resulted from lower participation levels as a result of staff reductions and a different mix of single/couple/family employee participation than budgeted.

Dental insurance continued to be offered through XYZ Dental Program. Two programs were offered—a dental maintenance organization (DMO) plan and an indemnity plan. These plans, which were fully paid for by the participating employees, had 400 participants in 1998. The 1998 premiums paid by the employees were $960,000.

Health Insurance Annual Review

Like any other large employer, and in many towns around the country, the health-care organization is the largest employer; RHMC provides health insurance for the town's employees. There are several interesting twists here. Because RHMC is both an employer as well as a healthcare provider, it knows better than most, the *costs* associated with providing care for its employees. That is the cost of care, not the price of the care.

Therefore, when negotiating with a health insurer to cover its employees, RHMC has both an advantage and a disadvantage. The advantage is that it knows its own prices for providing care, and as such, can use it as a measuring stick when the prospective health insurer makes its bid to service the medical center. The disadvantage is that RHMC will need to negotiate with these self-same insurers for managed care contracts over other employers. As such, it cannot reveal too much of its underlying cost structure or else it risks losing some of its negotiating leverage on its other contracts.

The other interesting twist is that RHMC has learned that the utilization of health services by its employees greatly exceeds the utilization by employees in any other industry. This is no fluke and no accident. It is, in fact, extremely logical. Because healthcare workers are exposed to these services, every day, as service providers, there is no mystery and no fear of its use. Healthcare workers, in general, are the greatest users of healthcare services in the country. But, because of this, the healthcare insurer wants to and needs to charge healthcare providers a higher monthly premium rate, due to use, than it would to workers in other industries.

Each year, the administration presents a wrap-up of the previous year's health insurance information for the finance committee so that it can assess the variances from budget and determine any potential variances in the coming year. This is particularly important if the organization is self-insuring its employees' medical coverage. Because RHMC had self-insured its medical coverage in past years, this report to the finance committee had become a habit. Thus, although RHMC currently offers a regular insurance coverage in the current year, it continues to present this report. A summary of this report is presented in Box 2–2.

3

CHAPTER

March

Sam Barnes was restless. He had just begun to prepare information for his organization's annual update of its strategic financial plan. But he was having a rare moment of doubt. In those times, he always did the right thing—he called his ex-boss in Florida for some advice.

"Jim, I've got a problem and I need your help," said Sam to his ever-understanding and patient colleague and friend.

"Yeah, what's up today," asked Jim Jordan, who just happened to be the chief financial officer (CFO) of a 600-bed academic medical center in the glorious state of Florida. Jim was always available to take a call from his former colleague.

"I'm about to start gathering information for the upcoming five-year strategic plan and it seems like we just finished the work from last year. I'm having trouble redoing this again year after year. I've forgotten what value we get from this exercise," said a frustrated Sam.

Now Jim, who was not only his facility's CFO but also the senior vice president for strategic planning, was a very patient man. He needed to be in order to untiringly listen to Sam's stream-of-consciousness, free association ramblings. And so Jim said, "Come on, Sam. Buck up. You've gotten into these funks before. It will pass; it always does.

"Let me remind you of something you told me just last year. You called me and you were very excited. As you were preparing last year's plan you realized that you had made an assumption that Medicare reimbursement would not go down as much as had been predicted by one of those consultants that your hospital retains. Your reading of the literature led you to a better prediction. And since your administration listened to you last year instead of the other guy, the hospital did not have to cut an additional ten employees."

"What?!?" cried Sam. "Oh my gosh, that's right. I did forget about that. Actually that was important for a number of reasons, particularly because the administration put more credence on my work for the first time. You are so right. As usual, you've been fabulous Jim. Thanks a lot. How do you always do that?" asked Sam, somewhat envious.

"Sam, Sam, Sam, I've told you this before. It is not a matter of talking. You just need to listen," said the always humble Jim.

———

The month of March opened in a very promising fashion in the Chicagoland region. The weather was unusually warm, allowing people to shake off their winter blues. Unfortunately, the blue period continued to extend to the healthcare industry. More than in previous years, events were intruding that looked to diminish both the reputation and finances of the industry. The federal government had recently embarked on a two-pronged attack of the industry and its financial and billing practices.

On the billing front, the Feds decided that they had probable cause to conclude that a great deal of the industry was filing erroneous Medicare and Medicaid claims within the statutes of the 1863 Civil War law dubbed the False Claims Act. In addition to believing that these erroneous billings constituted fraud, the Office of Inspector General of the United States and many state attorneys general believed that they could raise revenues using the fining powers granted under the False Claims Act.

On the financial front, the passage of the Federal Balanced Budget Act (BBA) in August 1997, which was effective in October 1997, was already affecting the financial bottom lines of all segments of the healthcare industry. The hospital segment was the first to feel the brunt of the $116 billion five-year payment reduction act. Home health agencies had already felt an immediate impact from the Interim Payment System segment of the BBA with 752 agencies shutting their doors in the first nine months.[1] Other segments of the industry, such as skilled nursing facilities and physician office practices, began to fully feel the implications as they budgeted for fiscal years beginning October 1, 1998. We explore the BBA and it's many industry implications in Chapter 4.

STRATEGIC FINANCIAL PLANNING—5-YEAR PROJECTIONS

Meanwhile back at Ridgeland Heights Medical Center, the accounting and finance staff were gearing up to present the implications of the BBA and several other significant operational changes to the organization's administration. They do this

---

[1] Ngeo, C. (1998). Trouble at Home. *Modern Healthcare*, July 27, p. 40.

through the annual preparation and presentation of a five-year strategic financial plan.

A healthcare organization's strategic financial plan can be defined as *the quantification of a series of strategic planning policy decisions.* Strategic financial plans are meant to quantify the tactics surrounding the organization's strategic plan. In order to be successful, it is important that any healthcare organization that wants to be financially competitive possess a number of critical attributes.

1. The chief executive has conceived a financial vision.
2. Management follows the simple rule "What gets measured gets done."
3. Management understands and applies principles of corporate finance.
4. Management has a sophisticated financial plan.
5. The organization favors a quantitative capital allocation process.
6. Management consistently applies quantitative decision-support tools.
7. Management sets annual financial goals and objectives, welcoming organizationwide inputs.
8. The organization has a visible operating plan and disseminates its financial goals.
9. The organization has a strategic plan that takes into account the requirements of the capital markets.
10. Management reduces expenses while improving service and quality.[2]

Ridgeland Heights Medical Center believes in these attributes and attempts to follow them as closely as possible. In particular, the center updates its five-year strategic plan every year in order to remain current with contemporary strategic and financial changes within the industry. Doing so helps them to carry out the attributes of items 1, 3, 4, 7, and 9 above.

Strategic Planning

In order to begin a successful strategic financial plan, management must finalize their strategic plan. This plan is updated every two to three years and presented for approval to the planning committee of the board of directors and then finally to the full board of directors. The strategic plan can be defined as *a statement of missions or goals (or both) required to provide guidance to the organization which incorporates a set of programs or activities to which the organization will commit resources during the plan period.*[3]

---

[2] Kaufman, K., Hall, M. (1994). *The Financially Competitive Healthcare Organization—The Executive's Guide to Strategic Financial Planning and Management.* Probus Publishing Company: Chicago.

[3] Cleverly, W. O. (1997). *Essentials of Health Care Finance* (4th ed.). Aspen Publishers: Gaithersburg, Md.

Strategic plans are imperative to the proper functioning of any successful organization. Yet in many organizations, the strategic plan is looked at as an added inconvenience. Many department heads, as well as many administrators, want to just "manage" (i.e., just operate their department or division without taking the time to determine just where they are headed). The strategic plan focuses the organization on the important changes in demographics, payor mix, payor reimbursement methodologies, physician recruitment and retention policies, new programs or other initiatives, and any other area that is pertinent to maintaining or improving the organization's financial position.

It is important to note that both strategic planning and financial planning are the primary responsibility of the board of directors. Certainly while the senior administration has a role in carrying out the plans, the future vision of the organization begins with the board. The vision of the organization's CEO is also highly pertinent. The CEO serves as a link between the board (as a member) and as head of the organization's management. The final link between the board and administration involves the board setting key financial policy targets. These targets should include debt policy and profitability objectives (e.g., operating margin percentages and return on net assets) as well as a capital plan.

The purposes of the strategic plan are to do the following.

- Identify key future issues and priorities
- Allow managers an opportunity to understand and contribute to the organization's direction
- Identify resource needs and guides on how they can get allocated
- Assure that the strategic plan supports board policy

In order to determine these strategies, it is necessary to do the following.

- Assess external environmental conditions
- Assess internal environmental conditions, such as current organization issues
- Describe the strategic gap from the desired to the current position relating to organizational and environmental variables
- Identify competencies and resources needed to close gap
- Determine strategic initiatives that can move the organization forward toward successful completion of the plan
- Allocate capital and/or operating dollars to each initiative

After the strategic initiatives are determined, the organization needs to determine the *tactics* they will use to activate the strategies. The tactics are the actual steps the various departments will take to implement those changes developed within the strategic plan. It is imperative that the organization's management is given and understands its accountability in carrying out the tactics. Without accountability the tactics have a great chance of not being achieved, thereby causing the strategic plan to fail.

Converting Vision (Strategic Plan) into Financial Reality—Market Share, New Services, and the Medical Staff

According to Professor William O. Cleverly, there are four steps involved in the development of a strategic financial plan.

1. Assess financial position and prior growth patterns
2. Define growth needs in total assets for the planning period
3. Define acceptable levels of debt for both current and long-term categories
4. Assess reasonableness of required growth rate in equity (net assets)[4]

RHMC generally follows these steps. After approval of the strategic plan, the finance department goes to work on the strategic financial plan. There are a number of specific steps taken to translate the organization's vision into financial reality. Some of these steps may be performed concurrently while others need to wait for previous steps to be completed.

At RHMC, the *first step* is for the finance officer to call a meeting of the senior administration. The objective of the meeting is to determine the volume changes over the next five years. This is often a result of market share analysis and the organization's current and proposed market share position. For example, suppose that the organization's current market share across all of its markets (primary and all secondary) is 12%. Also let us suppose that the organization has determined that for it to enjoy continued success, it needs to increase its market share to 18%, an increase of 50%. This is not the kind of change that can happen easily. The quickest way to increase market share in the short term is to buy it. This, of course, presumes that there is a willing seller in the market. There are many scenarios that can play out if acquisition is the desired method of choice.

The next most likely method for increasing market share is to determine the services that are most desired by the local market. A good way for the organization to make this determination is through surveys, both focused and general. These surveys help to determine the *demand* for any new or expanded services that are already being met, or alternatively creating demand for services that the market may not *yet* know it really wants.

Medical Staff Issues

There are many examples of what a demand analysis may uncover. For example, let's say that an organization is in an area where a majority of its residents favor alternative medicine such as chiropractics, acupuncture, and massage therapy. In fact, let's say that the survey reveals 43% of the population has already used at least one of these therapies over the past 12 months. In this case, what the organization can surmise is that a lot of healthcare is being administered to local residents, who are

---

[4] Ibid, p. 201.

prospective patients, without its input. However, while this might be an interesting finding, it may not allow this organization to do anything about it.

While a logical action plan might be to research these services and begin to offer them upon completion of an implementation plan, in the healthcare industry, nothing is quite so simple. This is particularly true because of the interdependence that the hospital shares with its affiliated medical staff. All community oriented hospitals and academic medical centers have bylaws that grant their medical staff a series of privileges to practice medicine in the facility, based on their academic and professional credentials.

The medical staff is charged with checking the credentials of physicians new to the staff as well as periodically reviewing existing credentials. This periodic review is usually at two or three year intervals, depending on the organization. A medical executive committee (MEC), sometimes called the medical board represents the organization's medical staff. The MEC is made up of elected and appointed physician representatives. Initial approval by the MEC is required for a physician to practice at the hospital, but, because of the interdependence mentioned earlier, final approval is required by the full board of directors of the healthcare organization.

One other privilege granted to the MEC is its ability to decide and determine the kinds of medicine that will be practiced in the organization. The MEC is made up of long serving members of the medical staff who understand the community they serve and the general needs and desires of its resident population. They have specific roles and responsibilities with regard to medical practice performed in the facility. Specifically, according to the bylaws of healthcare organizations such as RHMC, "subject to the authority of the board, the MEC shall determine all policy and shall have the authority to *make final decisions on all questions relating to the practice of medicine* within the institution."

In the above example, it is quite possible that there could be a major conflict between the organization's administration and its medical staff, as represented by the MEC. The administration is eager to add what it perceives to be needed services to its community (as well as increasing its market share) while the MEC may reject this addition because it does not perceive alternative medicine as in the best interest of the community or the medical staff. The MEC may reason that there has not been enough academic peer review in regard to alternative medicine, meaning that the efficacy of the treatments has not been proven. In addition, it may reject any treatments that may not have been approved by the state's Medical Professional Licensing Board. Any of this may stymie the organization in its desire to use alternative medicine, for example, as a way to increase its market share.

RHMC STRATEGIC FINANCIAL PLANNING

Volume Assumptions

In any event, the senior officers responsible for planning and implementation need to take the lead in determining the volume increases or decreases over the upcoming five years. Although the crystal ball may be somewhat snowy, it is an essential part of the administrative job responsibility to do this prognostication with the appropriate inputs. Following are the types of volumes that need to be reviewed for both current and proposed new programs.

Inpatient volumes
- Admissions
- Average lengths of stay
- Patient days

Outpatient volumes
- Emergency department
- Same day surgeries
- Observation days
- Home health services
- Other outpatients—defined as all other revenue producing services rendered to outpatients such as the following.
  - Laboratory services
  - Radiology services, such as general, ultrasound, CT scanning, and MRIs
  - Physical therapy, occupational therapy, speech therapy
  - Pharmaceutical (drug) sales
  - Renal dialysis
  - Other outpatient ancillary services

Physician office visit volumes
- Fee-for-service visits
- Capitated lives (or members)
- Relative value units (RVUs)

The volumes should be arrayed to show the trends over the past two to four years. This will enable the administrators to make more informed decisions on future volumes as they review their market share assumptions. The future volumes will generally be described as percentage increases or decreases of current volumes, by year. RHMC has conducted an analysis of its current market to determine the various volume assumptions. It has reviewed the following areas.

1. The demographics of the organization's service area (particularly the age trend)
2. The projected population growth rate of the area
3. The current age of the physician staff
4. The shifting criteria for inpatient admissions as dictated by the various insurance companies
5. The continuing shift from inpatient to outpatient care

Thus, RHMC's summarized volume assumptions looks like this.

- **We expect moderate declines in acute care volumes each year as follows:**
  - **Discharges decline 2% per year**
  - **Lengths of stay decline 4% per year**
  - **Patient days decline 6% per year**
- **Emergency department volumes are expected to increase 4% per year**
- **Other outpatient and physician volumes are projected to increase 8% per year**

Payor Mix

Another major set of assumptions project the percentage mix of third-party insurance companies that will make payments on behalf of its clients—the employers, employees, and individual subscribers. It is important to determine the potential mix of payors simply because each payor is likely to be paying a different amount to RHMC. This is usually based on each insurance company's ability to negotiate its best rates with the healthcare organization, usually called the provider of services, such as RHMC. The insurer's ability to negotiate better or worse rates with the provider is generally a function of unique market conditions and the provider's need to capture the volumes offered up by the insurer.

Payors vary dramatically, from the dominating nature of the Medicare and Medicaid programs to the control of the HMO providers of managed care to the somewhat more laissez-faire nature of the PPO providers of managed care. In addition, there is the unique reimbursement associated with worker's compensation and motor vehicle accidents to the diminishing role of commercial insurers. Finally, the industry constantly redefines the concepts inherent behind the patient-pay or self-pay patients, which often depends on the socioeconomic conditions of the community surrounding the healthcare organization. *In some communities, self-pay means "pay" while in other areas, it really means "no-pay."*

In the strategic financial plan, RHMC has once again performed a review, based on current year actual data. It has examined the current trends within various health insurance companies and employer fringe benefits areas. Based on this review, the RHMC administration has adopted the following payor mix assumptions (Table 3–1).

Rates and Reimbursements

The next major set of assumptions involve reimbursement rates, which represent the *net* revenues expected to be paid to the healthcare organization by the various payors throughout the industry. In the healthcare industry there is one dominant payor and it is the federal government. The two primary programs covered by the government

TABLE 3–1

The Payor Mix

	Current Year (Percent)	Percent Change, Each of Next 5 Years
Medicare	38	−0.5
Medicaid	6	0.0
HMO—managed care	16	+0.5
PPO—managed care	14	+1.0
Worker's compensation	4	0.0
Commercial insurers	8	−0.5
Other	12	−1.0
Capitation—Medicare	2	+0.5
Capitation—commercial	0	0.0

are Medicare and Medicaid. The federal government pays 100% of its agreed upon rates (not the organization's charges) for services rendered to Medicare recipients. In addition, the federal government pays at least 50% of the rates for services rendered to Medicaid recipients while each of the state governments pays a varying percentage that makes up the 100%.

Between Medicare and Medicaid, the government pays more than 50% of every healthcare dollar directed to providers. We review the Medicare and Medicaid programs in more depth in Chapter 4. Still, it is important to note that for purposes of the strategic financial plan, making the best guess on the direction of the Medicare and Medicaid programs into the near future, such as the upcoming five years, is essential to a quality outcome.

In addition to the Medicare and Medicaid programs, the next largest payor group is categorized as managed care. The term managed care is a catchall for a variety of health insurance that is designed to limit the cost of healthcare through a range of utilization and reimbursement techniques. The various managed care companies attempt to reduce costs by focusing on lowering the price paid to providers, limiting the volume of care rendered to their subscribers and reducing the intensity of services used.

Managed care concepts are reviewed in more depth in Chapter 4. For purposes of the strategic financial plan, it is important to recognize the implications of the reduction strategy used by these companies. Managed care methodologies favor reductions in admissions and lengths of stay, thereby further reducing the number of days that their subscribers spend as inpatients in healthcare facilities. Their methodologies will also cut outpatient visits wherever possible. In addition, managed care companies will negotiate very aggressively with providers to secure the best (i.e., lowest) prices possible.

T A B L E 3–2

Ridgeland Heights Medical Center
Managed Care Summary Percentage of Discount for Gross Charges

	Year 1	Year 2	Year 3	Year 4	Year 5
HMOs	30	32	35	38	42
PPOs	18	21	25	29	34
Medicare	46	48	50	52	54
Medicaid	68	69	70	71	72

There are over a dozen reimbursement methodologies that managed care companies may attempt to negotiate and impose. The easiest way to express the discount taken off of the provider's list price of services (usually called gross charges) is as an overall percentage. This will allow the provider to summarize a list of their various managed care contracts into one consistent number for calculation, analysis, and trending purposes. The summary for rate payors will usually be expressed as shown in Table 3–2.

Keep in mind that the percentages in Table 3–2 are fully blended between inpatient and outpatient rates. They will usually be determined and reported separately between inpatient and outpatient categories.

Capitation—Revenue Implications

There is one other concept that should be explored at this time, which began to have an affect on the revenue and rate structures of many healthcare organizations within the past 10 years. This is the insurance concept known as *capitation*. Capitation shifts the risk of coverage from the insurer to the provider of care. Capitation is defined as "a flat periodic payment per enrollee to a healthcare provider that is the sole reimbursement for providing *defined services* to a defined population. These defined services are specific to the contract between the provider and the insurer but may include coverages for the enrollee's entire assortment of healthcare needs. The word capitation is derived from the term per capita, which means per person. Generally capitation payments are expressed as some dollar amount per member per month (PMPM) in which the word "member" typically means enrollee in a managed care plan, usually a health maintenance organization (HMO)."[5]

Capitation can be paid to various providers of services at various different rates. Providers that typically accept capitation include primary care physicians (PCPs), specialist physicians, hospitals, and home health agencies. Again the rates

---

[5] A very concise overview of capitation concepts is presented in Gapenski, L.C. (1996). *Financial Analysis and Decision Making for Healthcare Organizations: A Guide for the Healthcare Professional*, Irwin Professional Publishing Chicago.

will vary depending on the provider and the age and sex of the enrollee. For example, a primary care physician may accept capitation from an insurance company on a large or small set of enrollees. The PCP may receive $12 PMPM for accepting the contract. Assume that the contract calls for the insurance company to supply 1,000 members, the PCP would receive $12,000 per month ($12 × 1,000 members) or $144,000 per year in net reimbursements. The PCP could then round out the practice by accepting more capitation from other insurers or preserving the rest of the practice for fee-for-service patients.

In the case of Ridgeland Heights Medical Center, capitation denotes the same concept but has a much larger consequence. RHMC only recently began accepting capitation contracts and is only now beginning to understand the financial impacts on its operations. Only two years ago, the organization accepted its first capitation contract, a Medicare HMO contract with one of the local health plans that is a certified Medicare HMO insurer. The insurer was required to contract with healthcare providers for the provisions of care and approached RHMC. RHMC was eager to break into the Medicare HMO capitation business as it foresaw a new and attractive revenue stream. It allowed the organization to learn the nuances of capitation on a small scale. After ascending the learning curve, RHMC wanted to move into capitation in a big way. It expected that it could provide the defined services at a cost below that of its premium revenues.

The Medicare HMO laws have one particular subtlety that make them unique. Medicare pays its insurers a PMPM depending on the specific county around the country in which the Medicare enrollee lives. These PMPMs vary from just over $300 to just under $800, a very significant difference. These PMPMs are based on the average adjusted per capita costs (AAPCC) within each of these counties. The PMPMs are a total for all healthcare services needed to be supplied by the insurer to assume the initial risk. The amount has to be parceled out to providers of hospital care, primary and specialty physician care, as well as skilled nursing and home health continuum of care. Because of the great variability of rates, it is clear that the Medicare residents of some counties are spending a great deal more money on healthcare than residents in other counties. In general, the counties where Medicare healthcare spending is highest, are populated with a disproportionately high share of Medicare age residents, such as Dade and Broward counties in South Florida.

Although RHMC is not in one of the higher level AAPCC counties, it still believes that it is capable of turning a profit on its Medicare HMO (or Medicare risk) business. In this case, RHMC has committed itself to building its Medicare HMO business. It has therefore projected that 4.5% of its payor mix would be Medicare HMO within the five-year strategic plan time frame. Because of this, the financial impact needed to be estimated and projected for both the premium revenues as well as the variable expenses. RHMC believes it can garner 1,500 Medicare members within a three-year time frame, thus earning an additional $300,000 per month ($200 PMPM × 1,500 members) or $3,600,000 a year. The $200 PMPM is the allocated hospital portion of the AAPCC in RHMC's home county. At the same time, the physicians, both primary care and specialists, will get to split as much as $150 PMPM (or a total of $2,700,000). The organization's administration considers this a considerable sum and well worth the trouble to achieve.

Operating Expense Implications

Projecting operating expenses over a five-year time horizon carries the same high risk of uncertainty as that of gross revenues. In the case of expenses, there are at least two main assumption sets that need to be determined—volume and inflation. Like revenues, all variable expenses are a function of projected volumes. Therefore, it is appropriate to use the projected volume changes that have already been previously accepted as one of the multipliers for the variable expense changes.

There is also a need to project inflation changes for all operating expenses, whether variable of fixed. Some may consider this nothing more than a guessing game. *Prior year* inflation rates, arrayed by major expense categories, can be found in a number of places. It is somewhat harder to find any company or service, whether proprietary or in the public domain, that will project inflation rates by category over the following five-year time frame.[6] However, RHMC has found a service that does these projections over five years and across the various healthcare organization major expense categories and has proven to have a reasonably good crystal ball. These external projections are then used as the source for inflation in the strategic financial plan.

An underlying and unyielding assumption that needs to be determined before finalizing the five-year plan is the *margin target* that the organization *requires* on an annual basis. This is necessary for the organization to determine whether its assumptions will produce the results that it desires. Every organization will use a different margin target depending on a variety of factors including but not limited to the following.

- Organization culture
- Board requirements
- Demographics of the organization's service area
- Payor mix
- Service mix
- Tax status—exempt or for-profit

RHMC has determined that the appropriate operating margin required for the five-year plan is 4%, a figure that has closely mimicked the average operating margin for the Fortune 500 organizations after taxes and before dividends. It therefore closely aligns with the kinds of financial returns generated by corporations in other industries and is supportable at the board level and within the community. The operating expense assumptions for RHMC is expressed in the strategic financial plan as follows.

---

[6] *Rate Controls Twice Monthly Newsletter*, Rate Controls Publications, (602) 995-9435.

- We expect salaries and wage to increase at a rate of 3.5% per year over the following five years.
- Controllable nonsalary inflation increases are assumed to be 3% per year.
- An additional $500,000 per year in nonsalary expense reductions need to be assumed in order to achieve targeted goals.
- As a result of net revenue reductions, in order to meet a targeted level of a 4% operating margin, staffing levels need to be reduced by 15%, from 1,000 full time equivalent employees (FTEs) to 850 FTEs at the end of the fourth year.

In addition to the assumptions listed in the strategic financial report to the finance committee and the board of directors, the organization's administration will also take the opportunity to supply an analysis and conclusion. In the case of RHMC, the summary and conclusion for the upcoming five-year period will appear as follows.

1. The ability to generate the targeted bottom line results will be compromised by the expected impact of managed care growth and capitated reimbursement plans. In addition, achieving the projected outpatient growth is a critical factor.
2. The anticipated onset of capitated reimbursement and declining noncapitated reimbursement requires dramatic reductions in operating expenses to maintain targeted margin and cash requirement levels. The magnitude of these cost reductions is consistent with those presented in the previous plan.
3. Compared to the prior plan, the level of planned capital expenditures has been reduced by over $5 million.
4. It needs to be noted that the baseline strategic financial plan is essentially an operating plan assuming current market share. Market share is an integral part of the strategic plan. If successful, increased market share dramatically improves the results of this financial plan.
5. Concerns about possible community reaction to real or perceived reductions in customer service or patient care quality as staff reductions occur may override the realization of cost reduction and margin targets.

RATIO ANALYSIS

The assumptions used by the organization's administration lead to several financial and operational conclusions. Specifically, in order to meet the 4% operating margin target, the strategic financial plan indicates a number of directions that the organization may take. If the organization is not able to improve its future financial condition through volume and revenue assumptions, then it needs to take appropriate actions on the expense side. In addition, the five-year future financial statements that are developed through this process create a series of financial ratios that are essential to the analysis and action plans being prepared. Finally, the analysis can be used to determine that future ratios will exceed the levels required by the bond covenants.

Ratios force users to take two seemingly unrelated bits of data and create a result that has deeper meaning. The result often allows the information user to trend and benchmark the result, shaping a direction for action. For example, a simple ratio that validates this notion is the net margin ratio. The net margin ratio is the result of dividing the net margin by the total revenues, both of which are taken from the statement of operations. The result, expressed as a ratio, has more meaning than the underlying two numbers.

Consider the following.

- In 1997, RHMC had a net margin of $5,300,000 on total revenues of $100,800,000. In 1998, its net margin is $6,400,000 on total revenues of $103,100,000. By itself, these numbers may not have much meaning.

- For example, if all you knew about the organization was that it earned $5.3 million or $6.2 million, would you think the organization did well financially? Well, perhaps it would be appropriate to know what base of revenues these earnings represented. Those earnings on $100 million in total revenues would be better than those earnings on $1 billion in total revenues.

- So developing a ratio that reflects the underlying value of the equation is important. In this case, running the numbers through the equation results in net margin ratios for 1997 and 1998, respectively of 5.3% and 6.2%.

- This is better but it still does not give us final information for decision making. For that we need to see these results over time (trends) and against competitors and peers (benchmarking). However, determining the ratio itself does complete the first step.

In healthcare, several external services use ratio analysis to make decisions for their clients or themselves. The most likely use of ratios for external users is to determine how well the organization did in relation to other organizations. This is always done by bond rating agencies such as Moody's and Standard and Poor's, usually on an annual basis and occasionally on a quarterly basis. The ratings are continually updated in order to evaluate the ongoing financial health of the organization with bonds that have been issued and are still outstanding.

There are literally dozens of ratios available to be computed. Perhaps the best source of healthcare ratio analysis that is available in the industry is published by the Center for Health Information Performance (CHIPS) in its annual *Almanac of Hospital Financial & Operating Indicators*.[7] This book, usually running upwards of 500 pages, presents current financial ratios against a wide variety of peer groupings. There is also commentary, analysis and explanation of the various ratios.

---

[7] Cleverly, W.O. (1998). *The Almanac of Hospital Financial & Operating Indicators*, 1998–1999 ed.

Bonding Related Ratios

For the healthcare *financing* community, as already mentioned in Chapter 2, the three most important ratios involved in bond repayment are long-term debt to capitalization ratio, debt service coverage ratio, and cash flow to total debt ratio.

These ratios were fully described and their calculations shown in Chapter 2.

Other Ratios

Still, there are other ratios that are always evaluated in the overall mix of bond rating because of their influence in the overall financial health of the organization (Box 3–1 shows the actual equations).

- Operating margin
- Net margin
- Current ratio
- Cushion ratio
- Days cash on hand
- Average age of plant
- Capital expenditures as a percentage of total expenses
- Days in accounts receivable
- Average payment period

There are benchmarks for all of these ratios. The benchmarks are usually reported as the median values of a list of organizations somewhat similar to yours. Medians are usually defined as the organization in the sample that is exactly in the middle of the pack when the values are arrayed highest to lowest. There are several rating organizations that collect and disseminate benchmarks. See Table 3–3 for some of the values reported by these organizations.

Operating margin and net margin—Both these ratios involve either the operating results or net results as a function of net revenues. These are widely used indicators of profitability. Unfortunately, these ratios are not always comparable. The controversy involving the placement of interest income "above the line" has already been discussed in Chapter 2. Still, the operating margin ratio can be considered useful when trended against itself. This allows the organization to determine if its financial direction is positive or negative. Meanwhile, the net margin ratio can be either trended against itself or compared to local, regional, and national benchmarks to determine whether the organization's financial outcomes are favorable or not.

Current ratio—This ratio describes an organization's ability to use its current assets to pay off its current liabilities. As long as the ratio is above 1.0 the liabilities should be able to be extinguished without problem. Still, a current ratio closer to 2.0 is considered good and clearly preferred. To achieve a higher current ratio (which is preferable), the organization needs to either increase its current assets or decrease its current liabilities.

B O X 3–1

OTHER FINANCIAL RATIO FORMULAS

Operating margin =

$$\frac{\text{(total operating revenue} - \text{total operating expenses)}}{\text{total operating revenue}}$$

Net (excess) margin (%) =

$$\frac{\text{(total operating revenue} - \text{total operating expenses} + \text{non-operating revenue)}}{\text{(total operating revenue} + \text{non-operating revenue)}}$$

Current ratio (x) = $\dfrac{\text{total current assets}}{\text{total current liabilities}}$

Cushion ratio (x) =

$$\frac{\text{(cash and cash equivalents} + \text{board designated funds for capital)}}{\text{estimated future peak debt service}}$$

Cash on hand (days) =

$$\frac{\text{(cash and cash equivalents} + \text{board designated funds for capital)} \times 365}{\text{(total operating expenses} - \text{depreciation and amortization expenses)}}$$

Average age of plant (years) = $\dfrac{\text{accumulated depreciation}}{\text{depreciation expense}}$

Capital expense (%) =

$$\frac{\text{(interest expense} + \text{depreciation and amortization expenses)}}{\text{total operating expenses}}$$

Accounts receivable (days) =

$$\frac{\text{(net patient accounts receivable} \times 365)}{\text{net patient revenue}}$$

Average payment period (days) =

$$\frac{\text{(total current liabilities} \times 365)}{\text{(total operating expenses} - \text{depreciation and amortization expenses)}}$$

Cushion ratio—A ratio that is used to determine the amount of cash and cash equivalents available to pay off future peak debt services (which is defined as the largest annual interest expense and principal payments on the existing debt). A higher ratio is always preferable.

Days cash on hand—Another ratio that is used in determining total cash available to liquidate or pay off annual operating expenses. The available cash includes

Ridgeland Heights Medical Center
Key Hospital Financial Statistics and Ratio Medians
As of September, 1998

Measure	RHMC — 1998 Actual	RHMC-2002 Strategic Financial Plan	Moody's All Ratings	Standard & Poor's All Ratings	HCIA and Deloitte & Touche	Data Advantage Corp	MECON
Sample size			308	78	2,865	3,156	407
Operating margin (%)	5.0%	1.2%	3.6%	3.1%	3.9%	1.2%	n/a
Net (excess) margin (%)	6.2%	4.1%	5.8%	5.7%	5.4%	6.6%	n/a
Current ratio (x)	1.27	1.9	1.90	1.97	2.06	1.92	n/a
Cushion ratio (x)	12.19	16.4	9.90	12.28	n/a	n/a	n/a
Days cash on hand (days)	525.87	643.45	151.20	167.00	n/a	98.29	n/a
Average age of plant (years)	6.55	9.2	8.50	8.00	9.34	8.03	n/a
Capital expenses (%)	18.8%	19.3%	n/a	8.7%	7.1%	8.4%	n/a
Accounts receivable (days)	63.31	55.00	60.70	59.60	65.82	63.07	61.40
Average payment period (days)	81.90	62.00	64.10	61.80	58.91	70.06	n/a
Long-term debt to capitalization (%)	64.6%	54.78%	37.8%	31.8%	31.0%	42.1%	n/a
Debt service coverage (x)	2.28	2.9	4.04	3.97	4.76	n/a	n/a
Average length of stay (days)	4.07	5.1	5.1	n/a	4.12	5.04	4.8

long-term investments that can be converted to cash in less than one year (generally without decreasing the value of the investment). Bond investment managers and bondholders of the organization's tax-exempt bonds are interested in its ability to meet its short-term obligations. If the benchmark is approximately 100 days of cash on hand, then it would be important for the organization to meet, if not exceed, this. A higher ratio is always preferable.

Average age of plant—An important and underrated ratio that represents the relative age of the organization's plant and its capital equipment. In this case, a lower result is preferable because it designates the equivalent of a newer or more modern physical plant. Even if the organization does not build a completely new plant, this ratio accounts for all capital renovations and equipment replacement that has taken place.

Capital expenses as a percentage of total expenses—A ratio that is linked to the average age of plant because any capital expenditures will effect both ratios. There are differing views on the value of this ratio.

One school of thought suggests that because higher expenses for capital lead to higher depreciation expenses and, thus, lower operating and net margins, *any* expended capital should pay for itself through a return on investment calculation. The thinking is that any capital that does not pay for its annual depreciation may well need to be paid for through decreased FTEs. Trading FTEs for capital purchases may be a good idea only if it is done with foreknowledge. However, it is not uncommon in this industry for capital purchases to be made without enough financial analysis.

Still, The Advisory Board has made a case that those organizations with higher than average capital expenses as a percentage of physical assets as well as higher capital expenditures per bed create an enduring advantage if the capital purchases are made to expand or establish new services.[8] In this case, The Advisory Board highlights Columbia/HCA and suggests that heavy reinvestment of profits in plant and equipment will likely magnify an advantage over time.

Days in accounts receivable—A ratio that is used by both bond rating agencies and internal operational management to assess the value of potential cash tied up in the accounts receivable. There are also numerous opportunities to benchmark this ratio. This allows the organization's administration to determine if their accounts receivable management is effective. The concepts behind accounts receivable management and the implications of this ratio are explored in Chapter 5.

Average payment period—This ratio is somewhat tied to those ratios that assess cash levels and the organization's ability to pay its debts. In this case, the debts being liquidated specifically refer to current liabilities. The largest current liabilities are usually the trade vendor payables. Bond rating agencies review this ratio to determine that the organization is in line with industry standards for payment periods. This is not a detailed review of the payable balances, but rather, a result derived from financial statement information. If either the investment manager or the organization is interested in getting behind the numbers, an external rating agency such as Dun and Bradstreet will provide details.

---

[8] The Advisory Board. (1996). *The New Competitive Standard for Hospitals*, The Advisory Board Company, p. 25.

Operating Ratios

There is more to ratio analysis than just bond rating. Ratio analysis can be extremely useful in understanding the organization's operations. Following are useful operating ratios.

- Full time equivalents (FTEs) per adjusted patient days (APDs)
- Salaries, wages, and fringe benefits as a percentage of net revenues
- Expenses per APDs
- Expense per adjusted discharges (EPADs)
- Revenue per FTE
- Length of stay

Box 3–2 shows the ratio calculations.

FTEs per APDs—The most common ratio used in the healthcare industry to measure overall productivity. FTEs represent the wages being paid to an employee that is designated as full time. Full time in most organizations means that the employee is paid (but does not necessarily work) for 2,080 hours (52 weeks × 40 hours per week). APDs are a calculation that attempts to convert the outpatient revenues into an equivalent inpatient day.

Some controversy surrounding this widely used equation has sprung up in recent years. FTEs/APDs has become an established benchmark throughout the

B O X 3–2

OPERATIONAL RATIO FORMULAS

$$\text{Adjusted patient days} = \frac{\text{Total revenue} \times \text{inpatient days}}{\text{Inpatient revenue}}$$

$$\text{Adjusted discharges} = \frac{\text{Total revenue} \times \text{inpatient discharges}}{\text{Inpatient revenue}}$$

FTEs per adjusted patient day = see Table 3–4

$$\text{Salaries, wages, and fringe benefits as a percentage of net revenues} = \frac{\text{Salary expenses} + \text{Total fringe benefit expenses}}{\text{Total revenues}}$$

$$\text{Expenses per adjusted patient day} = \frac{\text{Total expenses}}{\text{Adjusted patient days}}$$

$$\text{Expenses per adjusted discharge} = \frac{\text{Total expenses}}{\text{Adjusted discharges}}$$

$$\text{Revenue per FTE} = \frac{\text{Total revenues}}{\text{Total FTEs}}$$

$$\text{Average length of stay (days)} = \frac{\text{Patient days}}{\text{Total discharges}}$$

industry. Yet it is fraught with inconsistency. The numerator (FTEs) is highly susceptible to manipulation while the denominator is a poor equalization factor for converting outpatient services into an inpatient equivalent.

In the case of the numerator, the total number of paid (or worked) hours is divided by the number of hours in the period under study (e.g., a week would be 40 hours, biweekly would be 80 hours, and a year would be 2,080 hours). The problem is that most organizations only collect and report the hours paid to employees, but not the hours paid for contract labor or purchased services. So, if an organization wanted to manipulate the FTEs/APDs calculation in order to make its overall productivity look better, it could outsource many of its services to nonemployees.

Inpatient and outpatient revenues consist of different service components and differing levels of severity. They are not comparable! Most hospital charge masters (which generate the list price for every service and supply) are not completely based on established costing methodologies. Instead they have evolved over time without an ongoing review for consistency. Because of this, outpatient services may have become either overweighted or underweighted, making the denominator a poor factor for such an important benchmark.

In the case of the denominator, the equation used to convert the outpatient revenues into inpatient day equivalents is significantly flawed. This equation was created many years ago when 85% to 90% of hospital revenues were derived from inpatient services and the remainder was outpatient. At the time, this equation did a moderately fair job of conversion. But, in the current period of the late 1990s, when outpatient revenues have equaled or exceeded 50% of total revenues in hospitals and integrated delivery systems, the service equivalent no longer works.

Salaries, wages, and fringe benefits as a percentage of net patient service revenue—This is a better ratio to measure overall productivity. This ratio was popularized by Columbia/HCA, which saw the problems inherent in the FTEs/APD equation. With 350 hospitals, they needed a ratio that was reliable and consistent. This ratio removes the question of whether all outsourced *hours* have been accounted for and whether or not the APDs equation does a good enough job in converting the outpatient services.

The ratio includes all salary dollars paid out plus all dollars paid to contract labor and service companies for staffing expenses. Further, it includes all dollars paid out in fringe benefit because they are fully attached to salaries. The resulting ratio measures the level of labor costs in relation to the revenues being generated by the organization. A downward trend is preferred. Better financial performance will usually result when labor costs can be minimized.

RHMC decided to take the compromise position in the controversy. Although it is aware that the FTEs/APDs ratio has consistency problems, the organization still wants to capture the data and at least measure the trends against itself over time. Continuing to use the ratio against its own prior performance eliminates one of the two problems plaguing the ratio—the contract labor component. It does not, however, eliminate the problem that the conversion factor is flawed. At the same time, RHMC has adopted the salaries, wages, and fringe benefits ratio as an adjunct.

When it started to use the ratio, it went back three years to see whether it is trending favorably or unfavorably. In fact, although its FTEs/APDs were trending favorably downward, salaries, wages and fringe benefits as a percentage of net revenues were trending unfavorably upwards. This is another indication of the problem inherent with the former ratio. Table 3–4 summarizes the inputs and outputs of the two equations.

RHMC's FTEs/APDs in 1998 was recorded as 4.10. According to various reputable benchmarks published around the country, this would be considered very good, from the standpoint of productivity measures and cost containment. But as an

TABLE   3–4

Ridgeland Heights Medical Center
Analysis of FTEs per APD vs Salaries, Wages and Fringe Benefits as a
Percentage of Net Revenues for the Years Ended 1996–1998

	1996	**1997**	**1998**
FTEs per Adjusted Patient Days			
FTEs	880	1,000	980
Patient days	46,000	45,500	44,200
Inpatient revenue	$73,000	$74,000	$78,000
Outpatient revenues	$65,000	$69,000	$76,000
Total revenues	$138,000	$143,000	$154,000
Calculation of Adjustment to Patient Days			
$\dfrac{\text{Total revenue} \times \text{inpatient days}}{\text{Inpatient revenue}}$	1.89	1.93	1.97
Total adjusted patient days per year	86,959	87,926	87,267
Number of days in the year	366	365	365
Number of adjusted patients per day	237.6	240.9	239.1
Ratio — FTEs per adjusted patient days	3.70	4.15	4.10
Salaries, Wages, and Fringe Benefits as a Percentage of Net Revenues			
Salaries	$32,000	$34,000	36,000
Contract labor	$1,300	$1,500	$1,000
Fringe benefits	$4,900	$5,400	$5,800
Total staffing costs	$38,200	$40,900	$42,800
Net revenues	$92,800	$92,800	$93,400
Ratio — Salaries, Wages and Fringe Benefits as a Percentage of Net Revenue			
	41.2%	44.1%	45.8%

example of how this ratio often is falsely portrayed, it would be important to know that RHMC outsources its laboratory services. It has been estimated that these services provide the equivalent of 105 FTEs to the organization. If they were accounted for in the equation, the 1998 FTEs/APDs would increase from 4.10 to 4.54, still a respectable ratio but not as good as before. The salaries, wages, and fringe benefits as a percentage of net patient service revenue ratio is similarly affected because the expense is treated as a purchased service not as contract labor. This highlights some of the ways that any ratio could be distorted.

Expenses per adjusted patient days and expenses per adjusted discharges—These two ratios are closely related. The numerator is the same while the denominator is either inpatient patient days or discharges adjusted for outpatient services provided. Because this is primarily an operational ratio and not used by bond rating agencies, there are less external services that provide benchmarks. However, the EPAD ratio is available annually through the Mercer/HCIA Top 100 analysis published in the November/December time frame issue of *Modern Healthcare*. Expanded information and analysis is also available directly through HCIA. Other services like McFaul & Lyons provide proprietary expenses per APD ratios established through an analysis of over 1,000 clients.

These ratios are particularly important to the organization's administration because they demonstrate actual cost performance. In addition, because they can be both benchmarked and trended, they become extremely useful as an overall indicator of how well or poorly the organization is performing over time and against other like organizations.

Revenue per FTE—This is an interesting ratio because it is one of the few that cuts across other industries. Most other industries routinely capture and report revenue per employee as an operational productivity value. As a service industry, healthcare organizations will generally earn less revenue per employee, but that should not deter the evaluation of this ratio. By capturing the ratio, the organization can strive to continually improve its revenues.

Length of stay—This is one of the most ubiquitous ratios in healthcare. Almost every segment of the industry uses this ratio. Hospitals, psychiatric facilities, skilled nursing facilities, and children's hospitals all capture this measure and use it to continually compare themselves against prior years' measurements as well as against outside benchmarks.

It should be recognized however, that this ratio is only one component of operational understanding. Organizations have been attempting to and succeeding in reducing length of stay since 1983 when Medicare changed its method for reimbursing hospitals. They went from paying costs on a per diem (or per day) basis to paying for the type of diagnosis for which the patient was being treated. Because it was not in the organization's best financial interest to keep patients for longer periods of time, care plans were established to allow the patient to be discharged sooner.

Still, there is a big issue that needs to be analyzed when reviewing the length of stay ratio or when benchmarking length of stay against either other organizations or your own organization. The length of a patient's stay is often a function of the severity of a patient's illness. The industry has spent many years developing numerical equivalents for the patient's severity or acuity. The most common statistic used as a proxy for severity is called the Case Mix Index (CMI). CMI is the accumulation of the case weights for all the Medicare inpatients that have been discharged from the hospital over a defined time period. The average CMI is 1.00, but it varies from .40 for the most common labor and delivery case to over 16.00 for a tracheostomy. So when looking at length of stay statistics, it is also important to incorporate a severity indicator.

THE CAPITAL PLAN AND ITS RELATIONSHIP TO THE STRATEGIC PLAN

The annual strategic financial plan compels the organization to continually update its capital plan in order to determine capital requirements and its relationship to the organization's available cash and investments. These steps are performed concurrently with the operating projections. The process used to execute the capital plan is often organized in seven basic steps.

1. Defining the institution's capital position
2. Identifying ongoing capital requirements
3. Quantifying the debt capacity and identifying the level of risk capital
4. Defining the primary funding/financing problems and setting key goals
5. Developing and evaluating financing alternatives
6. Establishing a master capital plan
7. Preparing an implementation plan[9]

RHMC believes in these steps and follows them closely. It performs annual updates of the capital plan in conjunction with the strategic financial plan updates.

The centerpiece of the capital plan is the identification of its ongoing capital requirements (item #2 above). To do so, the medical center has to make a series of capital assumptions linked to the strategic plan and the strategic financial plan that are moving along just ahead of the capital plan. These assumptions relate to decisions on whether to purchase, lease, or build necessary capital. In any case, the dollar values associated with these acquisitions are the critical feature after the organization decides what to acquire.

Table 3–5 illustrates the RHMC's ongoing capital requirements. As can be seen, it is a five-year plan that summarizes various types of planned capital acquisitions. In addition to the budgeted routine capital items, special, nonroutine capital items are featured. These special line items consist of information technology and

---

[9] An excellent discussion of capital planning and its implication for healthcare organizations is presented in Kaufman, K., Hall, M. (1990). *The Capital Management of Healthcare Organizations.* Health Administration Press: Ann Arbor, Mich.

TABLE 3–5

Ridgeland Heights Medical Center
5-Year Capital Budget (in thousands)

	Budget 1998	1999	2000	2001	2002	5-Year total
Routine capital budget	$5,000	$6,000	$7,000	$ 7,000	$ 7,000	$32,000
Information technology	3,000	5,000	3,000	3,000	3,000	17,000
Facility improvements and upgrades	2,500	2,500	2,500	2,500	2,500	12,500
Property acquisitions	500	500	500	500	500	2,500
Physician recruitment	1,000	1,000	1,000	1,000	1,000	5,000
Physician medical office space	500	500	500	500	500	2,500
Total	$12,500	$15,500	$14,500	$14,500	$14,500	$71,500

facility upgrades, typically the two largest contributors to capital purchases. In addition there are separate budget categories for land acquisition as well as physician recruitment and physician medical office space.

Routine capital items—This line item generally consists of much of the equipment that is needed in areas such as the laboratory, radiology, and cardiology as well as the nursing floors. As stated in Chapter 2, this is applicable only for purchases where the price exceeds that of the organization's capitalization policy and has an estimated useful life greater than one year.

Information technology—This capital line has gotten much more respect over the past few years. Prior to the mid-1990s, the healthcare industry spent less than 2.5% of its capital for information technology. This compares unfavorably to the 5% to 7% spent by the manufacturing, insurance, and banking industries. Being behind these other industries meant that the right amount of information was not being collected, reported, or analyzed in either the financial or clinical sides of the healthcare business. This allowed opportunities for those in the healthcare industry to gain a competitive advantage through technology. Towards the end of the century, most of the healthcare providers got the message, aided by the Year 2000 problem.

At RHMC, the administration started to understand its lack of effective information technology support in 1996, when it began to allocate a greater portion of its scarce capital resources to IT. As such, it now makes it a point to separately break out this line and spend for IT in the most appropriate manner. Some of the allocated monies are projected to be spent on upgraded IT infrastructure such as new fiber optic cabling and distribution closets—costing $1.2 million. In addition, it plans to upgrade all Year 2000 noncompliant hardware and software. That is budgeted at $2.0 million. Finally the purchase of a new organization-wide clinical and financial system is expected over the next three years at a price of $9 million dollars. The issue of information technology in healthcare is discussed in great detail in Chapter 10.

Facility upgrades—Like other industries, healthcare needs to remain reasonably current with its physical plant. Thus, RHMC projects the amount of money it believes it will need to spend over the next five years to keep its plant modern. In addition, this line is used to allocate capital funds for new major projects that will involve the acquisition of new or expanded facilities—whether through construction, purchase, or capital lease. RHMC has allocated funds for projects such as major renovations for two of its medical/surgical units, projected to cost $2 million each, a new renal dialysis unit with 16 patient stations projected to cost $1.6 million, and a newly expanded emergency department projected to cost $2.5 million.

Land acquisition—This is an important and often overlooked line, particularly dependent on the location of the healthcare facility. In the case of RHMC, it is landlocked—surrounded on all four sides by residential housing. In order to expand, it needs to allocate funds to buy up all of the single family housing that comes on the market within the target area that has been designated by the administration and approved by the board. Its policy also allows it to solicit the homeowners in the target area to sell to the organization based on the appraised market value. RHMC's target area consists of two streets directly adjacent to its campus. It believes that once it acquires all the houses along the block it will be able to incorporate the area into the existing healthcare zone, tear down the houses, and expand service offerings. It is important to note that this is a very long-term strategy that has the opportunity to succeed *for the next administrator.*

Physician recruitment—Another line item that has sprung up since the early to mid-1990s when hospitals began in earnest to employ physicians. This helped to change the face of the industry in a fundamental way. Hospitals began to recruit and employ physicians in response to the rapid buildup of managed care health plans throughout the country. The defining feature of managed care plans was its insistence that its covered beneficiaries, known as members, always see a primary care physician (PCP) before any advanced care would be covered (i.e., paid for) by the plan. Hospital care, whether inpatient or outpatient, was considered specialized care. Hospitals wanted to remain in some control of their volumes and knew that physicians employed by them would refer their hospital business to them.

So, hospitals began to employ physicians, some in bigger ways than others. Following are the two primary ways to acquire physician practices.

1. Buy existing practices
2. Establish new practices by employing young physicians just out of residency programs

Each method has its own issues. However, the hospital will spend capital money in either case. The purchase of existing practices will require the transfer of funds from the hospital to the physicians in the group to pay for their existing assets. The establishment of new practices will require the hospital to fund significant start-up costs sometimes for as long as three to five years until the practices are self-sustaining.

In any case, the capital needs for physician recruitment have become significant for healthcare entities in the late 1990s and show no signs of slowing down any time soon. RHMC is caught up in the physician employment frenzy, as are their immediate competitors. And so they have found themselves needing to allocate considerable sums in their long-term financial plans. We examine physician practice management issues in greater detail in Chapter 8.

Physician medical office space—If your organization is going to employ physicians, you will obviously need to find them a place to practice. So, RHMC has allocated funds to either build or capital lease new facilities for their physicians to practice. Even if you don't employ physicians, organizations may want to build medical office space to attract physicians to practice at your organization.

Capital Affordability

An important aspect of this five-year capital budget is its cumulative total. This total will be used to determine if the organization can, indeed, afford all of it. There are several ways to determine how much money the organization can afford to spend on capital equipment. Two ways used by RHMC are the following.

1. Spending equivalent to annual depreciation expense
2. Spending equivalent to a percentage of annual depreciation expense

Spending equivalent to annual depreciation expense—This is a tried and true, time-honored method used by many organizations in many industries. Because depreciation is a noncash expense on the statement of operations, most administrators believe it is acceptable to spend the depreciation money on capital acquisitions. And many do. It is the equivalent of turning capital funding into operational funding on an annual basis.

Spending equivalent to a percentage of annual depreciation expense—Even though many healthcare organizations allocate and spend 100% of their annual depreciation expense on capital acquisitions, this may not be the most efficient or effective use of these funds. We saw earlier in the chapter that the RHMC administration is currently proposing a $5 million reduction in its current five-year capital expenditure plan because of the negative impact these purchases would have had on the organization's bottom line.

In fact, there are organizations that routinely spend only 70% to 80% of their depreciation expense on capital purchases in order to maintain a lower future depreciation expense. This is done knowingly because these organizations do not want to trade FTEs for depreciation, as we already reviewed earlier in the chapter. So, using either of these methods does at least allow healthcare organizations to make informed decisions regarding its use and implications.

In summary, the capital plan is the culmination of the strategic plan process, setting the stage for the approved capital acquisitions that the organization will be permitted to make throughout the upcoming years. RHMC's diligence in preparing and updating its strategic plan, strategic financial plan, and capital plan has allowed it to maintain healthy margins. It has also allowed it to project both the best and worst into the future. In doing so, it has turned plans into actions, with forethought. This is the mark of good management. With all the work that had been performed by the RHMC staff, and the quality of the analysis presented by its administration, the board of directors approved the updated five-year strategic financial and capital plan at its special March meeting. Specific application of the capital plan will be implemented during the annual capital budgeting process that will commence in June. See Chapter 6 for initiation of the annual capital budget.

CHAPTER

April

Sam Barnes panted as he lunged at a well-placed kill shot delivered with pinpoint precision by his opponent Joel Hogan.

"Ugh! Missed again," grunted Sam.

"Sam, what's the matter with you," asked Hogan, his friend and racquetball partner over the past several years.

"I don't know," answered Sam. "Well okay, maybe I do know. Even though you know that I love to play racquetball and it keeps me in decent shape, I've been unable to find enough energy to maintain my conditioning over the past several weeks."

"Well I have noticed that you seem to have lost a step or two over the past couple of months," said Joel with an air of pleasure in his voice. "So what the heck is going on with you?"

"Joel, I've been thinking a lot about what I do at work. And it sure seems like things are closing in on this industry. The biggest thing that's come down the pike over the past several years is this new Balanced Budget Act (BBA) passed by Congress and signed by the president last August. It seems as if nobody in the general public has any concept of the major changes that are going to take place because of this act. It's true that the Feds need to save a lot of money if they're going to keep the Medicare Trust Fund solvent. But by doing it primarily on the backs of the providers, it is likely that a variety of services will be cut, thereby making services less accessible to the very people who need it—the sick, the old, the poor."

"Okay, so the Feds are going to do this with or without your approval. Why are you letting this sap your energy?" asked Joel.

"Sometimes," said Sam, "I can't really help how I feel. You know that I'm pretty passionate about my work. It's more than a job with me. I care about the quality of the services we provide at Ridgeland. Just as important, I care about the perception of quality provided throughout the industry because if one provider gets a bad name, it usually paints a black mark on the rest of us. And I can't imagine that the quality will go unscathed as we get $116 billion cut out over the next five years."

Joel was perplexed. "So what do you plan to do about it? Are you planning to take any action or just wallow in pity and despair?"

"That's just the problem," said Joel. "At the moment I haven't quite figured it out but I know I'll keep working on it till I do. Right now though I plan to refresh myself by beating your sorry body at this game."

April Fools Day at Ridgeland Heights Medical Center. It should have been a time for some practical jokes and a little bit of frivolity, but at Ridgeland Heights, this was not so. The medical center was starting to reduce its expectations as a result of some significant decreases to its revenue. These lowered expectations were having negative impacts on employee morale. Although the organization's administration was trying to counter the prevailing mood by creating a positive environment, it was not working. While the administration made a point of staying in close touch with its staff to explain these revenue changes, the fact remained that these changes added new pressures to the organization.

It was obvious to many of RHMC's constituency that belt-tightening was upon them. The medical staff noticed. They perceived that there were fewer nurses on the floor to take care of patients. The nurses noticed. They recognized that nurses who resigned were not being replaced as fast as before. They knew this because they were being asked to work quite a bit more overtime. They believed this was the effect of the staff tightening. The remainder of the clinical staff noticed. They were aware that the nurses were more tired and critical as they worked more and more hours. The administration noticed. The prized patient satisfaction scores, which everyone in the organization was so proud of, were in decline. Over the past two years, the organization had managed to maintain its patient satisfaction scores in the range of the 90th percentile across a set of 400 peer hospitals. RHMC had in fact managed to move into the high 90s during several of those months, in all three of the rated areas, in-patient, outpatient ancillary services, and the emergency department.

Unfortunately, while the effects were obvious, the constituencies were misdiagnosing the causes. Coincidentally, in the middle of the revenue reduction efforts by many of the third-party payors, the industry was in the middle of its third major nursing shortage in the past 20 years. As RHMC's administration had assembled much of its staff over the past three months to explain the revenue reduction problem, it made a great effort to communicate its commitment to patient care and patient satisfaction. In fact the current year budget included *increases* to the nursing staff, not a decrease. However, its message was lost in the continuing depression caused by the ongoing overwork.

At RHMC, the reduction in revenue was a function of its payor mix. RHMC identifies its payor mix in order to analyze and understand the source of its revenues. Following is the RHMC payor mix based on gross revenues.

	Current Year
Medicare	38%
Medicaid	6%
HMO—managed care	16%
PPO—managed care	14%
Worker's Compensation	4%
Commercial Insurers	8%
Other	14%

In this case, RHMC is representative in all of its payor mix with the national averages except for Medicaid. Because of its location in a relatively affluent community, there are not as many Medicaid-eligible residents. Table 4–1 shows the RHMC payor mix and how it compares to the national averages.

Because RHMC has almost 40% of its total revenue stream coming from Medicare, it is extremely important for the organization's administration to understand the roots of the reimbursement reductions. Even more important, they must make decisions on how to operationalize changes that need to be made because of the current and continuing revenue reductions.

The roots of the revenue reduction were set many years ago during the creation of the federal Medicare and Medicaid programs as well as the more recent rise of managed care.

TABLE 4–1

Total Payor Mix—RHMC Compared to National Averages

	RHMC	National Average
Medicare	38%	33%
Medicaid	6%	15%
Other government	2%	13%
Private health insurance and other private funds	42%	36%
Out-of-pocket	12%	3%

Source: *Health, United States,* 1996–1997, United States Department of Health and Human Services, Table 125.

MEDICARE AND MEDICAID NET REVENUE CONCEPTS

The History of Medicare and Medicaid[1]

Medicare and Medicaid, known legally as Title XVIII (18) and Title XIX (19) of the Social Security Act, were enacted in 1965. Medicare was created to provide health insurance to most American citizens ages 65 and over and to certain disabled people under 65 years. Medicaid was created as a state-operated program to provide publicly financed healthcare coverage for the poor. These programs, which were signed into law by President Johnson on July 31, 1965, became effective on July 1, 1966.

Over the last three decades, the Medicare program has received considerably more publicity and press than the Medicaid program. This may well be the result of two particular factors—Americans over 65, through experience, have learned to use the system to their advantage, meaning that they have more political clout than Medicaid patients. In addition, the Medicare program costs more than the Medicaid program and is thus more likely to contain expenditure savings and entitlement impacts.

The Medicare program actually has two components. Part A (called the hospital insurance program) primarily covers inpatient hospital and surgery services, post-hospital skilled nursing care, home health services, and hospice care. In 1972, the Part A Fund also began providing coverage for patients with end stage renal disease (ESRD) and certain organ transplants. Medicare Part B (called the supplemental medical insurance program) primarily covers physician services, outpatient medical and surgical services, and independent laboratory services.

Each of these two coverage types is financed independently and differently. Part A services are paid through a Trust Fund financed through a special form of Social Security tax on earnings. These funds are accumulated and collected through employer and employee contributions. The Medicare tax is equal to 1.45% of salaries and wages payable by both the employer and the employee for a total of 2.9%. Self-employed individuals are required to pay both parts of the tax. In addition, while non-Medicare Social Security taxes have annual maximums above which the taxes end, there is no annual maximum for the Medicare contributions.

Part B services are financed through patient premiums and general federal tax revenues. When the Medicare program was started, 50% of the Part B services were financed through the premiums. Over the years, as the increases in patient premiums did not keep up with the increased cost of services, the percentage of the Part B services financed by these premiums has dropped to approximately 25%. Therefore the federal treasury now finances 75% of Medicare Part B services.

---

[1] An interesting and short history of the Medicare program with extensive bibliography and citation listings was reviewed for this section: Pearman, W.A., Starr, P. (1988). *Medicare: A Handbook on the History and Issues of Health Care Services for the Elderly*. Garland Publishing: New York.

Getting passage of the Medicare bill was the number one priority of President Johnson in 1964 and 1965. Several previous presidents had tried and failed to get some form of legislation passed that provided health insurance to various segments of the American population. President Truman proposed a national health insurance program during his term. It was defeated by Congress. Both Presidents Eisenhower and Kennedy advocated some form of national health insurance. In fact, President Kennedy campaigned on a promise that he would propose a national health insurance program that would protect the elderly regardless of their finances.

Given the long-standing advocacy by various presidents for national health insurance, and its lack of passage, it is obvious that there were heavy political forces arrayed against programs of this kind. The two greatest opponents to federalized health insurance were the American Medical Association, representing the nation's physicians, and the American Health Insurance Association (now known as the Health Insurance Association of America), representing the nation's private insurance companies. The physicians were concerned that federalization of health insurance would lead to a decline in quality of care while the private insurance companies were concerned that federalization would drive them out of business.

Still, President Johnson's landslide victory in the 1964 election and his single-mindedness in adopting his Great Society programs allowed him to push Congress hard for passage. Ultimately the Part A program was adopted to pay primarily for the hospital inpatient services while Part B was adopted as a way of separating physician payments from the hospital side. Finally, to appease a number of constituencies that wanted means-based health insurance, Medicaid was adopted as a state-operated, income-based supplemental plan.

Impacts of Medicare and Medicaid on Provider Net Revenues

One of the most interesting aspects of both the Medicare and Medicaid programs is that they literally had an explosive financial effect on the industry. Medicare and Medicaid were expansive and expensive. Prior to these programs, small hospitals and individual solo physician practices dominated a cottage industry. There was a lot of charity care given by healthcare providers because many patients were very poor and could not afford the care that they needed. The passage of the Medicare and Medicaid programs turned healthcare into an INDUSTRY!

All of a sudden (7/1/66), money was plentiful. It was as if a gigantic spigot opened. Dollars gushed. So much so that within six weeks of Medicare's birth, President Johnson ordered an inquiry into the rising cost of medical care. Figure 4–1 shows the rise of Medicare outlays and beneficiaries from 1967 through 1995, while Figure 4–2 shows the rise of Medicaid outlays and enrollees from 1972 through 1995. The only constant is a significantly upward slope on the cost lines. Medicare went from paying out just under $5 billion in 1967 to expenditures of $184 billion in 1995, a 37-times increase over this 28 year timespan.[2] Medicaid expenditures

---

[2] Health, United States, 1996–1997, United States Department of Health and Human Services, Table 138.

FIGURE 4–1

FIGURE 4–1

Medicare Expenditures and Enrollees 1967–1995

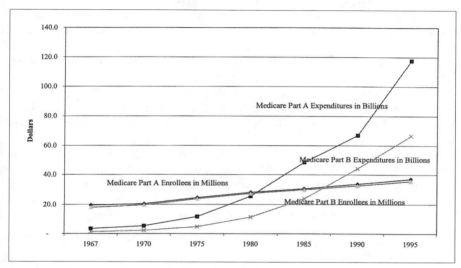

Source: Health, United States, 1996–1997, Table 138.

FIGURE 4–2

Medicaid Enrollees and Expenditures 1972–1996

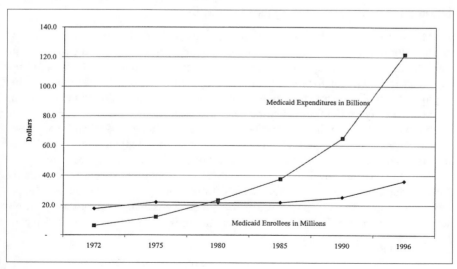

Source: Health, United States, 1998, Table 139.

meanwhile increased from $6 billion in 1972 to $120 billion in 1995.[3] This is a significant element in why healthcare is now the $1 trillion industry mentioned in Chapter 1.

In addition, it should be noted that the Medicare program calls for patients to pay a deductible to the provider of service for the healthcare rendered. Insurance deductibles are generally developed to discourage usage because these fees are supposed to be paid directly by the consumer of service out of their own pocket. The Medicare hospital deductible is meant to represent the cost of the first day stay in a hospital. Therefore, in order to further symbolize the caliber of hospital cost increases between 1966 and 1998, it is interesting to note that the original inpatient hospital deductible was $40 and in 1998 it is $764, a 19-fold increase over 32 years.[4]

Medicare and Medicaid fueled the great expansion of healthcare inflation in the country. As previously stated in Chapter 1, when it was the sleepy industry pre-1966, healthcare absorbed just 5.7% of the gross domestic product (GDP) in the country. In the intervening 32 years, the percentage of GDP has grown to 13.4%, a 235% increase.[5] And the beneficiaries of this increase have been the following.

- Providers who have been able to expand access to patient care (and make money doing so)
- Patients, most of whom have never had greater access to high-touch, high-tech healthcare
- Community, which has saved many of its most valuable resources, its residents, who, because of the increased access to medical care, no longer die prematurely

Implication to Ridgeland Heights Medical Center

RHMC's growth over the past 32 years imitates that of Medicare. Once a sleepy community hospital, RHMC, like many of its competitors, expanded exponentially once Medicare opened up the floodgate of money. Previously, hospitals could not count on full payment for many of its services. Now, Medicare was guaranteeing payment for basic services as well as a whole new set of care. Skilled nursing home care for 100 days and unlimited home healthcare services would now be reimbursed from a payor with seemingly unlimited resources (Medicare). Medicaid would now guarantee the rest of the skilled nursing home care, after depletion of the patient financial resources. In either case, the provider of care knew it would be paid.

In the case of physician services, the new revenue streams were enormous. Before Medicare, physicians often wrote off bills for the elderly because these patients could not afford to pay. Even worse, there were many patients who did not want to accept charity. They would therefore not present themselves for needed care.

---

[3] Ibid, Table 140.
[4] Health Care Financing Administration, Federal Register, November 3, 1997.
[5] Ibid.

FIGURE 4–3

Deaths Rates Per 100,000 Resident Population

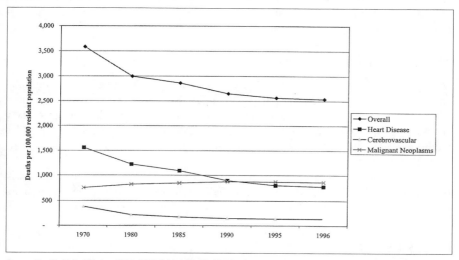

Source: Health, United States, 1996–1997, Tables 37, 38, 39, 40.

They would then get sicker and often die. In fact, the advent of Medicare in 1966 had a dramatic and positive effect on the death rate in America. According to government records, the death rate for all causes dropped by 29.1% between 1970 and 1996 for all persons aged 65 to 74. Figure 4–3 shows declines in the overall death rate as well as the death rates for heart disease, cerebrovascular causes (strokes), and malignant neoplasms (cancers).[6] Interestingly, as the population increased over this time period, and the death rates in some of the more intransigent diseases declined, the death rates for cancers increased.

CALCULATION OF MEDICARE AND MEDICAID CONTRACTUAL ADJUSTMENTS

With the advent of the Medicare and Medicaid programs in 1966, hospitals and other healthcare providers began to do something that they had never done before on their financial statement—they began to record contractual adjustments on their income statements and allowances for these contractual adjustments on their balance sheets.

Contractual adjustments are the discounts that the provider agreed to accept from the insurance company (also known as third-party payor) for providing healthcare to that company's beneficiary. Prior to 1966, the most prevalent third-party

---

[6] Health, United States, 1996–1997, United States Department of Health and Human Services, Tables 37–40.

payor was the Blue Cross plans across the country. Blue Cross provided "indemnity insurance" coverage for its beneficiaries, which meant that they generally paid the entire bill that was submitted without discount. Medicare changed the rules. If providers wanted to service Medicare patients, they were required to accept the payments being offered.

Medicare Net Revenue Concepts

Medicare started off as a cost-based payment system. They agreed to pay the total "cost" of services provided to their beneficiaries. But, there were no caps on these costs originally and so there was an incentive for healthcare providers to take on new costs and grow their businesses. And they did. Meanwhile Medicare developed a plethora of reimbursement methodologies for paying for the various disparate services that it covered.

Table 4–2 summarizes the many different ways that Medicare reimburses in the late 1990s. The biggest change, until 1997/1998, was in the inpatient reimbursement. As previously stated, Medicare originally reimbursed all services on cost. But

T A B L E   4–2

Medicare's Payment Methodologies Through 1998

Medicare Covered Service	Payment Method
Inpatient hospitalization	Diagnostic related groups (DRGs)
Capital related costs	Limited cost based through 2001, quasi-prospective reimbursement
Outpatient surgery, radiology, and diagnostic services	Blend of hospital-specific costs and national rates
Physician services	Resource based relative value scale (RBRVS)
Skilled nursing care	Cost based with "reasonable cost limits"
Home health services	Cost based with per visit limits
Organ transplants	Cost based
Hospice care	Four different types of reimbursement depending on the service
ESRD	Per treatment fee
Prospective payment system exempt hospitals and units such as	Cost based, but limited to the special target rates
• Psychiatric	
• Acute rehabilitation hospitals	
• Children's hospitals	
• Hospitals outside the United States	
• Distinct part hospitals	

as these costs quickly exploded, Medicare moved to put a cap on them. They were reasonably unsuccessful until 1983 when they adopted a very new prospective payment system (PPS) reimbursement methodology for inpatient services. It was called diagnostic related group (DRG) reimbursement.

DRG reimbursement had a dramatic effect on how the industry operated. It changed the provider's incentive. Prior to DRGs, Medicare reimbursed all of the provider's costs at the percentage of Medicare patient utilization. DRGs reimbursed the provider a fixed price per case, regardless of the cost of providing the care. Therefore providers needed to adapt to a new reality, become more cost-conscious, and really begin to understand their cost structure for the first time.

DRGs—How They Work

DRG reimbursement takes approximately 12,000 individual diagnoses available to physicians in America (available through the International Classification of Diseases, 9th edition, and Clinically Modified for the United States—also known as the ICD-9-CM codes) and looks at whether there was a surgery associated with the case. It also takes into account the patient's age, sex, and whether or not there were additional complications or comorbidities. Then through the use of a computer program, called a *grouper,* all of these data are crunched to determine into which one of the 490 DRGs the patient belongs.

Interestingly, DRGs were not originally developed to be used as a reimbursement tool for the Medicare program. It was instead developed by researchers at Yale University and Yale–New Haven Hospital in the middle 1970s in order to facilitate clinical analysis. All of the ICD-9-CM codes that fall into each individual DRG are supposed to utilize approximately the same amount of resources. They are supposed to act similarly. But, in actuality there are many DRGs that are not homogenous and therefore the average price assigned to a DRG by the Medicare program creates many problems for the provider.

Still, as we've now seen, the Feds were looking for a way to contain total Medicare reimbursement for inpatient services and move away from cost-based reimbursement. Ultimately they selected the DRG methodology and established the pricing equivalents for each of them. As we can see from Figure 4–1, this does not appear to have been successful in containing costs.

Under the PPS, case weights were assigned to each DRG. These case weights are then multiplied by each individual hospital's base rate to determine each of the DRG prices for each hospital. It does not matter what the hospital *charged* for all of the services rendered during the patient's stay. If the patient was a Medicare beneficiary, the hospital will be paid only the DRG rate. The difference between the gross charges (hospital prices) and the DRG payment (Medicare reimbursement) is recorded as the contractual adjustment on the income statement and as a Medicare contractual allowance (discount) to the accounts receivable on the balance sheet.

For example, assume that RHMC had a base rate of $4,000. Mary Smith, who is the patient, generated gross charges of $10,000 for her stay in the hospital. The DRG for her stay had a case weight of 1.5. Therefore, RHMC will expect to be paid

$6,000 (1.5 × $4,000) for her stay. Medicare will pay 100% of this DRG amount to RHMC minus Ms. Smith's annual deductible of $764.

The accounting debits and credits for this case are represented as follows.

| Dr. | Accounts receivable (balance sheet) | $10,000 |
| Cr. | Various gross charges (income statement) | $10,000 |

To post the various gross charges as the fee for services rendered to the patient

| Dr. | Contractual allowance (balance sheet) | $4,000 |
| Cr. | Contractual adjustment (income statement) | $4,000 |

To record write-down of Mary Smith's account to reflect the expected reimbursement, *at the time of billing*

Dr.	Cash—received from Medicare	$5,236
Dr.	Cash—received from Mary Smith (patient)	$ 764
Cr.	Accounts receivable—Mary Smith	$6,000

To record cash received from Medicare and the patient to zero out the patient's account.

As we have already seen previously in this chapter, DRGs are just one of many payment methods that may be used to reimburse healthcare providers. Medicare has several methodologies for various types of providers (Table 4–2, again). Medicaid, which is a state-run program, allows each state to determine the payment method to providers and uses many different ones depending on patient type (inpatient, outpatient, physicians, home health, skilled nursing care, etc.) Managed care payors also use a variety of payment methods when determining the provider's net revenues. Still, the concept of contractual adjustments remains the same. Once you know and understand that there are various reimbursement methods, it is simple to prepare contractual allowances on a monthly basis for the financial statements. We examine the various types of managed care reimbursement later in this chapter.

Medicaid Net Revenue Concepts

Over the years, Medicare has received considerably more press than Medicaid. This is primarily because Medicare is a national program administered with mostly consistent rules across the United States affecting a very politically astute constituency—the elderly, who have been known to vote politicians in or out of office. Medicaid, in contrast, is a national program but is controlled and administered by each of the 50 states in widely different ways. Although the federal government mandates the specific entitlements that each and every state must provide to Medicaid recipients, the states are allowed to determine the socioeconomic level of their residents who will be eligible. Because Medicaid is a program designed for the poor, beneficiaries are generally disenfranchised to a greater extent than politically connected Medicare beneficiaries.

FIGURE 4-4

Medicaid Recipients — Percentage by Categories 1972–1996

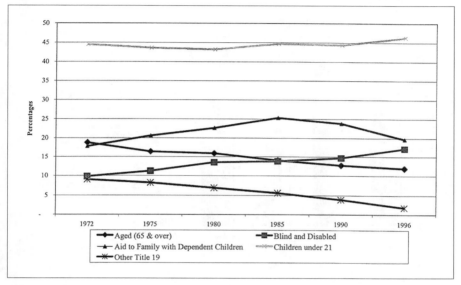

Source: Health, United States, 1998, Table 139.

Medicaid differs considerably from Medicare in its required benefits and level of payments to providers. Because it is state administered and financed, the States are continually struggling to balance the level of provider payments with their own budget constraints. In fact, the states have struggled with federally inspired "unfunded mandates," which require specific entitlements to be included in the Medicaid program but do not include any new monies coming from Washington.

There is one particularly surprising revelation surrounding the Medicaid program that is not generally reported. Figure 4–4 shows the 25-year trend of Medicaid recipients according to eligibility type as a percentage of totals. In addition, Figure 4–5 isolates the 1996 year and compares and contrasts recipients as a percentage of totals versus recipient payments. As can be seen, in 1996, patients 65 years of age or older make up only 11.9% of total Medicaid beneficiaries. Yet they account for 30.4% of the total Medicaid expenditures. The primary reason for this is that while Medicare will pay for only the first 100 days in a skilled nursing facility (SNF), Medicaid will pay for unlimited stays that are deemed medically necessary. It is often the case that persons of Medicare age, when they finally require chronic care in a SNF, will exhaust the assets that they have accumulated throughout their lives after Medicare pays for the first 100 days. They will then become Medicaid eligible. Because these chronic illnesses treated in SNFs are often costly and often last until death, Medicaid has become the largest individual line item in the budget of almost

FIGURE 4–5

1996 Medicaid Recipients and Payments as a Percentage of Total,
by Basis of Eligibility

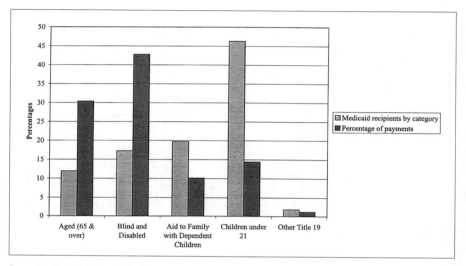

Source: Health, United States, 1998, Table 139.

every state, averaging over 14% of the total. On the other hand, children under the age of 21, who make up 46.3% of Medicaid eligible recipients, account for only 14.4% of Medicaid expenditures.[7]

In any event, Medicaid programs around the country have been notorious over the years for underpaying for the services rendered to their beneficiaries. Providers have had to scramble in order to make up the net revenue shortfalls engendered by providing services to Medicaid patients. Hospitals and physicians that are particularly affected are generally located in the inner cities and rural areas, where economically challenged citizens live. These hospitals may have a Medicaid payor mix approaching 40% to 60%. Added to their Medicare payor mix that could average 30% to 40%, they often suffer with maintaining operating margins that would allow for capital replacement or expansion or to properly pay to maintain their workforce. In some cases they may even have to close their doors, thus eliminating a major access to healthcare in their community.

RHMC, on the other hand, is in the enviable position of being located in a socioeconomic advantaged area. Their Medicaid payor mix is only 6%. They have been able to offset their Medicaid shortfalls relatively easily, thus, the expected net revenues from Medicaid and the ensuing contractual adjustments do not have a major detrimental effect on the organization's bottom line.

---

[7] Health, United States, 1998, United States Department of Health and Human Services, Table 139.

IMPLICATIONS OF THE BALANCED BUDGET ACT OF 1997

Despite Medicare's attempt to reign in its payments to providers, particularly with the advent of DRGs in 1983, it deemed itself unsuccessful. The continuing upward spiral of provider payments was having a detrimental impact on the Part A Trust Fund. Remember that the Part A Trust Fund is financed through a social security (Medicare tax) payment from employers and employees. It turns out that between 1966 and 1996, the Part A Trust Fund accumulated an excess of almost $120 billion. These were the net inflows from workers minus net outflows to providers. Still, Medicare prognosticators actuarially estimated that the Trust Fund would be depleted in the upcoming five years.

The problem was not particularly on the inflow side. It was estimated that the Medicare Trust Fund would continue to take in as much in the ensuing years as before. It was clear, however, that the outflows were about to dramatically increase because of the following.

1. Perception of provider fraud and abuse
2. Increasing healthcare options available to Medicare beneficiaries
3. Improving benefits for staying healthy[8]

Additionally, there was great concern over the growth in the over-65 population, characterized by the march of the baby boomers approaching Medicare eligible age. Consequently Congress came together to pass the most dramatic piece of health legislation since the inception of Medicare in 1966. Called the Balanced Budget Act (BBA) of 1997, it changed the way that Medicare reimbursed for all the services provided to its beneficiaries. This included outpatient services, home healthcare, skilled nursing care, hospice, graduate medical education, rural providers, and physicians. The BBA also changed some of the reimbursement concepts within the Medicaid program.

The legislation was designed to save the Part A Trust Fund $116.4 billion over the five-year period of October 1, 1997 to September 30, 2002. Savings were expected to be generated in the following areas.

• Hospitals	$44,100,000,000
• SNFs	16,200,000,000
• Home health agencies	9,500,000,000
• Beneficiary premium increases	13,700,000,000
• Medicare+Choice	18,500,000,000
• Physician services	5,300,000,000
• All other	9,100,000,000
• Total BBA savings	$116,400,000,000

The initial savings generated in the very first year have already had significant impacts. The three biggest changes were the following.

---

[8] Balanced Budget Act of 1997, http://www.hcfa.gov/init/bba/bbaintro.htm

1. *Zero increase in the annual update factor*—In 1983, at the advent of the DRG system, Medicare promised to update each provider's base rate by an inflation factor based on a market basket of healthcare goods and services. However, over the years, Medicare generally allowed for an increase in the market *minus* about 1%. At the advent of the BBA, in order to produce the needed savings, Congress determined that there would be no increase in the annual update factor for the 1998 fiscal year. Future year updates in fiscal years 1999, 2000 and 2001 are to be at the market basket *minus* 1.8%, 1.1%, and 1.1%, respectively.

2. *Correction of a formula driven overpayment (FDO)*—This item, included in the BBA, is the correction of a calculation error. It is expected to save over $2 billion alone. It was instituted immediately, on October 1, 1997, and reduced provider payment proportionately.

3. *Change in home health services reimbursement*—The BBA represented a significant change to the cost-based reimbursement system that existed for home health services for so many years. Although Congress ultimately wants home health services for Medicare beneficiaries to be reimbursed on a prospective system by fiscal year 2000, it created an interim payment system (IPS) beginning in fiscal year 1998 to begin capturing savings immediately.

Keep in mind that government figures show that of the 2.4 million home health patients in 1996, 72.5%, are 65 years of age or older.[9] Providers are therefore receiving a majority of their home health services reimbursement from the payor that cut their payments between 15% and 20%. In addition, the IPS puts new restrictions on the number of visits Medicare will reimburse and a new cost limit per beneficiary. The combined effect of these reductions are significantly hurting both the free-standing and the hospital-based programs through the closure of over 750 home health programs in the first nine month of the IPS.

The devastation of the home health services sector of the industry is evident. Congress has taken notice and currently believes that the legislation may have gone further than they envisioned. They are currently considering backtracking on some of the provisions to halt the continuing closure of home health providers.

Impact of the Balanced Budget Act on Medicaid

The BBA also had some effect on Medicaid reimbursement. Although not as extensive as the Medicare impact, there are a few changes worth noting. The most interesting change was the decision by Congress to repeal the Boren Amendment. The Boren Amendment to Medicaid administrative rules required state Medicaid

---

[9] Health, United States, 1996–1997, United States Department of Health and Human Services, Table 86.

programs to reimburse providers at "reasonable and adequate" rates. Over the last several years SNFs and hospitals have used the Boren Amendment to successfully sue states for higher Medicaid fees. The SNFs had the most at stake because Medicaid paid for almost 50% of all SNF care in 1995 while Medicaid paid for only 15% of hospital costs in 1995. As has been previously mentioned in this chapter, Medicaid has traditionally underpaid for services rendered to its beneficiaries and in the 1990s the Boren Amendment was the only tool that providers had to rectifying the situation.

Some other changes that the BBA made to Medicaid include a provision to pay providers at the lower Medicaid rate when patients have dual eligibility for Medicare and Medicaid and expansion of Medicaid eligibility and benefits. Finally, there is an increase of $4 billion dollars to extend health coverage to five million low income, uninsured children. Under this program, dubbed by some KiddieCare, the states will have significant discretion on how to spend this money.

Overall Impact of the Balanced Budget Act on Ridgeland Heights Medical Center

Most providers throughout the industry are feeling the pressure of lowered operating margins. A *Modern Healthcare* article reported that 1998 was shaping up as the first time in the 32-year history that Medicare outflows to providers would be *less than* that of the previous year.[10] As expected, the Medicare payment reduction was affecting all providers, but particularly those that had a high Medicare payor mix of patients. In addition, it was having a compounded negative effect on those organizations that provided inpatient and outpatient services, home health services, skilled nursing care, and physician services.

Ridgeland Heights Medical Center was just such a provider. It had been able to beat its 4% budgeted operating margin over the past years with some ease, given its location and favorable payor and service mix. Yet for the 1998 budget year, it recommended to its board that the operating margin be cut to 3% in order to account for the expected BBA revenue reductions. The organization's financial analyst estimated the reduction just from Medicare cuts would be over $1 million in the first year alone. This was just over 1% of their operating margin. In addition, the organization's administration was not able to devise expense reductions on the short notice given by the federal government for the 1998 budget year. The president signed the $116 billion payment reduction bill on August 5, 1997, just eight weeks before the start of the 1998 fiscal year.

MANAGED CARE NET REVENUE CONCEPTS

Medicare and Medicaid shortfalls from the BBA were not the only things impacting the bottom lines of many healthcare entities. The continuing rise of managed care in America was having negative financial consequences on many providers. Managed

---

[10] Weissenstein, E. (1998). A One-Year Dip, Medicare Inpatient Spending to Resume Climb in '99. *Modern Healthcare*, February 2, p. 12.

care is generally defined as a *range of utilization and reimbursement techniques designed to limit costs while assuring quality of care*. To reduce costs, managed care plans focus on price, volume, and intensity of service. These cost reduction techniques, which were itemized in Table 1–4, have played havoc with the operating margins of many healthcare providers.

Managed care type health insurance has overwhelmed and overtaken the traditional indemnity plans that were the primary form of health insurance in this country over the past 50 years. Although managed care plans have been around almost as long, it was mostly confined to the Kaiser plans in the western United States. Throughout the rest of the country, insurance companies were paying providers close to or at 100% of their submitted charges. However, as stated in Chapter 1, these charges by providers and payments by the insurance companies were having a detrimental effect on the real healthcare payors, the employers. In the late 1980s, employers revolted against the continuing rise of health insurance premiums and switched to managed care plans. The results, as seen in Figure 4–6, were dramatic. Managed care plans came from almost nowhere in 1976 to provide coverage for over 70 million Americans today.

Managed care plans have a variety of methods for reimbursing the providers that service the plan's enrollees. Box 4–1 highlights the methods used for reimbursing hospitals while Box 4–2 summarizes managed care reimbursement

FIGURE 4–6

Growth of Managed Care in America—1976–1997

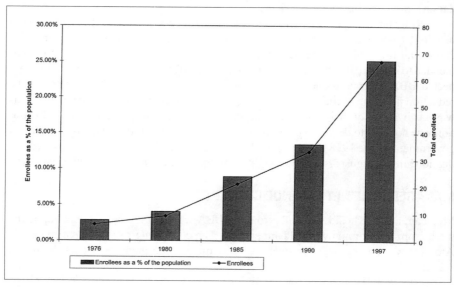

Source: Health, United States, 1998, Table 135.

BOX 4–1

METHODS FOR REIMBURSING HOSPITALS BY MANAGED CARE COMPANIES

- Charges (not common)
- Percentage of charges
- Per diems (defined dollar amount per day)
- DRGs
- Medicare plus $x\%$ (determined through negotiation)
- Carve-out of various services
- Case rates
  - Facility only
  - Bundled for hospital and physician services
- Bed leasing
- Capitation
- Periodic interim payments or cash advances (cash flow implications only)
- Penalties and withholds—to incentivize shorter stays or lower level of care
- Ambulatory patient groups (APGs) for outpatient care

BOX 4–2

METHODS FOR REIMBURSING PHYSICIANS BY MANAGED CARE COMPANIES

- Charges
- Percentage of charges
- Fee schedule by CPT code
- Medicare plus $x\%$
- Capitation—with carve-outs
- Capitation—without carve-outs
- Carve-outs
- Retainer
- Salary
- Hourly rates
- Global fees
- Bundled case rates
- Outpatient and professional DRGs or APG
- Withholds
- Penalties
- Changing schedules on the basis of performance
  - Quality measures
  - Patient satisfaction measures

methodologies for physicians. In every case, the reimbursement for services is *less than* the providers received previously.

Not only do managed care companies have all of the above ways to reimburse providers, but the providers could contract with dozens of different managed care companies during any given year. This means that the providers, whether they are hospitals, physicians, home health agencies, or SNFs, need a mechanism or tool to keep track of the various types of deals they have signed. Otherwise, they will not be able to prepare their monthly financial statements that include managed care contractual adjustments.

Providers have had to make significant adjustments in their operating structures to accommodate the decreased reimbursements from the managed care organizations (MCOs). Because the MCOs offer less expensive premiums to their subscribers, they have a need to procure services from providers at less expense. So they negotiate contracts with providers offering payments as shown in Boxes 4–1 and 4–2. At the same time, they offer plans to subscribers (beneficiaries) that generally limit the benefits. These plans generally come in three flavors.

1. Health maintenance organization (HMO) plans—This is a formally organized healthcare system that combines delivery and financing functions. The fixed monthly premiums paid to the HMO are generally lower than premiums for the traditional indemnity plans. In return for these lower premiums, the members of the plan must use the providers stipulated by the plan. It is a limited-choice plan for the members that requires a primary care physician be the gatekeeper for all other specialty services.

2. Preferred provider organization (PPO) plans—This is a healthcare financing and delivery program, which provides financial incentives to consumers to utilize a select panel of preferred providers. The difference between HMOs and PPOs is not always significant. Both lock the member into using their panel of providers, but PPO members are steered to use the primary care physician that they selected for their initial visit through lower deductibles and copayments. PPOs also often have a clause allowing the member to use specialist providers outside the preferred panel, but then the member has to pay additional fees for the services.

3. Point-of-service (POS) plans—Also called open-access products, the members (enrollees) are permitted to choose providers outside the main panel, without referral from a primary care physician. Coverage is offered under a financing mechanism similar to traditional indemnity and is available any time that service is desired. Benefits for services received outside the HMO network are typically less comprehensive than the HMO benefits and usually include deductibles and/or copayments.

The original managed care model was the HMO type of plan. In the early 1990s the PPO type of plan began to be offered as employers were looking for some additional choice in health insurance options for their employees. The POS plan began to be offered in the mid-1990s and have accelerated in the late 1990s as employees began to complain about the *lack of choice* offered in the provider panel plans. The most interesting aspect of this movement to POS is that it looks, feels, and operates very much like the traditional indemnity plans that employers rejected in the early 1990s because of the high price of the premium.

It is a simple equation.

The greater the choice = the higher the insurance premium
The more limited the choice = the lower the insurance premium

Still, the biggest difference between POS and indemnity is that under POS the providers no longer receive their charges as payments. There has been some kind of negotiated discount agreed to between the provider and the payor.

Regardless of the type of plan offered, the provider needs to be able to determine the final payment for the services that they rendered and record the difference as a contractual adjustment. The total of the contractual adjustments applied to the monthly gross charges will give the provider a clear idea if they are doing a better or worse job of negotiating contracts with the various MCOs with whom they do business. For example, suppose that an analysis of the managed care contractual adjustments looks like this.

	For the Year Ended	
	1997	1998
Managed care contractual adjustments	$28,000,000	$33,000,000
Total gross revenues	143,000,000	154,000,000
Managed care contractual adjustments as a percentage of total gross revenues	19.6%	21.4%

Providers can learn a lot about themselves by performing appropriate analysis of their managed care payor mix. For example, in the above summary data set, the managed care contractual adjustment increased by 1.8 percentage points. On first impression, this seems like a small amount. Yet the percentage increase between years is actually 9.2% (the percentage difference between 19.6% and 21.4%). That is, in fact, a substantial increase between years and negatively impacts the organization's bottom line by $2,816,000 ($33,000,000 − $30,184,000). The $30,184,000 is the amount of the managed care contractual adjustment that the organization would have discounted if they had been able to maintain a 19.6% contractual adjustment percentage.

So, there are many steps that the organization can take to analyze this increase. The ultimate purpose of the analysis is to make informed decisions on the need for the organization to meet its changing revenue streams. Following are some questions that could be asked.

1. Was the change in contractual percentage a result of a changing mix of the MCOs with which we contract?

2. Was the change a result of some poor inpatient utilization of services? For example, did the length of stay increase beyond the budget?

3. Was there a change in the mix between inpatient and outpatient utilization of services beyond the projections?

4. Are we, as an organization, being paid appropriately by the MCOs? Have the MCOs properly performed their own contract analysis?

Providers may be contracting with 2 to 200 MCOs. This usually depends on the level of managed care penetration in a particular geographic region. The greater the penetration, the more sophisticated the provider must be in order to be able to negotiate, bill, collect, and analyze the various contracts. Most providers have found that they need an automated system into which they can load the terms of the various contracts in order to get accurate and timely information on the net revenue that is expected to be generated per case, whether it be inpatient or outpatient.

These various automated systems usually called *contract payment analyzers* or *contract management systems* may be attached to the organization's main computerized billing system or they may be freestanding and interfaced with the billing system. The output from these systems is the primary source for the posting of managed care contractual adjustments. The difference between the gross charges and the contractual adjustments become the posted net revenue for all the managed care accounts. These systems also allow the providers to determine if the managed care companies have paid the net amounts expected accurately and timely.

PREPARATION OF THE MEDICARE AND MEDICAID COST REPORT

Who, why, how!!!

For a hospital that has a December fiscal year end, April is the month when the processing of the Medicare/Medicaid Cost Report heats up. HCFA rules require that the cost report be filed with the fiscal intermediary (FI) within 150 days of the end of the fiscal year. The purpose of the cost report is to allow Medicare to properly pay for outpatients, SNFs, and other specialty care services rendered by healthcare providers to Medicare beneficiaries.

Filing of the cost report has been required since the beginning of the Medicare program in 1966. It was particularly necessary because in 1966 Medicare reimbursed all of its services at cost. This remained true until 1983 when Medicare changed its reimbursement for inpatient services from retrospective cost based to the fixed prospective payment methodology called DRGs. The cost report continued to be necessary in 1983 because reimbursement for all of the other hospital services was still reimbursed at cost. The only way to determine the cost apportionment for these services was to continue to prepare the cost report. The big difference was that a year-end payable or receivable for *inpatient* services no longer applied.

The Medicare cost report is designed in a reasonably logical way to allow the preparer (Provider) and the payor (Medicare) to understand the development of each year's report. Table 4–3 shows the various major elements of the cost report. Each element assists in progress towards understanding an organization's Medicare cost.

The Medicare cost report has had a significant impact on the healthcare industry. While Medicare mandated provider preparation of the cost report in order to determine its required settlements, the cost report and its costing methodology became a de facto standard for cost accounting in the industry. Before 1966 and the advent of the Medicare system, most of the industry had no need for any type of cost accounting system, whether or not sophisticated. Most hospitals were small and much of their revenues were generated from a small set of charges and

T A B L E 4–3

Medicare/Medicaid Cost Report
Major Elements—Index of Worksheets

Worksheet	Purpose
A	Determine provider's total costs allowable by Medicare
B	Step-down costs of nonrevenue (overhead) departments to revenue producing departments
B-1	Statistics used to allocate overhead department costs
C	Determination of the ratio of costs to charges (RCC) used on Worksheet D to develop Medicare's proportionate cost
D	Determination of Medicare's total portion of provider's cost (including pass-through items, TEFRA limits, outpatient ancillary costs)
E	Determination of Medicare's "final settlement" with the provider
F	Calculation of return on equity capital—for for-profit providers only
G	Presentation of the providers audited financial statements
H	Determination of hospital-based home health agency final settlement
I	Determination of hospital-based renal dialysis costs
K	Determination of hospital-based hospice costs
L	Calculation of final capital payments
S	General information—including wage rates used to determine regional wage indices

a lot of donations. Medicare and Medicaid reimbursement ushered in the era of healthcare as a business nationally. And the Medicare cost report primarily required that hospitals use a very specific type of cost finding technique called *step-down*.[11] The very name step-down is representative of the way that the technique looks.

The step-down method of cost-finding organizes the healthcare facility's costs so that the overhead expenses will be properly allocated to revenue producing cost centers. Those departments that will most likely have costs (overheads) related to the other departments are allocated (or closed) earlier than others. The allocation is based on statistics that have been refined over the years to provide the best apportionment of the overheads.

Table 4–4 displays the step-down methodology. As can be seen, the actual step-down (worksheet B in Medicare parlance) looks like a descending staircase as it moves from left to right. This example is a summary of a complete step-down. It is presented to illustrate the way that the initial step-down methodology works.

---

[11] Cost reports using the step-down allocation methodology were developed by New York Blue Cross in its contracting with its providers in the 1950s and later adopted by Medicare in 1966.

TABLE 4-4

Ridgeland Heights Medical Center Step-down Costs For the 12 Months Ended December 31, 1998

Allocation Methodology	Salaries	Non-salaries	Total	Deprec.-Building Square Feet	Deprec.-Equipment NBV	Employee Benefits Gross Sal.	Operation Plant Square Feet	Accumulated Cost	Administration & General Acc Cost	Environmental Square Feet	Medical Records Gross Rev	Step-down Costs Total
Depreciation—buildings		$2,500,000	$2,500,000	$2,500,000								
Depreciation—equipment		2,000,000	2,000,000		$2,000,000							
Employee fringe benefits		1,572,000	1,572,000		$20,000	$1,592,000						
Maintenance and operation of plant	$400,000	300,000	700,000	375,000	50,000	97,221	$1,222,221					
Administration and general	2,000,000	4,000,000	6,000,000	500,000	20,000	486,107	287,581		$7,293,688			
Environmental services	300,000	200,000	500,000	50,000	30,000	72,916	28,758	$681,674	304,497	$986,171		
Medical records	200,000	150,000	350,000	25,000	15,000	48,611	14,379	452,990	202,346	15,654	$670,989	
Total nonrevenue departments	2,900,000	10,722,000	13,622,000	950,000	135,000	704,855	330,719	1,134,664	506,843	15,654	0	
Operating and recovery rooms	600,000	1,000,000	1,600,000	300,000	300,000	145,832	172,549	2,518,381	1,124,935	187,842	139,200	$3,970,358
Anesthesia	300,000	300,000	600,000	100,000	100,000	72,916	57,516	930,432	415,615	62,614	54,219	1,462,880
Laboratory	600,000	1,200,000	1,800,000	250,000	315,000	145,832	143,791	2,654,623	1,185,793	156,535	81,713	4,078,663
Radiology	600,000	800,000	1,400,000	250,000	400,000	145,832	143,791	2,339,623	1,045,085	156,535	90,961	3,632,204
Cardiology	300,000	200,000	500,000	175,000	200,000	72,916	100,654	1,048,570	468,385	109,575	28,178	1,654,708
Physical and rehabilitation medicine	250,000	150,000	400,000	75,000	100,000	60,763	43,137	678,901	303,258	46,961	9,362	1,038,481
Central supplies	200,000	1,000,000	1,200,000	175,000	150,000	48,611	100,654	1,674,264	747,877	109,575	91,987	2,623,702
Drugs	300,000	1,500,000	1,800,000	75,000	100,000	72,916	43,137	2,091,053	934,052	46,961	128,231	3,200,297
Emergency department	500,000	200,000	700,000	150,000	200,000	121,527	86,274	1,257,801	561,847	93,921	47,138	1,960,707
Total revenue producing department	3,650,000	6,350,000	10,000,000	1,550,000	i,865,000	887,145	891,503	15,193,648	6,786,846	970,517	670,989	23,622,000
Total costs	$6,550,000	$17,072,000	$23,622,000	$2,500,000	$2,000,000	$1,592,000	$1,222,221	$16,328,312	$7,293,688	$986,171	$670,989	$23,622,000

B O X 4–3

STATISTICAL ALLOCATIONS FOR NONREVENUE DEPARTMENTS

Nonrevenue Departments	Statistical Allocation Method
Building depreciation	Square feet
Employee benefits	Full time equivalent staff
Human resources	Full time equivalent staff
Information services	Total expenses
Plant operations	Square feet
Environmental services	Square feet
Cafeteria	Full time equivalent staff
Administration	Total expenses
Financial services management	Total expenses
Materials management	Supply expenses
Laundry	Laundry pounds
Patient accounting	Inpatient and outpatient units of service
Medical records	Inpatient and outpatient units of service
Planning and marketing	Total revenues
Medical staff	Total revenues
Central transportation	Adult admissions
Food services	Adult patient days
Care management	Nursing labor
Community services	Total revenue
Overhead	Total expenses
Bad debts	Total revenue

Box 4–3 shows a sample list of the nonrevenue type departments whose costs need to be allocated to revenue producing departments and their statistical allocation basis.

Ratio of Costs to Charges

The purpose of the step-down is to allocate overhead costs in order to create total costs for the revenue producing departments so that ultimately these total costs can be compared to the total charges for each of these revenue-producing departments. This comparison is known as the *cost-to-charge ratio (or the ratio of cost to charges often abbreviated as RCC)*. The charges for those services provided to Medicare patients are then multiplied by this cost to charge ratio to determine the *cost* of rendering care to Medicare patients.

A summarized version of this calculation works in the following way.

Cardiology direct costs (per Worksheet A)	$5,000,000
Cardiology allocated costs (per Worksheet B)	4,000,000
Total cardiology costs (final column—Worksheet B)	9,000,000
Total cardiology charges (per Worksheet C)	18,000,000
Overall cost-to-charge ratio	.50
Outpatient cardiology charges for Medicare beneficiaries	4,000,000
Outpatient Medicare cost for cardiology services	$2,000,000

Implications and Sensitivities of Medicare Cost Reporting

In the above example, outpatient services were used instead of inpatient services because, as we now know, inpatient services have not been reimbursed under a cost-based system since 1983. And by the year 2001, Medicare is supposed to phase out the last remnants of the cost-based system. The BBA requires Medicare to adopt prospective, noncost-based reimbursement for hospital-based outpatient (ambulatory) services, home health services, and SNFs services.

Yet it is certain that the Medicare cost report will survive. At the moment, this cost report is the most comprehensive financial statement *required* for every hospital provider in the United States. There is no other source that combines overall charge information with high-level cost and statistical information. These kinds of data are invaluable to competitors in tracking their neighbor's operation because it is fully available through the Freedom of Information Act to anyone requesting it. And coupled with billing information from the Medicare Medpar file, health policy experts and analysts are able to spot trends that would not be obvious without such data.[12]

Each year the RHMC financial analysts gear up to collect the required information. Cost and charge information is assembled from available figures on the hospital's books. Statistical information is collected and prepared using time-honored techniques. All information is double-checked for accuracy. Like a tax return filed with the government, the cost report is an official document that supports payment made to the provider by Medicare. The RHMC financial analysts take this preparation very seriously. They have had heavy-duty training, attending many continuing education seminars over the years. They study the literature and pay attention to all the new pronouncements issued by the Medicare program throughout the year. Most of these pronouncements are published in the Federal Register, now available on a daily basis on the World Wide Web at http://www.access.gpo.gov/su_docs/fedreg/.

---

[12] The Medicare MedPar file is an accumulation of all the financial and clinical data included on the bills submitted to the Medicare program for reimbursement.

Furthermore, the financial analysts and their bosses are well aware of recent government efforts to review cost report submissions for fraud. Cost reports have always been reviewed by each hospital's Medicare FI for reasonableness and completeness. Where errors were found during audit affecting the final annual reimbursement, either positively or negatively, changes were made by the intermediary, payments without interest were made, either by the healthcare organization or the government, and the cost report year was closed. Recently, however, the federal government has staged some high-profile raids on the corporate offices of major for-profit providers, alleging that two sets of books were being kept, the regular set and a "reserve" set of books.

Like income tax policy and practice, there are *gray* areas in the Medicare regulations. Many providers in the healthcare industry believe that it is permissible to submit a cost report that includes items that have not yet been deemed *black* or *white* by the government. Yet it is uncertain whether the submitted request for additional reimbursement will ultimately withstand government scrutiny. Conversely, Generally Accepted Accounting Principle (GAAP) requires that organizations take a conservative approach in the booking of revenues. This is essentially where the irresistible force meets an unmovable object. Most hospitals that take an aggressive or disputed position in filing of the cost report also book a reserve against the amounts that they are uncertain of receiving.[13] At the moment, it appears to be the government's position is that these reserves represent the equivalent of a second set of books, based on actions they are currently taking against a couple of large integrated delivery systems.

Thus, providers that believe the Medicare regulations allowing them to report certain disputed expenses would be well advised to send a cover letter with their annual cost report submission explaining that a disputed position has been taken. The industry is currently monitoring developments in these cases because of its applicability to most healthcare providers.

PRESENTATION OF AUDITED FINANCIAL STATEMENT TO THE FINANCE COMMITTEE

As the organization's administration continues to monitor and respond to the ongoing revenue reduction issues, the bimonthly finance committee is upon them. While operations are currently being maintained through a mix of some small expense reductions, the operating margin is nonetheless being negatively impacted.

Meanwhile the centerpiece of the April finance committee is once again the presentation of the previous year's audited financial statement by the partner of the external accounting/auditing firm retained by RHMC. The audit partner has a particular agenda that she wants to present to the committee. It is a tried and true format with

---

[13] Section 115 of the Provider Reimbursement Manual (HCFA Pub. 15-2—titled "Cost reports filed under protest") states that "You are permitted to dispute regulatory and policy interpretations through the appeals process established by the Social Security Act. Include the nonallowable item in the cost report in order to establish an appeal issue, and the disputed item must pertain to the cost reporting period for which the cost report is filed."

which the auditing firm is comfortable. It includes an overview of the healthcare industry as well as some of the current risks inherent in the business. The partner then reviews unusual circumstances, if any, surrounding the audit. Finally, the partner presents the financial results of the audit. From the point of view of the organization's management, the most important finding is the lack of any audit adjustment. This means that the financial statements that have been presented on a monthly basis by the finance administrator have been valid and fairly presented. This allows the board finance committee to continue to place its trust in its current management.

Implications of Management Letter Comments Proposed by the Auditors

Each year, as part of their scope, the auditors prepare a review of the internal controls of the organization. This review is made into a report and submitted to the finance committee commenting on any material weaknesses in financial controls that have been uncovered. This is an essential part of the audit and is given great weight by the board members. This is one of the few times that the board gets to "see behind the curtain" through independent eyes as to whether the management is doing what they say.

The management of RHMC is quite aware of the weight given to this report by the finance committee. But the finance administrators have always welcomed the publication of this report. These administrators have been trained to understand the importance of internal controls right down to the detail level (where the auditors dwell). They know that the best way to avoid any types of misappropriation is to maintain proper internal controls. RHMC's finance administrators have a history of having various types of operational and financial reviews performed, on a proactive basis, to understand their systems, uncover any problems, and fix them. Some of the operational reviews that have been performed in the recent past include the following.

- Information system risks and controls assessment
- Treasury management risks assessment
- Cost report risk assessment
- Materials management risk assessment
- Account payable audit and assessment
- Patient registration and accounts receivable process assessment

This year, as in the past several years, the auditors did not discover any significant financial or operational issues to present. This reaffirmed for the finance committee that the management was acting properly in preserving the assets of the organization. The auditors did however comment strongly on the organization's Year 2000 compliance. They firmly recommended that the organization finalize its plans to test, identify, and replace all equipment, clinical and nonclinical, that has a computer chip in it, for compliance with the Year 2000. This is reviewed, in depth, in Chapter 10. Other than that very important comment the auditor stated that they were pleased with the controls.

Finally, as is done every year, the organization's entire management, which includes the president and chief executive officer, the chief operating officer, the chief financial officer, and the chief strategy officer were dismissed from the meeting. This was done so that the audit partner could give the members of the finance committee, acting in their capacity as the audit committee, a private assessment of the organization's management. Because this particular management group had been together over 10 years, it is presumed that the audit partner was giving the board members the same clean bill of health in private as that given in public.

5

CHAPTER

May

Sam Barnes was working on a presentation to the finance committee when his phone rang. Angela Renfro, the organization's patient accounts manager, was on the other end of the line.

"Angela, what's up?" asked Sam.

"Sam, I've got this problem that I wanted to talk to you about," she said.

"Okay, tell me about it," said Sam inquisitively.

Angela was a little tentative. She was unsure of how she wanted to begin. "Well, I don't know if you've noticed but the accounts receivable balance has been going up the last several weeks," she quietly proclaimed.

Somewhat amused by the question, Sam said, "Actually Angela, I did notice. I was going to call you tomorrow to see what is going on. On my first quick review, I thought I noticed that the percentage of accounts older than 120 days from discharge was growing but I had not yet done a complete review."

"Sam, that is just my point," she fairly screamed. "It is not the older accounts that are the problem. In fact, if you look at the accounts stratified by age, you will find, as I did, that the receivable dollars in all the billed accounts are decreasing. The trouble is in the accounts where the patients have been discharged but no bills have yet been produced."

"What, oh my gosh," said Sam. "You know, I haven't been looking at the discharged, not-final-billed category recently because it had been doing so well. I just forgot about it for a while. Do you know why it all of a sudden went out of control?"

Angela was agitated. She was squirming in her seat now. "Well, ever since the organization restructured management and moved the medical records departments from your responsibility to the operations director, I've noticed that they lost some of their focus on the financial aspects of the medical records function. Then the manager told me that he lost some of his coding staff to out-of-state moves and pregnancies. With limited staff, they thought they would concentrate on some other clinical medical records issues, not the coding and abstracting completion, which I need before the bill can drop."

"Aaaarrrgghhhh!!!" thought Sam. Then he said, "I hate to use this expression but you know, I told them so. When they restructured I warned them this could and probably would happen. Management is really just a function of focus. Only when the finance division is responsible for all aspects of the finance function is there accountability. Okay, so how many receivable dollars are tied up just waiting for the coding to take place?"

Angela was ready with her reply, "Sam, it is already almost $3 million. This is just about six extra days in the accounts receivable balance at our average daily revenue of approximately $500,000 a day."

"Okay, so I better have a talk with the medical records manager and his boss to make sure we get a whole lot of focus back on this issue pronto. I sure do hate to have responsibility for something without the authority," said Sam.

"Yep," replied Angela. "I know what you mean."

———

May in the northern regions in the United States. A time of great promise. The frost of winter is finally gone. The April rains have subsided and the flowers are beginning to bloom in earnest. A reawakening occurs among the frigid-fingered inhabitants of the northern climes. At RHMC this reemergence from winter's cold usually is a cause for celebration. Men start to bring out their spring suits, shedding the wool of winter. Women are happy to put away some of their warm weather outfits and replace them with lighter weight and more flexible fashions.

The accounting and finance staff continues to do the jobs for which it is responsible. It is one of the two times during the year that there is a slightly lighter load of work. The year-end functions are behind them and the budget has not yet really begun. This is a purging month for the staff as they perform their own spring cleaning, rifling through the files, both electronic and paper, to delete and reorganize as appropriate. This however is not the case for staff and managers responsible for the billing and collection of patient accounts.

FUNDAMENTALS OF ACCOUNTS RECEIVABLE MANAGEMENT

The month of May typically holds no particular milestone in the world of accounts receivable management at RHMC. The management of accounts receivable is an hour-by-hour, day-to-day task that involves dozens of small but important transactions. Managers of the accounts receivable function are most often task oriented and driven to achieve the various goals set down by the organization's administration.

These goals are often an aggregation of important aspects of management. At RHMC these goals are the following.

- Improving patient service and satisfaction
- Improving employee satisfaction (morale)
- Improving the quality of the department's outcomes
- Reducing the dollars in the overall accounts receivable in relation to the net revenues being generated (called "days in accounts receivable")

Achieving these goals are hard, yet not unlike the goals of any other management position. One of the differences is that the accounts receivable manager is one of the few management positions that holds the fate of the rest of the organization in its hands. There are several healthcare organizations that live from "hand-to-mouth." Said another way, the only way that the organization may be able to meet its payroll or pay its vendors is for the accounts receivable manager to collect cash on the outstanding bills. So, no collections, no payroll!

The accounts receivable manager (hereafter called the patient accounts manager or PAM) understands this. This is true because accounts receivable production is constantly monitored by the administration, often on a daily basis. While the administration is primarily concerned about the daily cash receipts, the PAM has a significantly more complex set of productivity measures, which, once met, will turn the generation of patient bills into cash.

Box 5–1 represents a summarized listing of the major elements of accounts receivable management. Each and every one of these items has significant implications to the nature and quality of the ultimate cash collection.

Within all of the items listed in Box 5–1, there are six areas that need to be specifically highlighted because of their overriding importance.

1. Precertification, preadmission, and insurance verification
2. Documentation capture
3. Coding and reimbursement
4. Fraud and abuse issues
5. Managed care arrangements and negotiations
6. Monitoring results

Precertification, Preregistration, and Insurance Verification

Of all the important concepts in accounts receivable management, these are the most important. The quality and speed of the collection process at the time of billing and thereafter is *completely dependent* on the quality and skill exhibited during the precertification and insurance verification process at the time of preregistration. In a discussion that follows later in the chapter regarding which division the patient registration department should report to, the importance of overemphasizing these areas is demonstrated if the organization wants their days in receivables to be low.

B O X 5–1

ACCOUNTS RECEIVABLE MANAGEMENT ISSUES

A. Policy, planning, and evaluation
1. Establishing objectives and goals
2. Internal and external auditing policies
3. Performance standards and measurements
4. Third-party relationships (e.g., Medicare, Medicaid, managed care)

B. Admission and Registration Policy & Procedures (INPUTS)
1. Inpatient and outpatient registration policies and procedures
2. Precertification
3. Preadmission or preregistration
4. Insurance verification
5. Registration
6. Customer relations

C. Patient financial services, policies, and procedures (THROUGHPUTS)
1. Charge capture issues
2. Documentation capture
3. Coding and reimbursement issues (e.g., ICD-9-CM and CPT-4 coding)
4. Revenue maximization activities (e.g., lost charge recovery efforts)
5. Medical records, quality assurance, and utilization review issues

D. Post-discharge account management (OUTPUTS)
1. Bill preparation and mailing
2. Billing audits/fraud and abuse/ controls
3. Third-party and self-pay follow-up techniques
4. Patient cost sharing—inpatient and outpatient

E. Collections policy and procedures
1. Bad debts expense and charity care policies
2. Financial counseling issues
3. Financing of self-pay patient accounts
4. Payment policies
5. Selection of collection agencies
6. Monitoring performance of collection agencies

F. Legal aspects
1. Bankruptcy issues
2. Contract issues
3. Federal rules and regulations
4. Litigation policy
5. Workers' compensation
6. Patient and hospital rights/ obligations

G. Managed care organization (MCO) issues
1. Arrangements/negotiations between providers and MCOs
2. Contractual obligations between the two parties
3. Capabilities of the provider to meet managed care requirements
4. Competitive issues
5. Monitoring results
6. Future trends

Precertification and insurance verification is important because it has become imperative to recognize and capture the patient's or employer's policy information that is usually located on the patient's insurance card. The organization's registration department is responsible to determine the preauthorization requirements for every patient who presents for services, whether as an inpatient or outpatient and verifying the benefits with the appropriate managed care company. Determining the accurate demographic (name, address, telephone number, next of kin, etc.) and insurance information (guarantor's name, address, telephone number, exact policy number, etc.) is the most important function that the patient registration department performs. The patient accounting department relies completely on the quality of this information to be able to perform timely billing and collection activities.

Documentation Capture

The ability of the medical records department to assure optimal reimbursement within the revenue cycle for inpatient or outpatient accounts is wholly dependent on the quality of the documentation. Documentation is the *written* record of care provided during a patient's stay. There is a very old saying in the industry that goes, "If it isn't documented, it didn't happen." There is no better way to say this. Documentation of services and the distinctions made by the clinicians (physicians and nurses) contemporaneously during the stay are critical to the ability to maximize the organization's reimbursement.

This is also a legal distinction. More and more, healthcare organization's coding for its services are being challenged. There will be a much stronger presumption of innocence if the organization is able to document the level of clinical services required by the patient and provided by the organization.

One of the best ways to assure the capture of quality documentation is to provide *ultra* training for all the people involved in this effort. The most important people involved in documentation are the floor nurses, the utilization review nurses (sometimes called care managers), and the physicians. The toughest group to train is the physicians, because of the following reasons.

1. They usually do not work for the organization.
2. They may believe that they have no stake in improving the documentation.
3. They were never taught in medical school that documentation equals better reimbursement and generally do not want to learn it now.

But it is absolutely necessary to make sure that this training is carried out in an appropriate and effective way. The difference between, for example, a DRG without a comorbidity or complication (cc) versus a similar case with a cc could be several thousand dollars. Physicians who understand these distinctions are actually creating a better medicolegal record of the case. So any documentation training needs to emphasize that improved documentation is always worthwhile for all the participants involved.

RHMC is fully aware of these distinctions and understands that improved documentation equals improved reimbursement. It is also aware that the best way to improve documentation is to invest heavily in training. Therefore several years ago, they hired an outside consulting firm that specializes in documentation training and they then provided it on a mandatory basis to the utilization review nurses and the medical records coders. They also included a number of physicians who have substantial practices at the hospital in the training. In addition, they made sure to provide this same training to any new employees who started in these areas subsequent to the original training.

Finally, they contracted with this same consulting firm to perform quarterly reviews on a sample basis to determine that all documentation was properly included and that the coding for reimbursement purposes was accurate. The consulting firm used the same coding books and rules employed by the Medicare program to do so. Because it had taken these steps, RHMC was comfortable that it had complied with the difficult billing requirements required by the Medicare program, even though the reimbursement for its inpatient cases had *improved*. It was a case study in how to do better by doing better.

Coding and Reimbursement

One of the primary functions of the finance division is to maximize reimbursement. The best way to do this is to maximize the quality of the clinical documentation. This allows the coders to have the best opportunity to apply for the highest level of reimbursement, where appropriate. In addition, each healthcare organization needs to provide the coders with the best available tools, such as up-to-date coding books and automated software.

It is absolutely appropriate for every healthcare organization to maximize reimbursement. Notwithstanding the federal government's current focus on what they characterize as healthcare billing fraud, it is legal, moral, and proper to apply for the best available reimbursement so long as the documentation is reflective of the care provided, it supports the coding, and the coding supports the billing.

There are many technical aspects to the coding function. However, the most important detail is the ability to convert the clinical documentation into clinical coding. Coding comes in many different forms. Following are the most prevalent coding formats.

- ICD-9-CM—*International Classification of Diseases*, 9th edition, Clinically Modified (for the United States). In Chapter 4, we saw that ICD-9 codes are the single most important element in the creation of the diagnostic related group (DRG), and the DRG is the way that Medicare reimburses hospitals for inpatient stays.
- HCPCS—HCFA's Common Procedure Coding System. HCFA is the acronym for the Health Care Financing Administration, which is the regulatory body that the Medicare program falls under. While ICD-9-CM creates the reimbursement for Medicare inpatients, HCPCS

is a uniform method for healthcare providers and medical suppliers to code for their professional services, procedures, and supplies.

- RBRVS—Resource based relative value scale. This is the method that Medicare has defined to reimburse for physician office services. It is based on the HCPCS codes mentioned above.
- CPT-4—*The Physicians Current Procedural Terminology*, 4th edition. This is a systematic listing of procedures and services performed by physicians. It is the most widely accepted coding methodology in America.

Whether the coder works for a hospital, a physician's office, or any other healthcare entity that gets any part of its net revenues from the use of coding, it is always important to remember its primary significance to reimbursement maximization. So when the patient accounting staff prepares to send out a bill to any third-party payor that reimburses for services using these codes, they are always aware of the revenue implications of coding.

Timeliness of Coding

There is one other very specific and very critical aspect within the coding cycle of patient accounting and billing. The patient's bill cannot be sent out to the third-party payor until the coding is completed and validated. The specific steps involved in this procedure include the following.

1. The physicians documentation of the patient's final diagnosis
2. The completion by the various service units (radiology, laboratory, cardiology) and receipt by the medical record coders of all the written (documented) test results
3. The abstracting from the medical chart of all clinical information relevant to the most proper coding of each patient's stay. Often information that becomes available just after the patient's discharge from, say, a lab test, can add significantly to the severity of the case by the inclusion of an additional ICD-9 code. This extra code could make a big difference in the final DRG that may improve the organization's reimbursement.
4. The coding itself, which is performed by the coder who now has all of the relevant information

The management of this medical records function (coding) has a great bearing on the ability of the billing department to send out a timely bill. Another truism of the healthcare industry is that the PAM is responsible for the entire accounts receivable balance, whether or not they have control over all the functions described in Box 5–1. In many cases, the PAM does not always have control over all those functions. Therefore, he or she has to use his or her best management skills to become "best friends" with the manager of medical records and the coding supervisor in order to accomplish the primary goal of timely billing. The reality is that untimely coding can cause unbilled accounts to skyrocket and add millions of dollars and many days to the accounts receivable. (There is a further discussion on the issue of timeliness and control, particularly related to patient registration issues, later in this chapter.)

Fraud and Abuse Issues Related to Billing Issues

The issue of fraud and abuse in the billing of services is multifaceted and complex. The Medicare and Medicaid programs want to be sure that they are paying only for the services required for and used by their beneficiaries. Yet they have estimated that several billion dollars are being squandered in payment to providers. The Office of Inspector General, which is an arm of the Department of Health and Human Services, has created a work plan of what they believe are the biggest area of fraud and abuse in claims processing. In effect, these are the areas that this enforcement agency has identified as having the greatest risk of fraud and abuse. These are the areas that they have targeted for substantial review in 1999. A summary listing is presented in Table 5–1.

So, it is pretty obvious that the government is serious about billing fraud and abuse. The list in Table 5–1 is not comprehensive. And yet some of the areas on the list will be given weights greater than other areas. It is not known which of these areas is considered higher weighted but some suppositions can be gleaned from the Office of the Inspector General's (OIG's) work of the recent past and the probability of a greater monetary return for the government.[1] Still, the PAM and the organization's billing staff needs to be aware of all the billing rules all the time in order to stay legal in this very important operation.

Following are some areas that probably represent the risk of greatest exposure.

1. *Upcoding of patient bills*—This usually involves inpatient and emergency department cases and is a function of claiming higher reimbursement than is deserved because the clinical documentation does not support the claim. This is unlike the situation mentioned above involving RHMC, where their improved documentation lead to higher reimbursements.

   Upcoding was prominently featured when a *Wall Street Journal* article in early 1997 highlighted how upcoding works and why it can cost Medicare so much money.[2] In a nutshell, the article explained that the DRG system, and the codes needed to drive it, is so cumbersome that the DRGs, codes, and guidelines fill two volumes totaling more than 2,600 pages, thus making it extremely difficult to claim proper reimbursement. In fact, healthcare providers often downcode as well as upcode because of these difficult issues.

---

[1] Gardner, J. (1998). Budget Battle Looms—Clinton Uses Fraud Fines, User Fees to Pay for Programs. *Modern Healthcare*, February 9, p. 2.

[2] Lagnado, L. (1997). Hospitals Profit by 'Upcoding' Illnesses. *Wall Street Journal*, April 17, p. B1.

T A B L E   5–1

Department of Health and Human Services,
Office of Inspector General, Fiscal Year 1999 Work Plan
Selected Areas of Review in Billing and Claims Processing

Area of Concern	Issue
Hospitals	
Monitoring DRG coding	Assessing the extent and quality of HCFA's monitoring of DRG coding by hospital. In a 1996 sample of hospital abstracts, an 8%–10% variation was found between initial hospital coding and the data abstraction coding.
Outpatient psychiatric services	Determining whether psychiatric services rendered on an outpatient basis are billed and reimbursed in accordance with Medicare regulations
Home Health	
Physician case management billings	Determining the reasonableness of physician claims for home healthcare
Home health aides	Examination of claims for home health aide services provided to Medicare beneficiaries in residential care facilities in one state
Skilled Nursing Home Care	
Ancillary medical supplies	Ongoing determination if skilled nursing facilities (SNFs) have claimed unallowable costs for ancillary medical supplies
Nursing home implementation of consolidated billing	Examining early implementation of consolidated billing in nursing homes. The Balanced Budget Act legislated a new billing method for all Part B services provided to Medicare beneficiaries residing in nursing homes, effective July 1, 1998. For nursing home stays not paid by Medicare Part A, nursing facilities will be responsible for submitting bills to Medicare contractors for most Part B services. Outside entities will no longer be able to directly bill the program. This is known as consolidated billing
Physicians	
Accuracy and carrier monitoring of physician visit coding	Assessing whether physicians are correctly coding evaluation and management services in locations other than teaching hospitals and whether carriers are adequately monitoring physician coding

The federal government is currently reviewing the issues of upcoding for pneumonia cases involving DRGs 89 and 90 and the significant difference in their case weights. The article pointed out that DRG 90—simple pneumonia, which has no secondary complication—

TABLE 5–1

Department of Health and Human Services, concluded

Area of Concern	Issue
Physicians	
Physicians with excessive nursing home visits	Identifying and auditing the billings of physicians with excessive visits to Medicare patients in SNFs
Automated encoding systems for billing	Determining if errors found in Medicare billings for physician services are associated with providers' use of automated encoding software
Hospitals	
Billing service companies	Determining whether (1) Medicare claims prepared and submitted by billing services companies are properly coded in accordance with the physician services provided to beneficiaries and (2) the agreements between providers and billing service companies meet Medicare criteria
Medical Equipment and Supplies	
Duplicate billings for medical equipment and supplies	Determining if duplicate billings for medical equipment and supplies are being made to both durable medical equipment regional carriers and regional home health intermediaries
Hospice Part B billings	Determining appropriateness of selected durable medical equipment Part B billings on behalf of hospice patients
End Stage Renal Disease (ESRD)	
Clinical laboratory tests provided to ESRD beneficiaries	Identifying inappropriate Medicare payments for clinical laboratory tests for ESRD patients. Providers may be either separately billing for laboratory tests that are included in the monthly composite rates or are providing laboratory tests that do not conform to professionally recognized standards.
Medicare Managed Care	
Duplicate fee-for-service billings	Determining whether fiscal intermediaries and carriers improperly reimbursed Medicare providers for services provided to beneficiaries enrolled in risk-based managed care plans during calendar years 1995–1997

Source: Department of Health and Human Services, Office of Inspector General, Health Care Financing Administration Projects, Work Plan, Fiscal Year 1999.

might have a reimbursement rate of $2,791 while DRG 89—pneumonia with complications—may have a reimbursement rate of $4,462, a difference of $1,671 or 60%! This additional amount can be achieved by adding an additional complication to the patient's chart and it is often only an issue of the provider, be it the physician or the utilization review nurse, paying a little more attention to some of the secondary clinical issues and test results. So, healthcare organizations have been hiring consultants to teach documentation and coding maximization in order to improve their reimbursements. As the chief financial officer of a major academic medical center said in the article, "It is like hiring a tax expert to make sure you took all your deductions."

2. *Nursing home implementation of consolidated billing*—This is a developing area, possibly ripe for fraud and abuse because of the potential for double billing. A major change in the billing rules rendered by the 1997 Balanced Budget Act mandated that for nursing home stays not paid by Medicare Part A, nursing facilities will be responsible for submitting bills to Medicare contractors for most Part B services. Except in a very few specialized areas, only the SNF will be able to directly bill the Medicare program. The possibility of other providers continuing to bill the Medicare program, while these services are now bundled into the consolidated bill, is the concern of the OIG. They plan to monitor this area closely.

3. *Accuracy and carrier monitoring of physician visit coding*—Like the coding issues described for inpatient hospitalization above, Medicare also reimburses physicians through the use of codes. In this case, the codes are called evaluation and management (E&M). Also like DRGs, there is the ability for physicians or their staff to code the visit at a higher level than is permitted based on the documentation. The OIG believes they have done enough sampling to indicate that this is a high-profile area to pursue.

4. *Billing service companies*—This is an expansion of the government's efforts to review the upcoding of patient bills submitted to Medicare. In this case the OIG particularly wants to review that Medicare claims prepared and submitted by billing service companies are properly coded in accordance with the physician services provided to beneficiaries. In some case, physicians use professional billing companies in place of their own personnel to code and bill for services. This review is a way for the OIG to put these billing companies on notice that they should be prepared to defend their coding choices in the event they are taking aggressive positions.

It is imperative that healthcare financial managers who have responsibility for billing or the reporting of the gross and net revenues and receivables should go to at least one, and probably several, continuing education classes and seminars held around the country on the fraud and abuse billing topic. Along with staying abreast of the current literature, these are the best ways to maintain knowledge and expertise in this highly volatile area. There is be an expanded discussion of the nonbilling fraud and abuse areas in Chapter 6.

Managed Care Arrangements and Negotiations

At this moment in the healthcare industry, managed care volumes may amount to 20% to 50% of an organization's net revenues. This may very well be the case in any of the large industry segments—hospitals, physician practices, SNFs, and/or home health agencies. Many of these organizations are large enough to have different personnel responsible for negotiating the managed care contracts and patient registration and billing. In those organizations, it is imperative that the departments responsible for these patient financial services be given a seat at the negotiating table. Their job at the table should be to ascertain that the negotiator agrees only to terms and conditions that can be appropriately administered by these departments. If this is not done, there is a very good chance the that organization will be stuck with the following.

- Lost revenues
- Increased accounts receivables
- Increased bad debts

These problems are the result of the organization's failure to properly precertify, preauthorize, and/or bill in a timely manner, which may be the result of a lack of coordination between the managed care negotiator and patient financial services personnel.

Monitoring Results

There have been several accounts receivable management processes highlighted in this chapter that suggest ways to improve department outcomes. Yet, while these may seem terrific in theory, the results may be quite different in practice. The primary method that is used to determine whether improvements have, in fact, been made is to first determine the baseline of the process you are measuring and then monitor the process outcomes on a periodic basis (daily, weekly, monthly). These outcomes will allow the PAM and the administration to understand which direction the outcomes are heading—up or down.

Earlier in the chapter, RHMC's goals for its patient accounting department were presented. The goals were to do the following.

- Improve patient service and satisfaction
- Improve employee satisfaction (morale)
- Improve the quality of the department's outcomes
- Reduce the dollars in the overall accounts receivable in relation to the net revenues being generated

Each of these goals can be numerically measured and monitored. One of the PAM's job requirements is to help set these goals and then achieve them. The best way to set goals in these areas is to use benchmarks, which can be used in various ways. In setting initial goals, for example, measuring the current year's results against prior years' results would be a good use of benchmarking. This is particularly appropriate if the organization is unable to find external benchmarks against which to measure. The advantage of this process is that it allows the organization to gauge the direction of its results. In other words, it can at least determine if it is getting better or worse against its own prior performance. The disadvantage of this process is that it does not allow organization to determine if its own performance is poor, good, or excellent against the results of its peers.

RHMC has set specific numerical goals in all four of the categories it has chosen to measure. Table 5–2 presents a summarized list of the various goals for RHMC's patient accounting department. These goals have been set in the following way.

T A B L E 5–2

Ridgeland Heights Medical Center
Balanced Scorecard Measures, Patient Accounting Department

Measure	Goal
Improving Patient Satisfaction and Service	
• Reduce patient complaints received	• < 6 patient complaints/unit/year
• Improve scores on patient satisfaction survey	• > 93 percentile in all categories
• Improve closure on every patient query received by the department	• > 98 percentage
• Improve employee productivity in collection unit	• 40 quality calls per day per employee
Improving Employee Satisfaction	
• Improve employee satisfaction scores	• > 80% score on employee opinion survey
• Reduce disputes brought to resources department	• Zero disputes brought to human resources
Improving Quality	
• Reduce billing errors	• Less than 2% error rate
• Reduce time taken to post cash	• Post all cash on day of receipt
• Improve timely posting of contractual adjustments	• 98% of contractual adjustments are posted within 24 hours after billing
Reducing Days in Accounts Receivable	
• Reduce net days in accounts receivable	• Less than 55 days

- *Improving patient service and satisfaction*—RHMC subscribes to a customer survey service company. Over 400 healthcare organizations from around the country are part of the benchmark group. Three of the questions asked on the survey that goes to all inpatients and outpatients who have been discharged relate to the patient accounting functions. The goals are set high to achieve a ranking in the top 10% of the group. The results are monitored monthly, feedback is presented to the staff, and improvements are constantly sought in order to improve the rankings.

- *Improving employee satisfaction (morale)*—RHMC also subscribes to an employee opinion service benchmarking group. In this case, employee morale is measured through an ongoing survey process. The PAM is able to measure the satisfaction of the staff in two ways. First, the satisfaction can be measured against the scores from prior periods to determine the direction of the morale. Second, the satisfaction can be assessed against the national norms that are published. RHMC's goal is to achieve an 80% satisfaction rating from its own employees.

- *Improving the quality of the department's outcomes*—These goals are extremely important to the organization's patient accounting department manager. This is one of the primary ways for the manager to set goals that will improve the department's processes, thereby improving the outcomes. Management has identified error rates as a critical quality outcome driver. Reductions in error rates always improve outcomes and productivity by reducing rework. Therefore, major emphasis is always placed on identifying and then correcting areas where errors are caused. For example, a significant area of focus is the production of clean claims (bills) to third-party payors. Clean claims get turned around and paid in a much more expedited manner. So the patient accounting department spends time monitoring both its electronic and manual claims production for errors. In general, the department strives to keep its error rate under 2%.

- *Reducing the dollars in the overall accounts receivable in relation to the net revenues being generated*—This is one of the most commonly cited measurement and benchmark in the healthcare industry. There are many sources for the measure popularly known as *days in accounts receivable*. The problem with this benchmark is that there are so many ways to calculate it. Accounts receivable is often cited as both gross receivable and net receivable. Either one may be used as the calculation's numerator. In addition, it is also possible for the denominator to be calculated using daily gross or net revenues. Finally, some organizations report only *some* of their receivable pay classes as gross and other pay classes at net. It makes for a very confusing measurement and benchmark.

RHMC has solved this problem by using the only days in accounts receivable measure that is considered reliable as a benchmark—*net* accounts receivable divided by daily *net* revenues. These net amounts are available on almost every healthcare organization's monthly balance sheet and income statement. In addition and more importantly, the net figures are reported on the annual audited financial statements. On these audited statements, the gross revenues have been reduced by contractual adjustments to its net expected value and the gross receivables have been reduced by the allowance for doubtful accounts (ADAs) and the allowance for contractual adjustments (ACAs) to its most likely value. Because these are audited figures, this is the most reliable set of measures available to create benchmarks for days in accounts receivable. RHMC's goal is to achieve 55 days in accounts receivable, which according to several of the benchmark services would place the organization favorable to the industry median.

PATIENT REGISTRATION—WHICH DIVISION SHOULD IT REPORT TO?

There is one issue that is not ordinarily discussed in print but which has a major impact on the management of accounts receivable. The question relates to which division in the organization the patient registration department should report. The answer will often go a long way in establishing the level of the days in accounts receivable. Around the time that Medicare came into being (1966) many of the patient registration departments reported to the operating division, not the finance division. There was good reason for this. As a cottage industry, the primary means of cash receipts was either from the patients themselves or a handful of third-party payors. The identification of the payor was extremely easy and did not require much training. In addition, there were no great financial implications to not properly identifying the correct payor because there were no preauthorization requirements or billing deadlines that would cause coverage denials for services rendered.

As already noted in Chapter 4, the commencement of Medicare turned the healthcare-providing services from a cottage industry into a major industry. Concurrently, the identification of the actual payor became more critical because many payors, including the indemnity insurers, sold different coverages to different employers under the same policy name.

Many administrators throughout the industry recognized that with these changes came a shift in the responsibility of the patient registration department. Although still extremely concerned about customer satisfaction, it was clear that the capture of insurance and demographic information became *the* critical aspect in effective accounts receivable management.

Over the next 10 to 15 years, many healthcare organizations, particularly hospitals that usually separated the registration function from the billing function, moved the reporting responsibility of patient registration from the operating division to the finance division. It is a truism of the industry that the best way to turn accounts receivable into cash is to perform correctly, accurately, and quickly the preregistration and registration functions. Put another way, the front end of the receivable cycle is considerably more important than the back end.

Precertification, preregistration, insurance verification, and registration represent the front end, while bill production, bill submission, third-party follow-up, and collection activities represent the back end. Good back-end processing is possible only if the front-end systems and procedures are faultless. Current contracts between providers and payors demand that the providers capture lots of specific data at the time of the patient's registration. Without the correct capture, there is a very good chance that the payor will delay or deny the claim (i.e., not pay it because the provider did not meet the technical specifications of the contract).

The PAM is fully responsible for the collection of the accounts receivable and the level of bad debts being generated. When the patient registration function does not report directly either to the PAM or to a finance director, there is a very good possibility that the accounts receivable will not be at the level required by the organization's administration and/or board.

Yet, anecdotally, there appears to be a disturbing trend in recent years. Hospital administrators are moving the reporting responsibility of the registration department back under the operations division. The most often cited explanation is that the admissions/registration function is performed at the front door of the hospital for many patients and, as such, the patient's experience as a customer begins here. Therefore, the reasoning goes, only the operations division can provide the kind of positive patient experience so highly sought after.

The two big fallacies in this argument are that the following occurs.

1. The operating division can collect demographic and insurance information equal to or better than the finance division.
2. The finance division cannot provide customer service and satisfaction equal to or better than the operating division.

Neither of these is true. Most healthcare finance professionals will tell you that the collection of accurate insurance information is extremely difficult. The reason for the difficulty is related to the number of managed care companies that currently populate the landscape. Every managed care company has a set of coverage provisions for its beneficiaries that are often different than its competitors. Thus, a different set of preverification steps and standards need to be followed. Making things even worse, within the same managed care company, there can be, as was shown in Chapter 4, several different kinds of plans. Because of this, when a registrar is presented with a patient's insurance card, there is no guarantee that payment is ensured. Different plans mean different benefits. Even the same employers may have three or four different plans.

The first priority of the registration manager must be the accurate and timely collection and processing of the patient's demographic and insurance information. The best way to accomplish this priority goal is through relentless insurance training of the staff. This training should consist of all nuances of the information contained on the insurance card. Additionally, the training should emphasize the implications of various preauthorization, precertification, and second opinion requirements contained in the diverse insurance plans within the organization's service area.

Although customer service must always be emphasized, there is an inherent conflict between properly collecting a patient's demographic and insurance information and the patient's desire to get immediate treatment. Healthcare organizations would like to register patients in the same manner as a hotel. But, it is important to recognize that *an insurance card is not a credit card.* The finance division will constantly try to balance the customer service requirements with the needs to collect information timely and accurately. Unfortunately, the operating division simply does not share the seriousness of the financial implications inherent in maintaining vigilance in this area as they generally place the patient's desire for speedy registration ahead of the requirements imposed by the insurance industry. Thus, the level of the organization's accounts receivable will be influenced by the decision of which division will be responsible for this information collection effort.

CALCULATION OF ALLOWANCE FOR DOUBTFUL ACCOUNTS AND BAD DEBT EXPENSES

These are key aspects of accounts receivable management. One of the aspects that have significant implications to the organization's income statement is the calculation of the ADA. The ADA is a *contra* account on the balance sheet to the accounts receivable asset line. It reduces the gross receivable by the amount calculated to be uncollectible. Sometimes referred to as the *Reserve for Bad Debt,* the ADA calculation encompasses some interesting twists and, as stated in Chapter 2, is one of the six extremely sensitive items most likely to receive an audit adjustment if it is done poorly.

Bad debt expense is the other side of the double-entry bookkeeping to the ADA calculation. (Bad debt expense is another of the six most sensitive financial statement items.) Most healthcare organizations use the four-sided approach to ADA and bad debt reporting. The four financial statement accounts that are always involved in this calculation are the accounts receivable, ADAs, bad debt expenses, and bad debt write-offs.

The ADA is the key to the entire set of equations. Every healthcare organization needs to perform a detailed analysis each month to determine the proper ADA balance. The ADA calculation attempts to measure the projected amount of the recorded accounts receivable that would not be able to be collected at that month's end. For financial statement purposes, it is the generally accepted accounting principle method used to write down the gross receivable to its estimated realizable value.

Table 5–3 represents an ADA calculation used by Ridgeland Heights Medical Center. The most important features of the calculation are its use of the aging schedule and the stratification by major pay classes. These concepts value accounts by the length of time they have been outstanding and the quality of the payor class with which each patient was registered. In the latter example, it is a truism of the industry that some payors will surely convert the receivables of their beneficiaries to cash once the claim has been determined to be proper. This is the case even if the account ages beyond a reasonable period. RHMC has also stratified its receivables

TABLE 5-3

Ridgeland Heights Medical Center, Detailed Analysis of Allowance For Doubtful Accounts (ADA)
For the Month Ended December 31, 1998

Inpatient Accounts

	Unbilled	Less: Allowance for Contractual Adjustment	Adjusted Unbilled	0–30 Days	31–60 Days	60–90 Days	91–120 Days	121–150 Days	151–180 Days	Over 180 Days	Total Billed	Total
Medicare receivable	1,782,084	(1,015,788)	766,296	852,582	264,409	161,301	73,747	59,881	21,606	257,328	1,690,854	2,457,150
Allowance percentage			5.00%	5.00%	5.00%	10.00%	20.00%	25.00%	35.00%	50.00%		15.80%
Medicare allowance			38,315	42,629	13,220	16,130	14,749	14,970	7,562	128,664		276,240
Medicaid receivable	107,285	(432,972)	(325,687)	36,451	122,285	118,464	39,360	37,500	40,208	116,979	511,246	185,559
Allowance percentage			5.00%	6.00%	10.00%	15.00%	20.00%	30.00%	50.00%	60.00%		17.50%
Medicaid allowance			(16,284)	2,187	12,228	17,770	7,872	11,250	20,104	70,187		125,314
Managed care receivable	878,541	(556,180)	322,361	1,440,125	1,117,852	558,417	429,685	230,325	161,410	989,547	4,927,361	5,249,722
Allowance percentage			4.00%	6.00%	10.00%	15.00%	17.00%	25.00%	25.00%	30.00%		11.20%
Managed care allowance			12,894	86,408	111,785	83,763	73,046	57,581	40,352	296,864		762,694
All other receivable	256,895		256,895	118,947	64,698	103,719	53,770	18,899	16,491	137,418	513,942	770,837
Allowance percentage			30.00%	30.00%	40.00%	50.00%	60.00%	70.00%	85.00%	98.00%		63.30%
All other allowance			77,069	35,684	25,879	51,860	32,262	13,229	14,018	134,670		384,669

TABLE 5-3

Ridgeland Heights Medical Center, Detailed Analysis of Allowance For Doubtful Accounts (ADA), continued

Inpatient Accounts

	Unbilled	Less: Allowance for Contractual Adjustment	Adjusted Unbilled	0–30 Days	31–60 Days	60–90 Days	91–120 Days	121–150 Days	151–180 Days	Over 180 Days	Total Billed	Total
Total inpatient receivable	3,024,805	(2,004,940)	1,019,865	2,448,105	1,569,243	941,901	596,562	346,604	239,715	1,501,272	7,643,403	8,663,268
Inpatient reserve			111,993	166,908	163,113	169,522	127,930	97,030	82,036	630,385		1,548,918
Total inpatient reserve percentages			10.98%	6.82%	10.39%	18.00%	21.44%	27.99%	34.22%	41.99%		17.88%

Outpatient Accounts

	Unbilled	Less: Allowance for Contractual Adjustment	Adjusted Unbilled	0–30 Days	31–60 Days	60–90 Days	91–120 Days	121–150 Days	151–180 Days	Over 180 Days	Total Billed	Total
Medicare receivable	1,239,377	(2,335,665)	(1,096,288)	703,717	933,793	408,121	249,968	185,515	89,856	436,316	3,007,286	1,910,998
Allowance percentage			5.00%	5.00%	6.00%	13.10%	20.00%	25.00%	50.00%	70.00%		15.80%
Medicare allowance			(54,814)	35,186	56,028	53,464	49,994	46,379	44,928	305,421		536,584
Medicaid receivable	95,464	(264,174)	(168,710)	33,418	46,354	52,374	17,530	21,100	3,385	54,593	228,754	60,044
Allowance percentage			5.00%	5.00%	6.00%	9.00%	12.00%	18.00%	23.90%	44.80%		17.50%
Medicaid allowance			(8,436)	1,671	2,781	4,714	2,104	3,798	809	24,458		31,899
Managed care receivable	1,501,256	(900,256)	601,000	1,225,365	1,395,822	751,254	648,952	482,541	315,965	2,152,748	6,972,647	7,573,647

TABLE 5-3

Ridgeland Heights Medical Center, Detailed Analysis of Allowance For Doubtful Accounts (ADA), concluded

Outpatient Accounts

	Unbilled	Less: Allowance for Contractual Adjustment	Adjusted Unbilled	0–30 Days	31–60 Days	60–90 Days	91–120 Days	121–150 Days	151–180 Days	Over 180 Days	Total Billed	Total
Allowance percentage	4.00%			6.00%	10.00%	14.00%	18.00%	30.00%	35.00%	41.00%		11.20%
Managed care allowance	24,040			73,522	139,582	105,176	116,811	144,762	110,588	882,627		1,597,108
All other receivable	925,652		925,652	475,812	544,813	364,785	287,596	215,874	135,896	842,095	2,866,871	3,792,523
Allowance percentage	30.00%			30.00%	40.00%	50.00%	60.00%	70.00%	85.00%	98.00%		63.30%
All other allowance	277,696			142,744	217,925	182,393	172,558	151,112	115,512	825,253		2,085,191
Total outpatient receivable	3,761,749	(3,500,095)	261,654	2,438,312	2,920,782	1,576,534	1,204,046	905,030	545,102	3,485,752	13,075,558	13,337,212
Outpatient reserve			238,486	253,122	416,316	345,746	341,466	346,051	271,836	2,037,759		4,250,782
Total outpatient reserve percentages			91.15%	10.38%	14.25%	21.93%	28.36%	38.24%	49.87%	58.46%		31.87
Total receivables	6,786,554	(5,505,035)	1,281,519	4,886,417	4,490,025	2,518,435	1,800,608	1,251,634	784,817	4,987,024	20,718,961	22,000,480
Total reserves			350,479	420,030	579,429	515,267	469,396	443,081	353,872	2,668,144		5,799,699
Total reserve percentages			27.35%	8.60%	12.90%	20.46%	26.07%	35.40%	45.09%	53.50%		26.36%

between inpatient and outpatient accounts because of the different payment methodologies that may be employed.

Importantly, the results of this monthly analysis are the amount of dollars that will be recorded as the ADA on the balance sheet. Because of this, it is imperative that the patient accounting manager and the finance administrators review the changes in the ADA on a monthly basis to determine causes for any significant changes to the ADA. This review may well highlight good or bad changes within various payor categories that need to be corrected immediately.

Meanwhile, Table 5–4 represents the analysis of a complete ADA, bad debt expense, bad debt write-off, and recoveries of bad debts. This schedule is prepared following the completion of the detailed ADA calculations. There are some significant implications in this schedule. It is important to note that *the bad debt expense that will be reported on the income statement is a function of the other three columns— the calculated ADA, as well as the actual bad debt write-offs and actual recoveries of the bad debt write-offs.*

To prepare this schedule, the organization must have already recorded the actual write-off of patient accounts, according to their bad debt write-off policy. In addition, it must also record any cash collected by the collection agencies engaged by the organization to perform more intensive collection work on accounts of patients who did not pay their bills. Using this methodology, the result of the equation yields the actual bad debt expense (also called provision for bad debts) that is recorded on the income statement.

RHMC management and finance administration review these schedules in detail every month because of its importance to both the balance sheet and income statement. In addition, it is the best set of summary schedules available for administration to determine the adequacy of the reserve for its bad debt as well as the performance of the collection agencies that are being used to back up the organization's regular set of in-house collectors. Because these schedules involve two of the six most sensitive types of accounts, this is a critical monthly review that is heavily weighted in importance.

CALCULATION OF ALLOWANCE FOR CONTRACTUAL ADJUSTMENTS

The other major allowance that reduces the gross receivable is the ACA. Like the ADA, the ACA is an estimate. In this case, the estimate is a result of a determination of the amount of money in the gross receivable that will not convert to cash because of stipulations in the contracts with the organization's various payors, particularly, Medicare, Medicare, and managed care. Generally accepted accounting principles require that "the provision for contractual adjustments and discounts be recognized on an accrual basis and deducted from gross service revenues to determine net service revenues."[3]

---

[3] AICPA Audit and Accounting Guide, Health Care Organizations, Revised June 1, 1996, Section 5.03, p. 55.

TABLE 5-4

Ridgeland Heights Medical Center
Analysis of ADA, Bad Debt Expenses, Bad Debt Write-Offs
For the 12 Months Ended December 31, 1998

	Opening Balance— ADA	Ending Balance— ADA*	Total Change in ADA	Add: Write-offs	Less: Recoveries	Subtotal: Net Write-offs	Provision for Bad Debts aka Bad Debts Expense
January	5,600,000	5,650,300	50,300	381,284	71,483	309,801	360,101
February	5,650,300	5,680,244	29,944	366,704	59,648	307,056	337,000
March	5,680,244	5,734,135	53,891	397,964	82,288	315,676	369,567
April	5,734,135	5,849,672	115,537	325,659	81,815	243,844	359,381
May	5,849,672	5,726,047	(123,625)	347,965	66,027	281,938	158,313
June	5,726,047	5,870,367	144,320	398,836	62,172	336,664	480,984
July	5,870,367	5,806,077	(64,290)	395,683	48,892	346,790	282,500
August	5,806,077	5,916,173	110,096	396,589	76,539	320,050	430,146
September	5,916,173	5,884,859	(31,314)	365,754	70,494	295,260	263,946
October	5,884,859	5,700,357	(184,502)	520,376	57,874	462,502	278,000
November	5,700,357	5,752,043	51,686	521,569	86,546	435,023	486,709
December	5,752,043	5,800,000	47,957	446,987	101,098	345,889	393,846
Totals	5,600,000	5,800,000	200,000	4,865,370	864,877	4,000,494	4,200,494

*As calculated by the detailed allowance for doubtful accounts worksheet.

Again, as stated in the Healthcare Audit Guide, "amounts realizable from third-party payers for healthcare services are usually less than the provider's full established rates for those services. The realizable amounts may be determined by the following.

- Contractual agreement with other plans (such as Blue Cross plans, Medicare, Medicaid, or HMOs)
- Legislation or regulations (such as workers' compensation or no-fault insurance)
- Provider policy or practices (such as courtesy discounts to medical staff members and employees or other administrative adjustments)"[4]

TABLE 5–5

Ridgeland Heights Medical Center
Anaysis for Allowance for Contractual Adjustments
For the Month Ended December 31, 1998

Inpatients	Medicare	Medicaid	Managed Care
Unbilled accounts (inhouse and discharged, not yet billed)	$1,782,084	$107,285	$878,541
Billed accounts	not applicable*	511,246	710,544
Subtotal	1,782,084	618,531	1,589,085
Contractual adjustment discount rate	57%	70%	35%
Allowance for contractual adjustment	$1,015,788	$432,972	$556,180
Outpatients			
Unbilled accounts (discharged, not yet billed only)	$1,239,377	$95,464	$1,501,256
Billed accounts	3,007,286	234,754	1,961,267
Subtotal	4,246,663	330,218	3,462,523
Contractual adjustment discount rate	55%	80%	26%
Allowance for contractual adjustment	$2,335,665	$264,174	$900,256

* No allowance is necessary for Medicare inpatient billed accounts because 100% of these accounts are automatically contractualized at the time of billing by the computer system's DRG grouper.

---

[4] Ibid, Section 5.02, p. 55.

Table 5–5 is the analysis that RHMC uses to determine its monthly ACA. There are several points that need to be made regarding this schedule.

1. The Medicare portion of the unbilled account is higher than the other categories because of very specific rules and regulation involved in billing Medicare inpatient accounts. The largest portion of the unbilled category, in this case, is known as discharged, not yet billed. The unbilled category is made up of two different types of accounts.

   - Patients who are in-house (e.g., in their hospital bed) at midnight of the balance sheet date
   - Patients who have been discharged, but the bill has not yet been produced by the organization

2. The total inpatient managed care billed accounts are not being written down to the ACA because many of these accounts have already been written down to their estimated contractual net expected receivable at the time of billing. RHMC uses a special software program that generates the actual net revenue. The software emulates the actual provisions of each managed care contract then reviews each inpatient discharge for those provisions and automatically calculates the reimbursement. Therefore, no additional accrual for ACA is needed because the account has already been written down.

3. The contractual adjustment discount rate is supposed to represent the actual average of all the accounts that have been processed over the past month. These amounts will change from month to month but on a very small scale. A large change may occur if a high-volume managed care contract is signed at a discount rate that is significantly higher than the average. The other big reason a change may occur is a large change in Medicare reimbursement rules. This would usually happen on October 1 of any year, which is the beginning of the federal fiscal year.

4. There is no in-house category for outpatients because, by their very nature, they are meant to receive services on the day they are registered, and should not be categorized as occupying a bed.

5. Finally, it is clear that there is no ACA for the accounts called "all other receivables" on the ADA schedule. These are primarily self-pay accounts and, as such, there are no formal discount contracts between the organization and its patients. Thus, there is no allowance, provision, or need for self-pay contractual adjustment.

The results of the monthly ACA are used to reduce the total balances on the ADA schedule before an allowance for bad debts is calculated. If this were not done, then the organization would be double-counting some of its discounts against its gross receivable.

Once again, RHMC staff and management spend significant time on this analysis each month because of its effect on both the balance sheet and the income statement. Variance analyses are also performed across time periods and against various pay classes to establish whether there have been any measurable changes, and if so, where.

In summary, the management of accounts receivable is a crucial part of the overall management of any healthcare organization. The responsibility to collect cash on a timely basis, in an efficient manner, and under significantly strict regulatory requirements is not for the faint of heart. RHMC has had the good fortune to have retained the same PAM for the last several years. The PAM has maintained her technical ability to manage through constant reading of industry literature and attendance at continuing education seminars throughout the year. The rapid pace of change in the industry has demanded continued vigilance, particularly in this area. RHMC has been reasonably successful, thus far.

6

CHAPTER

June

Rick Samuelson, the president and chief executive officer of Ridgeland Heights Medical Center, was in a quandary. His 35 years of experience in healthcare organizations in general, and 10 years at RHMC specifically, were not helping him at the moment. The organization was about to begin its annual budget process and he already knew he faced a dilemma.

"Sam," he barked at his finance officer, "What's our chance of doing good financially next year? I'm pretty concerned about some of the trends that you've been reporting over the last six months. This Medicare Balanced Budget Act certainly seems to be having an impact on our hospital net revenues, but it appears to be having an even worse impact on our skilled nursing facility and home health services revenues."

"Well Rick, you're right," said Sam empathetically. "It's absolutely true that our bottom line is eroding because of the issues you just mentioned. In fact, as you know, the Medicare BBA issues are only a part of it. We are having more and more problems negotiating what we feel are appropriate rates with managed care companies. We know that those companies are having their own problems with the claims they are paying for medical services. So they're trying to make it up by asking us for additional payment reductions."

"Yeah, okay, but what are we going to do about the current financial issues and the future budget planning we have to do now?" lamented the CEO.

Sam was happy to respond to the question. "There are only a few ways that we can have a positive impact on the bottom line. They're all tried and true methods, but none of them are easy. The best ways to improve our operating margin, now and in the future, are to enhance our inpatient admissions and outpatient volumes. This will generate additional gross and net revenues. As long as our variable expenses are less than these net revenues, our margins will improve."

"But, Sam, we haven't been able to make the kind of progress in the area we've wanted," said Rick.

Sam had heard it before and said, "Rick, I know that. First of all we need to be more innovative in this regard. More volume means we need to gain market share from other providers, especially since the population of our service area is not growing. Secondly, we have not tried hard enough to implement cost reductions in a logical way, using some very specific cost analysis tools that highlight some very possible areas of improvements. Finally, we haven't attempted to perform process improvements in a meaningful and effective way. This could free up many of our revenue producing departments to accept additional volumes, leading to additional income."

"Okay," said the CEO resignedly, "you're right. We have had this conversation more than once. But in the past you wanted to do this while we still had a pretty decent bottom line and so it was hard to convince our stakeholders to take either of these three issues seriously."

"Yeah, well, if we had done some of these things previously, because the strategic financial plan predicted it, we'd be in better shape for the near future. In any case, those three areas I highlighted are what we do need to do in order to survive and thrive now and in the future," said Sam emphatically.

———

June, in northern Illinois, is lovely. Spring has sprung with full force and warm breezes are being easily felt on the bare arms and legs of the joggers and pedestrians strolling leisurely through the parks around the region. Summer is just three weeks away and summer vacation plans are in full swing. It is sometimes hard to get people to concentrate on their jobs as they discuss their upcoming destinations.

That, however, is not the case at Ridgeland Heights Medical Center. Because its fiscal year ends on December 31, June is the month that the budget process starts in earnest for the upcoming year. The finance division and its staff, which is responsible for the entire budget process, has geared up for the initialization of this very important function. The amount of work ahead is daunting when taken as a whole. As a result, the process is broken down into smaller pieces that are more easily digestible. Starting in June, the budget process will keep the finance and accounting staffs occupied until just before New Year's Day.

BUDGET PREPARATIONS—THE BEGINNING

June is the month that RHMC begins its annual rite of passage, the operating and capital budgets. In its logical sequence, the annual budgets follow the strategic financial plan (which was discussed and described in Chapter 3), which follows preparation of the strategic plan. The logic of the sequence allows for the organization to do the following.

- Express its vision and long-term goals in the strategic plan
- Express its best numerical forecasting in the five-year strategic financial plan
- Develop this into a projection or budget, one year into the future

There are several steps that the organization needs to take in order to prepare and present its annual budget. Table 6–1 is a representation of the steps usually needed in preparing an operating budget. These 24 steps will take the organization between four and six months to complete, depending on philosophy. It will involve managers in every facet of the organization's operations. In addition, a critical set of stakeholders who must be accessed, solicited to, and appeased are the physicians who are linked to the organization, either in an employment capacity or in an affiliation relationship.

TABLE 6–1

The Process of Preparing an Operating Plan and Budget

Item #	Task	Reasoning/Thinking for Task
	Strategic Planning Segments	
1.	Environmental statement	Analysis of the organization's current operating environment
2.	General objectives and policies	Provides the budgeting effort a uniform direction for the optimal use of available resources. Objectives assume a macro view focusing on broad goals. Policies have a narrower focus, aiming at clarifying the details of budget preparation and establishing basic internal operating parameters.
3.	Assumptions	Statements that project future events and the resulting future environment
4.	Operating policy decisions	The setting of program priorities and the establishment of funding guidelines
5.	Operating objectives	Translates operating priorities into specific measurable goals that are obtainable within the budget period
	Administrative Segments	
6.	Budget preparation manual	Describes the mechanics of preparing the operating plan and budget

Continued.

The Process of Preparing an Operating Plan and Budget *(Continued)*

Item #	Task	Reasoning/Thinking for Task
	Administrative Segments	
7.	Projection package	Package of information that is transmitted for purposes of communicating either the raw data necessary for decision or actual decisions between different levels of management
8.	Projection package approval	Volume estimates are reviewed from the above perspective and the impact of such factors as the following.
		• Changes in the demographic character of the organization's service area
		• Technological changes
		• Historical trends
		• Managed care penetration and stage of development
9.	Administrative package	Basic package for communicating budget preparation instructions and information to departmental line management
10.	Administrative package approval	Sign-off of administrative package to assure that revisions are included and the package is complete
	Communications Segments	
11.	General budget meeting	Introductory meeting designed to formally initiate the annual planning and budget preparation process for departmental management
12.	Technical budget meeting	Focuses on the specific mechanics of the budget procedures and budget preparation; this usually involves a series of meetings with the revenue producing services areas
	Operational Planning Segments	
13.	Administrative meetings— revenue producing department level	Translates the environmental statement, assumptions, operating policies, and objective decisions into projects and activities at the revenue producing department level

The Process of Preparing an Operating Plan and Budget *(Continued)*

Item #	Task	Reasoning/Thinking for Task
Operational Planning Segments		
14.	Decision package preparation	Departmental management develops decision packages that identify the new activities being requested with their costs and alternatives based on the decisions made in #13 above
15.	Rank order of decision packages	Involves a series of consecutive meeting wherein succeeding levels of management integrate and rank-order the various decision packages prepared in #14 above
16.	Revenue budget preparation	Data from the projection package are used to calculate the initial revenue budget, using the current charge structure
Budgeting Segments		
17.	Detailed specifications	Department management specifies in detail the resource needed to carry out approved projects and these resource needs are converted into actual dollars
18.	Tentative budget completion	Organizes and aggregates the data developed in step #17 above; basically a clerical and computational step. These expense totals now need to be compared to the projected revenues. Expense or capital budgets may now need to be revised.
19.	Final administrative review	Senior administration makes a series of decisions, bring the two sets of budgets into balance
20.	Budget completion	Clerical steps needed to generate the final revenue, expense, and capital budgets. A cash flow budget should also be generated from this step.
21.	Board approval	Presentation to the finance committee and the board of directors for approval to carry out this operating and capital plan in the following year
22.	Communication of budget approval to department management	Involves feedback to the department managers of their final approved budget for the following year. They will be expected to meet the goals set for the following

The Process of Preparing an Operating Plan and Budget *(Concluded)*

Item #	Task	Reasoning/Thinking for Task
		Operational Planning Segments
		• Volumes
		• Gross revenues
		• Net revenues
		• Expenses
		• Departmental operating margins
23.	Implementation	Turning the budget into reality
24.	Feedback	Periodic feedback (usually monthly) back to the department managers in the budget year that follows; this feedback involves the following.
		• Statistical reports
		• Financial reports
		• Performance reports
		• Variance reports

BUDGET CALENDAR

The planning tool that RHMC uses to design and maintain this annual project is a budget calendar. There are separate calendars prepared for both the operating budget and the capital budget. The calendars make the time-frame expectations clear to all those individuals participating in the project. Table 6–2 is a representation of the operating budget calendar used by RHMC. It is divided into four columns, each having an important function.

1. Responsible parties—This column tells the reader who will be involved in each individual budgeting step.
2. Activity—This column represents each of the budgeting steps that will be followed.
3. Date—*The critical column.* Each of the dates listed *must* be met or else the whole budget process will be unsuccessful, and that is never allowed to happen. This column is monitored incessantly in order to avoid any slippage.
4. Meeting time and location of meeting—This column lets the responsible parties know when and where to show up.

There is a critical reason that the dates on the budget calendars are never allowed to slip. The budget is a plan designed by the management that needs to be

T A B L E 6–2

Ridgeland Heights Medical Center
2000 Budget Calendar
Operating Budget

Responsible Party	Activity	Date	Meeting Time/ Location
Executive and administrative staff Selected nursing and ancillary department managers Finance staff	Kick-off meeting for volume	June 1	Meeting Room 1 2:00–3:30 PM
Executive and administrative staff Finance staff	a. Approve projected 1998 and budgeted 1999 admissions, length of stay, and patient days by service b. Approve projected 1998 and budgeted 1999 outpatient trends by ancillary service	June 26	Meeting Room 1 2:30–4:00 PM
Finance staff	Issue 2000 operating budget calendar	July 1	
Finance staff	Compute gross revenues and contractual adjustments	July 11	
Executive and administrative staff Finance staff Accounting staff	Review salary and nonsalary assumptions a. Merit increase percentage b. FTE target level c. Benefit costs d. Inflation by category	July 14	Meeting Room 1 10:00 AM– 12:00 PM
Finance administration Finance staff	a. Review gross revenues and contractual adjustments b. Validate payor mix	July 15	Finance dep't. conference room 12:30–2:00 PM
Executive and administrative staff Finance staff	a. Review 2000 budgeted income statement developed by finance based on prior high-level assumptions b. Determine price increase targets c. Revise salary and nonsalary assumptions	July 18	Meeting Room 1 8:00–10:00 AM

Continued.

Ridgeland Heights Medical Center
2000 Budget Calendar
Operating Budget *(Concluded)*

Responsible Party	Activity	Date	Meeting Time/ Location
Finance staff	Issue 1999 projected/2000 budget worksheets to department managers	July 25	
Finance staff	Budget training	Various	Accounting dep't. conference room
Department managers	Complete budget worksheets and return to appropriate vice presidents/administrators	August 15	
Appropriate vice presidents/ administrators	Review and finalize departmental budget revisions	August 18–28	
Appropriate vice presidents/ administrators	Return budget worksheet to finance	August 29	
Executive and administrative staff Finance staff	a. Validate or adjust 2000 budget projections b. Preliminary approval of budget	Sept. 9	Meeting Room 1 1:00–3:00 PM
Executive and administrative staff Finance staff	a. Final review/approval of 2000 budget b. Review human resources committee packet	Sept 17	Meeting Room 1 9:00–11:00 AM
Finance staff Executive and administrative staff (as appropriate for document/ packet review)	Prepare drafts for human resources committee a. First draft—September 12 b. Final comments— September 14 c. Final draft—September 19 d. Mailing date—September 26 e. Committee meeting— October 3		
Finance staff Executive and administrative staff (as appropriate for document/ packet review)	Prepare drafts for finance committee a. First draft—September 30 b. Final comments—October 2 c. Final draft—October 7 d. Mailing date—October 14 e. Committee meeting— October 21		

approved by the board of directors, to allow management to operate the organization on a day-to-day basis. The board and the finance committee of the board have their own calendars with future agendas that also are strictly adhered to. In the case of RHMC, the calendars have been designed so that all affected parties are aware well in advance of the crucial meeting dates and activities so that they can clear their calendar accordingly.

Which Month Should the Budget Be Presented to the Board of Directors for Approval?

An important concept to note in the preparation of the budget calendar is the actual and total times required to prepare the budget. Ultimately, the preparers and the reviewers have to have the budget ready for the designated finance committee meeting that precedes the board meeting where final approval will be requested.

An interesting question that this often raises is, "Which month before the beginning of the new year is most appropriate to present to the board for approval?" The answer is, "It depends on the particular culture and needs of each individual organization." Still, there are some guidelines and issues that can be raised in order to try to answer the question.

The most common time frames used by healthcare organizations are to present their budgets in the first, second, or third month before the new budget year begins. There are pros and cons to each of these time frames. Table 6–3 highlights the particular pros and cons of each of the three time frames. The organization's culture, in this regard, can be conservative or liberal, either from the perspective of the board, the senior administrators, or the finance division preparers.

The board may be more or less comfortable having the budget approval under their belts earlier so that they can get on with other important business. Or they may like to know that the budget package they are approving is based on the absolutely latest volume information available. The finance preparers, on the other hand, aware of the mountains of data that went into the preparation, and the amount of work still required to produce reports for the department managers, will opt for the greatest amount of time available before the new year begins. Finally, the senior administrators are usually neutral, opting for the time frames that will cause the least disruption on the part of the department managers, without denying the wishes of the board.

Budget Calendar Time Frames

Once it is clear which month the budget needs to be ready by for the finance committee and the board, it is important then to determine all the steps that need to be taken in order to prepare and complete the budget. The RHMC budget calendar lists all the summarized major activities that need to be completed.

Now, to determine when the very first budget steps need to be started in any given budget year, it is imperative to know three things.

1. The date that the budget needs to be presented to the board

2. The amount of time needed between each budget activity

3. The amount of time needed during each activity

A *key concept* in budget timetable preparation is knowing the date the budget is needed and then calculating backward from that date. So, in the case of RHMC, which has a fiscal year end of December 31, the key dates will revolve backward

---

T A B L E   6–3

Which Month Should the Budget Be Presented to the Board of Directors for Approval?

Presenting the Budget 70–90 Days before the Next Budget Year Begins	
PROS	**CONS**
1. There is a greater amount of time to prepare and deliver the results of the approved budget back to the department managers. 2. There is a greater amount of time that can be used if the finance committee or the board decides not to approve the budget for any reason.	1. The data and information used to prepare the budget, particularly the volumes, are not as current as most of the managers and administrators would like in projecting subsequent year financials.
Presenting the Budget 40–60 Days before the Next Budget Year Begins	
1. There would be a reasonable amount of time available for the finance division to prepare and deliver the results of the approved budget back to the department managers. 2. The data and information used to prepare the budget, particularly the volumes, would be appropriately current, yet not too stale.	1. There may not be enough time before the new year begins to produce a remedial budget plan and package if the board of directors decides not to approve the budget.
Presenting the Budget 10–30 Days before the Next Budget Year Begins	
1. The data and information used to prepare the budget, particularly the volumes, are the most current available.	1. There is no time to prepare and deliver the results of the approved budget back to the department managers before the new year begins. 2. There is no time remaining to produce a remedial budget to the board before the new year begins if the proposed budget is rejected.

from the month that the board wants to approve it. At RHMC, there is a tradition of going to the board for approval during the October finance committee/board cycle. There is a very practical reason for this. At RHMC, the board and its committees meet only every two months, beginning in February and continuing through April, June, August, October, and December. Therefore, the only possible choices for this organization are October or December and they have concluded that the December time frame does not afford them enough time to prepare the budget results after board approval.

The boards of healthcare organizations may be constituted to meet every month, every two months (like RHMC), or as little as every three months. Again, it depends on the organization's needs and culture. For boards that meet monthly, the most likely approval point is the November meeting, which has the most balanced set of pros and cons. It is also possible for Boards that meet every other month to set their schedule so that the cycle constitutes January, March, May, July, September, and November. That would obviously allow the organization to use the more practical November meeting for presentation of the budget. Finally, it is possible for the board and finance committees to hold a special meeting once a year, in November, with an agenda devoted only to the budget, if they so choose.

Budget Calendar Steps

So, now the end date is known and all the designated budget activities have been counted backward to determine the start date. It is important to know that there is a definite order of activities that needs to be followed in order to produce the best possible budget results. Certain activities must be performed before other activities. This is required because the subsequent activities need the results of former activities for their processing. In order to proceed, several budget steps need to be accomplished in the kick-off month of June. The calendar lists these opening month activities in June.

June 1   Kick-off meeting for volume projections (hold meeting)
June 26   a. Approve projected 1998 and budgeted 1999 admission,
                   length of stay, and patient days by service
                b. Approve projected 1998 and budgeted 1999 projected
                   outpatient trends by ancillary services (hold meeting)

These activities are discussed later in this chapter.

VOLUME ISSUES

There are many activities listed on the budget calendar. The most important activity is determination of the projected and budgeted inpatient and outpatient volumes. Absolutely no other projection will be as crucial to the overall budget outcome as the volumes. All of the gross and net revenues, as well as all of the variable expenses, will be a function of the increases or decreases budgeted for volumes.

There are several methods that can be used to budget volumes in a healthcare institution.

1. Historical trends
2. Demographic changes
3. New services
4. Physician issues and inputs
5. Wishful thinking

Historical Perspective

The most common method used to project and budget volume changes is to review the current volumes and the volumes of the recent past (e.g., the previous two to three years) and extend that trend line into the future. This forecasting can be done with the use of regression analysis. Although this is the most common method used by healthcare institutions, it can be fraught with danger. As they say in mutual fund advertising, "Past results are no guarantee of future earnings." The same is true of volume budgeting. Nothing that happened in the past, including just last month, may have any bearing on the future. It is important to be aware of past volumes but the organization also needs to add many other characteristics to its analysis, such as demographic changes, new services, and physicians inputs, to be more confident that the budgeted volumes have a reasonable chance of being attained.

Demographic Changes

Adding any known or suspected demographic changes to the historical volume trends contributes significantly to refining the validity of the budget. It is imperative that the organization is aware of the population changes in its service areas. This is necessary in order to redetermine the community needs and evaluate which, if any, programs need to be expanded, contracted, established, or closed.

Demographic changes can have wide-ranging impacts on an organization's volumes and the success or failure of its various program offerings. For example, let's say that a real estate developer just bought up a 1,000 acre tract of farmland in an organization's service area with the express intent on building 2,000 single family housing units that are intended to be marketed to young, growing families. It would be important for the organization to be aware of this development. They then could attempt to determine inpatient and outpatient volume increases that may accrue to their pediatric, obstetrics, and labor room services and budget accordingly.

Another example of a demographic change that could cause volume decreases would be the closure of a major assembly plant in town. The healthcare organization, which may have come to rely on the volumes and revenues generated from these plant employees, may now have to downsize their services to reflect the possible reduction in the area's population. Any and all known demographic changes should be reflected in the organization's short-term budgeting. It is essential that the organization employ an individual or individuals to monitor these shifts and report them back to the administration and the finance staff in a timely manner.

New Services

Another set of major items that needs to be considered in the historical perspective are volumes for any new services or programs, such as diabetes, sickle cell anemia, or chest pain clinics, that the organization has planned to add in the upcoming budget year. For example, the addition of a magnetic resonance imaging system (MRI) is supposed to add new volumes to the radiology department. Because most new services are required to present a pro forma projected profit and loss statement before approval of the service, the volumes will be available to add to the budget. In reviewing the pro forma for the MRI in Chapter 1, it was shown that the volume projections were the critical drivers of the revenues and expenses. Critical evaluation was performed to determine the most likely volume projections. This is necessary for any new services proposed and accepted.

Physician Issues and Inputs

Another highly critical element to successful volume budgeting is an awareness of current physician satisfaction and any issues that may be affecting their usage of the organization's services. All patient volumes are a function of physician referrals to the healthcare organization. Physicians are, by their very nature, analytical and skeptical. Their long years of training and their responsibilities affecting a patient's life or death make them very demanding. They want the healthcare organization to be highly efficient and provide them with the latest state-of-the-art equipment to help them provide the highest level of patient care.

Physician issues can often complicate the completion of the operating budget. It is important for the organization's administration to constantly monitor the state of its employed or affiliated physician office practices for any demographic, managed care or structural changes. These could have an impact on the ability of the physician to continue the former referral pattern to the organization. Additionally, there are many physicians who split their practice between two or more healthcare providers. It is important for the organization to know which physicians are splitters. Because splitters often have to drive between their practices, which can take a lot of time and effort, some of these physicians eventually decide to give this up. It is a great advantage for an organization to be the recipient of the splitters full-time attention. This could have major positive effects on the upcoming budget year volumes. Conversely, should the competitor organization get all the business, the budget volumes would have to be adjusted downward.

Wishful Thinking

A concept that is sometimes used in volume budgeting is wishful thinking. This is often employed as the means to balance a budget that did not come out right the first time. When the budgeted bottom line will not meet board expectations using the techniques described above, wishful thinking may be employed to boost the volumes and revenues accordingly. Unfortunately, because it is not based on any of the established methods, it is unsupportable. However, that does not always stop healthcare administrators from using it. Finance managers and their staff should be ever vigilant in attempting to discourage this form of volume budgeting. If used, it will only delay the inevitable decisions to properly size the institution.

June 1—Volume Kick-Off Meeting

With the information described above as a backdrop, the finance division staff assigned to the budget calls a meeting with administrative staff and selected ancillary department managers to discuss upcoming volume issues. The first thing that they look at is the trend of historical inpatient and outpatient volumes. The key inpatient volume drivers are admission and length of stay statistics, which result in the total number of patient days. The key outpatient driver is usually the number of tests or examinations performed.

During this meeting, the clinical managers and the finance staff will review the historical trends, discuss the current status, and speculate on the near-term future prospects for volumes. The primary issues that will be discussed include the following.

1. Any changes in physician practices involving physicians currently on active staff
2. Any known additional physician practices that may be entering the service area
3. Any additional services that may be added based on newly acquired technologies
4. Any other change in services that will either add or subtract volumes

All of these items are instructive but not definitive. They will aid the department manager in projecting next year's volumes. Still, the organization's administration may well desire a very specific set of budgeted volumes in order to achieve a certain measure of profitability. If all of the items above do not equal the desired changes, the managers will need to determine additional steps to achieve them. Generally this may mean greater marketing and promotion within or outside the service area, more focused managed care negotiations leading to additional patient loads or improved service levels, and customer satisfaction necessary to attract patients to the institution. All of these issues are discussed and debated during the volume kick-off meeting on June 1. No specific conclusions are drawn, but the meeting provides a framework for subsequent actions.

TABLE 6–4

Ridgeland Heights Medical Center
1999 Projected and 2000 Budgeted Inpatient Volumes

		Admissions			Patient Days			Length of Stay		
	No. of Beds	1998 Projected	1999 Budget	Percent Variance	1998 Projected	1999 Budget	Percent Variance	1998 Projected	1999 Budget	Percent Variance
Medical/ surgical	120	2,700	2,800	3.7	13,000	14,000	7.7	4.81	5.00	3.8
Intensive care	24	1,800	1,900	5.6	6,500	7,220	11.1	3.61	3.80	5.2
Pediatrics	10	600	660	10.0	1,500	1,716	14.4	2.50	2.60	4.0
Maternity	24	2,000	2,200	10.0	4,000	4,400	10.0	2.00	2.00	0.0
Births	26	1,950	2,145	10.0	3,900	4,290	10.0	2.00	2.00	0.0
Psychiatric	20	1,000	1,200	20.0	6,500	8,160	25.5	6.50	6.80	4.6
Skilled nursing facility	30	800	840	5.0	8,800	8,400	−4.5	11.00	10.00	−9.1
Totals	254	10,850	11,745	8.2	48,186	48,186	9.0	4.07	4.10	0.7

June 26—Approve Projected 1999 and Budgeted 2000 Inpatient and Outpatient Volumes

Subsequent to the kick-off meeting, the finance staff will hold several one-on-one type meetings with various clinical managers to solicit specific feedback regarding where the managers believe volumes in their departments are heading. All of this input will be incorporated into the analysis that will be presented to the administration during the June 26 budget meeting to approve subsequent period volumes. The finance administrator will present the analysis developed by the staff to the assembled members. The clinical managers' assumptions are summarized, distilled, and explained at this time.

These assumptions will be debated and discussed. Some assumptions may appear to be too high or too low based on the assembled members knowledge and experience. The administrators are always interested in understanding any new service lines or physician ideas that have been projected by their clinical managers. In general though, the budget assumptions presented by the finance staff will be approved. Any changes generated at the meeting will be incorporated into the next iteration of the budget package.

Table 6–4 is a representation of the organization's 1999 projected actual volumes as well as the volumes that they are budgeting for 2000 by inpatient unit. Similarly, Table 6–5 illustrates the 1999 and 2000 budgeted outpatient visits. This is the result of discussions involving all of the items described above.

Overall, the clinical managers, along with the organization's administration, believe that their overall inpatient days will increase 9% next year while outpatient

TABLE 6–5

Ridgeland Heights Medical Center
1999 Projected and 2000 Budgeted Outpatient Visits

	Visits		
	1999 Projected	**2000 Budget**	**Percent Variance**
Emergency department	19,000	20,000	5.3
Outpatient surgery	4,500	5,000	11.1
Same day surgery	3,700	4,000	8.1
Observation patients	1,950	2,000	2.6
Home health services	26,000	30,000	15.4
Other outpatients	112,000	120,000	7.1
Totals	167,150	181,000	8.3

visits will increase 8.3%. These volume changes will be fully incorporated into the upcoming gross and net revenue budgets as well as the variable expense budget calculations. The one warning that always emerges from this meeting is that these projections and volumes are subject to change depending on the budgeted operating margins that emerge from the use of these numbers.

CAPITAL BUDGETING—JUNE

In the meantime, while the operating budget time line is being established and on its way to implementation, the capital budget process has also commenced. Because the operating budget bottom line includes depreciation expense, it is essential that the capital budget be completed prior to completion of the operating budget. The capital budget determines the capital equipment that will be acquired; the buildings that will be renovated, built, or leased; the amounts that will be spent; and the estimated useful life that will be assigned to each of these assets. These elements will allow the finance staff to determine the depreciation expense that needs to be included in the following year.

In Chapter 3, capital plan development concepts were reviewed in some detail as they relate to the organization's strategic financial plan. The various types of capital assets available for acquisition were discussed in that chapter. During the strategic planning process, the amounts of money available for the annual capital budgets were determined. Because the funding amounts and sources are already known, the main purpose of the annual capital budget is to identify the specific capital items to be acquired. The problem in almost all healthcare organizations is *which capital projects should be funded*. It is a classic question and there have been few good solutions over the years. The issue is to determine, in a reasonable and efficient

TABLE 6–6

Criteria-Based Strategic Capital Budgeting Process Summary

Step 1	Evaluate decision criteria
Step 2	Classify proposed expenditures
Step 3	Collect information
Step 4	Evaluate proposals
Step 5	Set strategic priority weights
Step 6	Calculate value scores
Step 7	Sort proposals on benefit-cost ratios

manner, how to allocate the organization's scarce resources—money available for capital.

The most common method used in past and present is characterized by the decision-making in the *smoked filled room*. Administrators would get together once a year with a wish list of items requested by department management. This list should include requests from various physicians that spend their time in those particular departments. Despite the amount of money being requested here, there may be no financial analysis performed or required. In general, the administrators with the most clout, the loudest voice, the most enthusiastic performance may get their pet project approved, while the most worthy projects are bypassed because of a less than optimal back room performance by its administrative champion.

This is not, nor has it ever been, a good situation. Yet it has always persisted because 1) the powerful have had no incentive to change it and 2) no really good alternative that incorporated financial and nonfinancial criteria had been presented to the industry. At RHMC, the finance administrators were tired of the infighting and lack of consistency usually exhibited at these annual rites of frustration. They were on the lookout for a better way to develop and control the capital funding process. A couple of years ago they were lucky enough to attend a seminar through the Healthcare Financial Management Association (HFMA) titled, Strategic Capital Budgeting: Optimizing Capital Decisions in Today's Healthcare Environment. This seminar highlighted the problems with the traditional approaches to capital budgeting. It also presented unique, simple and sensible solutions to these problems.[1]

The steps involved in this new capital budgeting methodology are summarized in Table 6–6.[2] In a nutshell, the solutions involve innovative organizational processes

---

[1] This seminar is offered periodically throughout the year by the Healthcare Financial Management Association at various locations around the country. It is taught by Catherine E. Kleinmuntz, Ph.D., and Don Kleinmuntz, Ph.D.

[2] In addition, these methods are further discussed in a January, 1999 unpublished paper titled *Strategic Appror Allocating Capital in Healthcare Organizations*, authored by Catherine E. Kleinmuntz, Ph.D., and Don Kleinmuntz, Ph.D. It can be obtained at www.decisiontechnology.com.

with supporting quantitative evaluation tools. It aids healthcare organizations in their need to allocate capital to maintain state-of-the-art clinical and facilities equipment while concurrently developing ambulatory facilities, physician networks, and information technology. It also involves many decision makers from across the organization as part of an ongoing strategic planning process. Finally, it allows the organization to *objectively* evaluate the capital proposals against established criteria and against proposals competing for the same scarce resources.

Table 6–7 represents RHMC's budget calendar that incorporates all of these concepts. In addition, the calendar is designed to run concurrently with the operating budget and finish in time to be presented simultaneously. The key characteristic of the budget is its incorporation of the organization's key strategic plan criteria. These criteria become the key drivers of the capital decision process. Rather than decisions based on the gut, in the old smoke filled rooms, the organization now has a *criteria-based capital decision process.*

In the case of RHMC, the administration has to first validate its strategic plan criteria. While an organization with board-approved strategic plan criteria should be making operational decisions based on them, this is not always the case. Very often healthcare organizations give only lip service to its strategic plan without providing financial resources to achieve its stated goals. In the criteria-based capital decision process, the strategic plan criteria provide the foundation for the ultimate outcomes—which capital asset will be funded.

The remaining budget steps in the June capital budget calendar involve training the various staff, both technical and administrative, on their roles. If the individual is a proposal reviewer, they will be trained to ensure that each capital proposal contains all of the data required before it can be moved on to the proposal evaluators. The proposal reviewers care about the technical aspects of the capital request, such as whether it will involve the following.

- Require additional considerations (e.g., electrical, facilities)
- Need any special computer hook-ups or special training for the technical staff (information technology)
- Necessitate any special negotiations on price or contract terms (materials management)
- Create any special funding requirements (accounting)

The proposal evaluators care about each of the proposals, how they stand up on their own merits, how they compare with all the other projects on a criteria basis, and whether the organization is well served in its total commitment to its strategic plan.

Both groups will be trained in the month of June on the use of the software that resides on their desktop personal computer. The software itself is on a computer server attached to the organization's local area network (LAN). Every individual

T A B L E 6–7

Ridgeland Heights Medical Center
2000 Budget Calendar
Capital Budget

Parties Involved	Activity	Date	Meeting Time/ Location
Executive and administrative staff Finance staff	Validate strategic plan criteria	June 1	Meeting Room 2 9:00–10:00 AM
Proposal Reviewers Accounting staff Facilities management Information systems management Materials management	Training for all staff assigned to *review capital proposals*	June 10	Meeting Room 2 2:00–4:00 PM
Proposal Writers All department management	Review the capital budgeting software Train all department management on the data elements required for a clean capital budget request	June 13 June 20	Meeting Room 2 3:00–4:00 PM
Proposal Writer All department management	Allow department managers access to the capital budget software upon completion of training	June 20	
Proposal Writers All department management	Submission of 2000 capital budget by department managers through electronic software located on managers' desktops	July 11	
Finance staff	Review all capital proposals for completeness of all required information fields	July 12–23	
Proposal reviewers	Capital proposals reviewed within the established time frames; review performed online at the reviewer's desktop	July 24– August 6	Reviewer's office computer
Proposal evaluators	Detailed discussion of all proposals over $100,000 and training of all proposal evaluators	August 11	Meeting Room 2 1:30–5:00 PM

Continued.

Ridgeland Heights Medical Center
2000 Budget Calendar *(Concluded)*

Parties Involved	Activity	Date	Meeting Time/ Location
Pool evaluators	**Discussion of pool proposals** Information systems 9:00–10:30 AM Construction/renovations 10:30 AM–12:00 PM Patient care 12:30–2:00 PM Medical technology 2:00–3:30 PM Market development 3:30–5:00 PM	August 12	Meeting Room 2
Proposal evaluators	Evaluate proposals online at the reviewer's desktop	August 12–15	Evaluator's office computer
Pool evaluators	**Pool consensus meetings** Information systems 9:00–10:30 AM Construction/Renovations 10:30–12:00 PM Patient Care 12:30–2:00 PM Medical Technology 2:00–3:30 PM Market Development 3:30–5:00 PM	August 22–25	Meeting Room 2 Various times—see attachment
Proposal evaluators	Proposal consensus meeting—All proposals over $100,000	August 25	Meeting Room 2 3:00– 5:00 PM
Proposal and pool evaluators	Revise ratings, if necessary, on the reviewers desktop	August 26–28	Evaluator's office computer
Proposal evaluators	Meeting to discuss results of evaluations Final review of 2000 capital budget	September 4	Meeting Room 2 9:00–10:00 AM

involved in the process will complete his or her role by accessing the LAN. The use of this software at RHMC creates a highly efficient situation. Everyone has access to the same information, in a timely manner. Because this process eliminates paper, all proposals are more consistently presented to the evaluator, easier for the accounting staff to administer and facilitates the ongoing updating of each project between the proposal writer and the evaluators.

As the month of June moves forward, these initial steps in the capital budget will be performed. In later months, the meat of the capital budgeting process will become more evident.

The training steps allow the finance staff to properly instruct the department managers in how to use the system to input all the required elements for each capital request. Upon completion of this training in June, the managers will be given access to the actual software on their PC. They will then be expected to submit all of their capital budgets back to the finance staff by July 11.

ACCOUNTING AND FINANCE DEPARTMENT RESPONSIBILITIES

Lost in the shuffle of all the fundamental issues that have been reported is some of the very routine business performed by the accounting and finance department. In many healthcare organizations, as highlighted at the end of Chapter 5, the accounting department is responsible for the preparation of the financial statement in an accurate and timely manner. In addition, they are also responsible for preparing and paying the organization's employees through the payroll function and all the trade vendors through the accounts payable function. They are also accountable for all financial analyses, which usually includes the cost accounting function, the maintenance of the price list, which creates the gross revenue, the reimbursement function, which includes the preparation of the Medicare Cost Report and the budget. Box 6–1 is a summarized list of the major responsibilities of the accounting department.

While it is hard to say which of the items on the list is the most important, it would be no understatement to suggest that being late with the payroll checks, even by 10 minutes, is the quickest way to lose the confidence of the entire organization. This would be true of the chief executive officer all the way down to the nonskilled staff. Missing a payroll deadline causes all kinds of trouble between the organization and its employees. Even when there is clear and direct communications about the cause of the problem, rumors begin to run rampant. So, it is extremely advisable to not miss a payroll. There are only a few reasons why the payroll would ever be late. Following are the two most common reasons.

1. *The computer breaks down.* This is not likely, but it is possible. Payroll systems are extremely mature and stable. They were one of the first applications designed for computers over 40 years ago. So, breakdowns almost never happen. Still, it has been known to happen.

   Good management suggests building redundancies into these systems. That could mean paying for a duplicate system and keeping it available if and when the initial system goes down. Or it could mean creating manual down-time procedures that would typically be less expensive than an automated solution but will cause more work in the event it needs to be used.

2. *The organization runs out of money.* It has been known to happen in some organizations that were having temporary or long-term financial

difficulty. This is a much more problematic situation than just having the computer break down.

Not paying its employees in a timely manner has numerous detrimental impacts on the organization as well as for the employees. Most employees count on their paychecks to meet the basic needs for themselves and their families, such as paying for rent, food, clothing, and transportation. When their paychecks are not available as expected, particularly when the employees already know that the organization is having

BOX 6–1

RIDGELAND HEIGHTS MEDICAL CENTER
Major Responsibilities of the Accounting and Finance Department

General Accounting

1. Capture of all of the organization's financial transactions during each accounting period (usually monthly) (This may be carried out through the use of paper accounting transactions or through electronic interfaces to subsidiary ledgers and journals.)
2. Production of accurate and timely organization-wide financial statements
3. Collection of information and completion and submission of all IRS-type tax returns, whether for-profit or not-for-profit returns
4. Preparation and facilitation of financial analysis for the external auditors
5. Facilitation of all appropriate internal auditing functions

Accounts Payable

1. Collection of all invoices from trade vendors on a timely basis
2. Three-way matching of purchase orders, receiving dock receipts and invoices to validate that all goods were authorized for purchase, received, and are being billed by the vendor correctly
3. Timely payments to the organization's trade vendors within payment terms, or sooner if a discount for prompt payment is being granted

Payroll

1. Collection of all payroll hours being requested and authorized for payment during each of the organization's payroll periods (This may be carried out through paper time cards or electronic time and attendance systems.)
2. Validation and verification of all payroll hours and determination that all payroll policies and procedures were applied correctly by all of the department managers
3. Timely payments of salaries and wages to the organization's employees
4. Timely payment to pension plans

Budgeting

1. Development and timely completion of the organization's *operating, capital, and cash budgets*
2. Compilation and submission of all board-level budget packages

financial difficulties, they begin to question the long-term viability of the organization. This inevitably leads to the staff looking for new jobs in other organizations, which begins a negative cycle of staff defections that weaken an already shaky situation.

Good management in this situation suggests that the payroll is always the first payment priority. This seems obvious, but as practical matter, it is not always easy. For example, while it is possible to delay payments to the trade vendors that supply the organization with medical and surgical supplies, there are times when

---

Major Responsibilities of the Accounting and Finance Department (Concluded)

Strategic Financial Planning

1. Development of the five-year strategic financial plan
2. Development of the five-year capital needs analysis and plan

Reimbursement

1. Completion of the Medicare and Medicaid annual cost reports
2. Coordinate all government audits and reports, including census reports
3. Model all new and revised managed care contracts in order to improve negotiations
4. Monthly analysis of organization's contractual adjustments
5. Maintain highly accurate net revenue calculations for financial analysis
6. Maintenance of the organization's charge master (price list), and annual analysis of potential and actual price increase

Financial Analysis and Decision Support

1. Development and maintenance of the organization's cost accounting system, including determination of variable and fixed costs, and direct and indirect costs
2. Maintenance and reporting from the decision support system (This allows the organization's operating managers to have the financial information needed in order to make proper decisions.)
3. Development of all pro forma financial analysis
4. Development of all other financial analyses
5. Coordinate the gathering of all data required by various healthcare associations and rating agencies such as the American Hospital Association, state and/or local healthcare associations, Standard and Poor's and Moody's

Other Responsibilities

1. Processing of the organization's property and casualty insurance programs
2. Monitoring of the pension plan and program; accounting coordination with the actuary assigned to the plan

those vendors will demand payments or else not ship those supplies that may be needed for surgical cases on the schedule for tomorrow.

The other situation that a financially stressed organization should never allow itself to become involved in is to avoid paying the government for the payroll taxes withheld by the organization. It must always be remembered that when the organization collects these payroll taxes for the various government agencies, it is acting as its agent. These funds cannot be used to pay for anything else, including medical supplies or the payroll itself. Payroll taxes are usually owed to the government within two to three days of payroll distribution. Penalties and interests will be assessed immediately following that time period. Also, it is important to note that the administrators and any other staff who are responsible for making the decisions when to pay the payroll taxes *are personally liable for the taxes, penalties, and interest* if the organization is unable to satisfy the debt. This is true even if the organization or the individuals successfully discharge its other debts in a bankruptcy proceeding.

JUNE FINANCE COMMITTEE SPECIAL AGENDA ITEMS

Human Resources Report

There are several reasons for presenting the report of the board-level human resources committee at the June finance committee meeting. The two most important reasons are to allow management to present analyses of local and regional salary levels and employee fringe benefit levels to this committee. The committee is charged with making recommendations and approving annual changes in these areas.

It is important for organizations to have goals related to these two items. There are significant issues that surround recruitment and retention policies. Ridgeland Heights Medical Center strives to maintain a certain level of compensation and benefits compared to the rest of the region. It is able to make this decision by accessing a variety of sources maintained by local and regional healthcare associations and other nonhealthcare labor bureaus. It is then able to determine whether or not it is maintaining its desired percentile compensation level.

The human resources committee along with the RHMC's human resources administrator are aware that it is in the organization's best interest to maintain a competitive position in the market place. In fact, many human resource professionals would prefer that their organization take an aggressive position in the market place, especially if it can be afforded. This allows the organization to recruit the best potential candidates, which will help to reduce the turnover rate, reduce the cost of help wanted advertisements, and improve overall employee morale.

The report given to the human resources committee in June is preliminary. It allows the committee to understand the current levels in the market place and ask any relevant questions. They will come together again in September to be asked to approve the levels recommended by management in the final development of the budget.

Pension Status and Actuary Report Review

Once a year, RHMC's management provides an update on the organization's pension plan to the finance committee. This is important because the board has a fiduciary responsibility to its employees to maintain the pension funds in a sound manner while assuring that the funds will earn returns appropriate to the pension portfolio's risk. The finance committee is interested in whether or not the market value of the organization's pension assets continues to exceed the present value of all accrued benefits. As long as this is the case, the organization is not in an underfunded position with respect to its defined benefit pension plan.

Box 6–2 highlights the items of major interest to the finance committee. Presented in this format every year, the finance committee relies on this report to understand various aspects of its pension obligations. This includes minimum and

---

B O X   6–2

RIDGELAND HEIGHTS MEDICAL CENTER Pension Status
1999 Actuarial Report

The report of our actuarial consultant was updated effective January 1, 1999, for the defined benefit plan. The following key items are highlighted compared to the prior year's results.

1. Market Value of Assets increased by $3,000,000 from $23,000,000 on 1/1/98 to $26,000,000 on 1/1/99.
2. Present Value of All Accrued Benefits is composed of the following.

	1/1/98	1/1/99
Active Vested Employees	$7,000,000	$7,400,000
Active Nonvested Employees	1,000,000	1,100,000
Retired Employees	8,000,000	8,300,000
Terminated Vested Employees	4,000,000	4,200,000
Totals	$20,000,000	$21,000,000

3. Assets over Accrued Benefits increased by $2,000,000 from $7,000,000 to $9,000,000.
4. Normal Cost (defined as the amount that is required to fund the benefits expected to be earned in the current year) increased by $40,000 from $680,000 to $720,000.
5. Normal Cost as a percentage of compensation decreased by 0.10% from 2.40% to 2.30%.
6. The minimum required contribution for 1997, 1998, and 1999 is $400,000, $700,000, and $0, respectively.
7. Actual beneficiary payments in 1998 were $800,000. Expected beneficiary payments in 1999 are $840,000.
8. Pension expense for the accounting years ending December 31, 1998 and 1999 were, respectively, $600,000 and $750,000.

maximum funding requirement established by the federal government's ERISA laws. It also includes the actuarially determined net periodic pension costs that need to be recorded on the organization's income statement as stipulated by the Statement of Financial Accounting Standards (SFAS) #87 as well as the present value of accumulated plan benefits stipulated under SFAS #35.

Because the ERISA and SFAS methodologies are very different, very technically complex, very complicated, and very required, the annual report to the finance committee is meant to be a simplified analysis. RHMC's finance officer verbally reports on some of the key assumptions used as inputs by the actuary to produce the results. Some of the key assumptions are the discount rates used, the expected rate of return on the plan's investments, and the expected rate of compensation increases.

In this case, the finance committee is pleased that the annual pension report shows an increase in the assets over accrued benefits. They are additionally pleased to learn that based on the previous funding level and interest income earnings over the past year, they will not be required to pay any cash into the pension fund next year.

7

CHAPTER

July

"Dad, you were right. This is a long story. Is it over yet?" asked Susie, the reasonably perplexed eight year old child.

Sam Barnes took a deep breath. He wanted to explain the story in the simplest of terms but apparently was not succeeding at the moment. Yet all he could say was, "Oh come on honey. This story is just getting interesting. There is so much more to it than I've already told you."

Susie was smiling. She sure was a cute kid.

She said, "Dad, I am glad that you've been telling this to me as a bedtime story. It sure has helped me get to sleep a lot easier. And I think I understand some of what you've told me. I guess I never knew how your place made money. I didn't know that your company had to make money so you could get paid. That's pretty cool. But I still don't understand why your company doesn't get paid all the money you charge to people when you take care of them. I know that when we go to the supermarket we have to pay the lady at the checkout counter for the food and stuff we have in our cart."

"Susie, you are so right, and that's pretty perceptive of you," declared Sam.

"Dad, what's perceptive mean?" asked Susie.

"Oh never mind, don't worry about that," Sam said to his precious little princess. "In any case, I do have to pay the lady at the checkout counter the amount of money that she rang up on her cash register. But what you're forgetting is that some of the things we bought were already discounted by the store or by the people who made the food and gave it to the store to sell. My company is doing the same thing. We are agreeing to discount our services to the people who are paying for the services, the insurance companies. The big difference between the supermarket and us is that we don't have any shelves to put our discounted prices on. Another difference is that we may only give those discounts to certain people who have insurance from companies that want to make a deal with us, not to everybody. It's kind of like people in the supermarket who have coupons. They pay less than other people for the exact same food because they have the coupon."

"Dad, I think I get some of it. But from the way you've been telling the story, it still seems unfair. It sounds like they just want to pay you a lot less than you want from them," said the still perplexed youngster.

"Yeah, it's true that some companies want to pay us less. But that's probably okay for our family. You see, part of the reason that my company pays me is to make sure that they know how much money we can discount and still have a certain amount left over at the end of the year," stated Sam with certainty.

"Yeah, well I sure am glad that you like doing it, because I'm not sure it sounds like a lot of fun to me," said Susie, with even more certainty.

———

Warm breezes wafted off of Lake Michigan blowing thin wispy clouds against a high light blue sky. Sunbathers and sunburners are lying out across a hot white sand beach. Summer is in full swing in the northern climes. Young and old alike enjoy the nice change in the weather. They know that it is fleeting. Winter is always just around the corner waiting to bring its cold arctic blasts down on the town.

So there is always great enjoyment this time of the year. Schools are out, temperatures are in the 80s and for many, vacations have begun or will begin soon. The reality rarely meets or exceeds the expectations but the psychology of summer is having its dazzling effect. People around town are smiling more easily; the pace of life has slowed as many stop to enjoy the weather. That is, all but the finance staff at Ridgeland Heights Medical Center.

BUDGET PREPARATIONS—THE MIDDLE MONTHS

July is the month when the budget becomes the top priority of the accounting and finance department. While June was devoted to preliminary work, July is when the heavy lifting begins. There are several critical meetings scheduled to take place that will shape the financial prognostications for the upcoming year. The July operating budget calendar is abundant with weighty issues.

July 1	Issue 2000 operating budget calendar
July 11	Compute gross revenues and contractual adjustments
July 14	Review salary and nonsalary assumptions (hold meeting)

July 15   Review gross revenues and contractual adjustments and validate payor mix (hold meeting)

July 18   Review 2000 budgeted income statement, determine price increase targets, and revise salary and nonsalary assumptions (hold meeting)

July 25   Issue 1999 projected/2000 budgeted worksheets to department managers

All of these steps require a great deal of effort and the finance staff is prepared to perform their tasks with rigor and vigor.

Which Is a Better Budgeting Technique—Top Down or Bottom Up?

Meanwhile as the organization continues its annual budget process, an age-old question is once again revived, "Which budgeting technique is better for the organization, top down or bottom up?" The answer usually depends on who is responding and the stake they have in it. It is a highly charged issue, of particular concern to department managers who have to live with the consequences of either answer.

Top down budgeting is defined as revenues and expense levels imposed by the administration and directed down to the manager who is expected to achieve them. Bottom up budgeting is defined as revenue and expense levels determined by each department manager that is aggregated to establish the organization-wide budget.

There are several implications to the use of either technique. Table 7–1 highlights the pros and cons of both techniques.

The key issue is control—who's got it and how are they going to exercise it? As is common in any hierarchical organization, the control is held at the top. But in this case, control is not really the most important issue. The really big issue is information management. Who's got it and how is it going to be used? The overriding problem in budget management is achieving a targeted operating margin that will be acceptable to the finance committee and the board. When department managers are given control of their own departmental budgets, they often have no good way to know what amount of departmental bottom line is needed by the administration to achieve the financial targets.

Now the next logical question is, "Well, why doesn't the administration just tell each department what type of bottom line is needed and then just let the managers go and achieve it?" Of course, the answer is obvious. If administration tell managers this information, they are effectively mandating the bottom line, which is once again top down budgeting. It is a circular argument. While managers want to be able to control their budgeted volumes, revenues, and expenses, allowing them to do so may potentially compromise the organization's bottom line.

There is another possible problem when managers are given control of producing their budget assumptions, particularly the volumes. Managers are hard working, diligent, loyal, and smart. And like all human beings, they are also focused on their own welfare. Whether or not the managers are permitted to participate in an

TABLE 7–1

Top Down or Bottom Up Budgeting Technique
Pros and Cons

Top Down		Bottom Up	
Pros	**Cons**	**Pros**	**Cons**
Administration maintains control on the assumptions that determine the targeted operating margin.	Department managers are not invested in the budget outcomes because they do not have any input into the process.	Managers who set their own budget will be more invested in process and the future outcomes.	Managers have no incentives to set aggressive or "stretch" budget targets for their own departments.
There will be less chance of the managers needing to redo their budgets one, two, three times in order to "balance the budget" as the assumptions change.	Administration is perceived as autocratic, not participative.	The budgeted volumes may be closer to reality, therefore causing less budget variances in the upcoming year.	Managers have no idea of the overall hospital budget targets and therefore no way of knowing the amount of bottom lines required from their departments for the organization to succeed as a whole.

organization's incentive compensation plan, they all have an annual review of their performance for the purpose of determining their annual pay raise. The managers will always be evaluated against established goals. Obviously, managers will attempt to establish goals that are easily achievable in order to maximize their accomplishments during the annual review. Therefore, the budgeted volumes, which drive the budgeted revenues, will not be aggressive. This will generally make it more difficult for the formulated budget to produce the targeted volumes required by the board.

So, what's the answer? In order to minimize manager frustrations caused by being asked to constantly change their own assumptions throughout the budget process, the top down technique is favored. Top down budgeting also measurably shortens the process by six to eight weeks because it minimizes the *rework* caused by unusable volume and revenue assumptions. Managers are often willing to accept and cooperate in the top down budget process when the pros and cons are explained to them and the ongoing budget process is constantly communicated. They still may not like it but they learn to live with it.

July 1—Issuance of the Budget Calendar

Although there was some considerable amount of preliminary work performed in June, which was facilitated by the finance staff with inputs from many of the clinical managers, the budget calendar is first issued on July 1. As explained in some detail in Chapter 6, the purpose of the budget calendar is to provide expectations of the duration and timing of the project for all involved participants. This is done through the establishment of meeting times and places for the various get-togethers that are required for good communication of some very complicated and demanding issues. The calendar sets the agenda for the next four month's work.

July 11—Compute Gross Revenues and Contractual Adjustments

Between June 28 and July 11, one of the key steps in preparation and execution of a valid budget process is being performed in the back room of the finance department by some of its most valuable members, the financial analysts. The calculation of the current and subsequent year's annual gross revenues and contractual adjustments are being developed based on the volumes approved at the June 26 budget meeting. At RHMC, the finance staff members with the expertise in these areas are determining volumes, gross revenues, and net reimbursements.

This determination is based on many assumptions. In addition to the inpatient and outpatient volume assumptions, the following items need to be projected in order to develop a valid and viable revenue budget.

1. Detailed payor mix, highlighting the mix across
   a. Many of the various clinical service areas
   b. The inpatient and outpatient service mix side
2. The payment levels for the entire payor mix. Every conceivable known change in payment levels is essential for this process to succeed. The financial analyst may need to rely on other individuals in the organization for help. For example, many organizations now have a full time employee to negotiate managed care contracts. This individual will have to provide his or her best guess on the discount levels projected for the upcoming year. It will be the best basis on which the organization has to develop the net revenue budget.
3. The gross revenues are broken down by inpatient and outpatient services. This is required in order to develop the projected contractual adjustments. As always the calculation for contractual adjustments is as follows.

Gross revenue − Net revenue (or expected payment) = Contractual adjustment

So, in order to determine the actual contractual adjustments, it is necessary to know the gross revenues, segregated into actionable categories.

The organization takes the various available financial and statistical elements and arranges them into usable criteria for analysis. The output of this extensive analysis is a summary sheet that will be used by the finance administrator at the budget meeting scheduled with the entire administration for July 18. Table 7–2 shows the summary gross revenue, contractual adjustment, and net revenue worksheet. Some of the key features of the worksheet are the following.

T A B L E 7-2

Ridgeland Heights Medical Center
Revenue and Contractual Analysis
1999 Projected and 2000 Budget (In Thousands)

	Gross Revenue					Percentage of Gross Revenues					Contractual Allowance Dollars					Contractual Adjustment				
	1998 Actual	1999 Budget	6/99 Actual	1999 Projected	2000 Budget	1998 Actual	1999 Budget	6/99 Actual	1999 Projected	2000 Budget	1998 Actual	1999 Budget	6/99 Actual	1999 Projected	2000 Budget	1998 Actual	1999 Budget	6/99 Actual	1999 Projected	2000 Budget
Inpatient																				
Medicare	36,000	38,000	19,000	38,500	40,000	48.6	48.7	48.0	48.2	47.6	16,500	21,000	10,000	19,500	24,000	45.8	55.3	52.6	50.6	60.0
Medicaid	2,000	2,000	1,050	2,000	2,400	2.7	2.6	2.7	2.5	2.9	1,500	1,500	800	1,500	1,800	75.0	75.0	76.2	75.0	75.0
Managed care	30,000	31,500	16,200	32,600	34,000	40.5	40.4	41.0	40.9	40.5	8,200	10,700	5,200	11,000	13,500	27.3	34.0	32.1	33.7	39.7
All other	6,000	6500	3,300	6,700	7,600	8.1	8.3	8.3	8.4	9.0	1,200	2,000	900	1,700	2,000	20.0	30.8	27.3	25.4	26.3
Total	74,000	78,000	39,550	79,800	84,000	100.0	100.0	100.0	100.0	100.0	27,400	35,200	16,900	33,700	41,300	37.0	45.1	42.7	42.2	49.2
Outpatient																				
Medicare	23,000	26,000	13,000	26,200	30,000	33.3	34.2	32.9	33.7	34.9	12,000	14,500	7,300	15,000	19,000	52.2	55.8	56.2	57.3	63.3
Medicaid	1,000	1,000	520	1,050	1,000	1.4	1.3	1.3	1.4	1.2	800	800	400	800	800	80.0	80.0	76.9	76.2	80.0
Managed care	36,000	38,000	20,000	39,000	42,000	52.2	50.0	50.6	50.2	48.8	7,000	8,500	4,000	8,700	10,000	19.4	22.4	20.0	22.3	23.8
All other	9,000	11,000	6,000	11,500	13,000	13.0	14.5	15.2	14.8	15.1	800	1,000	400	800	900	8.9	9.1	6.7	7.0	6.9
Total	69,000	76,000	39,520	77,750	86,000	100.0	100.0	100.0	100.0	100.0	20,600	24,800	12,100	25,300	30,700	29.9	32.6	30.6	32.5	35.7
Total																				
Medicare	59,000	64,000	32,000	64,700	70,000	41.3	41.6	40.5	41.1	41.2	28,500	35,500	17,300	34,500	43,000	48.3	55.5	54.1	53.3	61.4
Medicaid	3,000	3,000	1,570	3,050	3,400	2.1	1.9	2.0	1.9	2.0	2,300	2,300	1,200	2,300	2,600	76.7	76.7	76.4	75.4	76.5
Managed care	66,000	69,500	36,200	71,600	76,000	46.2	45.1	45.8	45.4	44.7	15,200	19,200	9,200	19,700	23,500	23.0	27.6	25.4	27.5	30.9
All other	15,000	17,500	9,300	18,200	20,600	10.5	11.4	11.8	11.6	12.1	2,000	3,000	1,300	2,500	2,900	13.3	17.1	14.0	13.7	14.1
Total	143,000	154,000	79,070	157,550	170,000	100.0	100.0	100.0	100.0	100.0	48,000	60,000	29,000	59,000	72,000	33.6	39.0	36.7	37.4	42.4
Gross revenues											143,000	154,000	79,070	157,550	170,000					
Less: grand total contractual adjustments											48,000	60,000	29,000	59,000	72,000					
Net revenues											95,000	94,000	50,070	98,550	98,000					
Contractual adjustment as a percentage of gross revenues											33.6	39.0	36.7	37.4	42.4					

- Total gross revenues segregated by inpatient and outpatient areas, without any price increase
- Total contractual dollars projected for the upcoming budget year
- Total contractual dollars as a percentage of gross revenue for prior years, projected current year, and upcoming budget year
- Net revenues projected for the current year and budgeted for the upcoming year

This is a significant worksheet. A considerable amount of time will be devoted to reviewing this worksheet both at the July 15 meeting with the finance administrators and then at the July 18 meeting when the finance administrators will present it to the assembled administration.

July 14—Review Salary and Nonsalary Assumptions

While the organization's reimbursement specialist is concentrating significant time and effort on the gross and net revenue calculations, a couple of other finance members are working on the expense side of the equation. At this administrative meeting, the only issues that will be discussed involve projecting upcoming expense increases. This will be somewhat similar to some of the techniques used during the strategic financial planning meetings held in March (see Chapter 3). The finance administrators will use this meeting to facilitate a series of discussions on four specific expense topics in order to be able to complete the preliminary budget.

1. Full time equivalent (FTE) levels
2. Wage and salary increases/decreases
3. Fringe benefits levels and increases/decreases
4. Controllable nonsalary expense changes

Full Time Equivalent Levels

This is always the most important part of the meeting. Healthcare is an extremely labor intensive industry. Labor costs, defined as all salaries, wages, contracted labor and fringe benefits, make up between 45% and 55% of all expenses in healthcare organizations. On the hospital side of the industry, some providers have as much of 60% of their expenses tied up in labor costs while others may spend as little as 40% on the same set of expenses.

The most important driver of labor costs is the amount of staff utilized. Labor costs are a product of pay rate times the number of people employed. Each of these two products has significant impacts on the total salary and fringe benefit costs. But, of these two components, only the number of employees is controllable by management. Pay rate is almost always a function of labor market conditions. As an employer, the healthcare organization will have to pay the going rate in the market place for its employees, or else it will not be able to recruit or retain staff. On the other hand, management has greater control over the number and mix of staff in every department of the organization.

Because labor costs are so substantial, it is of paramount importance that the organization attempt to properly *size* its workforce to maximize results. In healthcare, the challenge is to provide the best possible patient experience coupled with excellent clinical outcomes without overspending for those services. This spending objective is continually challenged not only by the clinical staff spearheaded by the nursing administration but often provoked by many of the organization's staff physicians.

Determining the right staff size is not easy. Healthcare, like other industries, has adopted benchmarking techniques into their arsenal of analysis tools. In healthcare however, benchmarking FTEs is fraught with peril. As was already explored in Chapter 3, FTEs per adjusted patient day, the most common industry benchmark, is highly susceptible to manipulation and produces a poor benchmark. The alternative benchmark, salaries, wages, and fringe benefits as a percentage of net patient service revenues, is a better measure of productivity. In order to use it in the annual budget analysis however, the dollar value of the projected FTEs needs to be converted into this percentage. This can be easily accomplished and at RHMC, the percentages associated with alternative models are always presented.

During this meeting, the prior year trends of total FTEs; FTEs per adjusted patient days; and salaries, wages, and fringe benefits as a percentage of net patient service revenues are presented along with the values associated with the current projected year and the upcoming budget year. These organization totals are supplemented by detailed departmental information. This allows the administrative reviewers to identify staffing trends within the various departments in order to make informed budgeting decisions. Table 7–3 displays the divisional FTE summary page used in the budgeting process by RHMC. This page is backed up by department totals within the various divisions.

Wage and Salary Increases

These increases are often less problematic for healthcare organizations to calculate. In a nonunion shop, the organization will access benchmark information from the healthcare industry around its region as well as increases predicted for other industries within the region that may be competing for the same pool of employees. This information is available through national and local hospital associations and other labor organizations. The finance staff merely calculates the impact of two or three potential increases being proposed by the human resources division and reports the projected results on the income statement to the administration.

In a union shop, the organization can easily perform this step if they are in the middle of a multiyear contract that does not expire in the upcoming budget year. They need only to use the amounts approved in the contract and they are essentially done. Budgeting for the remaining nonunion employees in the organization, often

Ridgeland Heights Medical Center
Divisional FTE Summary
For the Budget Year Ending December 31, 2000

	1999 Budget			2000 Budget			2000 B vs. 1999 B
	Regular	Overtime	Total	Regular	Overtime	Total	Incr (Decr)
Patient care services (nursing)	480.4	14.8	495.2	484.4	16.8	501.2	6.0
Clinical services (ancillary services)	215.8	5.0	220.8	218.6	7.1	225.7	4.9
Medical administration	11.0	—	11.0	12.0	—	12.0	1.0
Financial management	105.4	2.0	107.4	104.7	2.0	106.7	(0.7)
Human resources management	23.7	—	23.7	25.0	—	25.0	1.3
Facilities management	86.0	2.9	88.9	87.0	4.3	91.3	2.4
Information systems management	60.1	2.0	62.1	66.0	3.0	69.0	6.9
Administrative services	14.0	—	14.0	13.0	—	13.0	(1.0)
Total	996.4	26.7	1,023.1	1,010.7	33.2	1,043.9	20.8

FTE and salary trends

Total FTEs			1023.1			1,043.9	
Overtime FTEs			26.7			33.2	
Overtime FTEs as a percentage of total			2.6%			3.2%	
Salaries, benefits, and contract labor as a percentage of net revenues			47.05%			50.53%	
FTEs paid per adjusted patient day			4.17			4.00	
Net revenue per paid (total) FTE			$91,193			$91,005	

just the management, becomes relatively easy because it involves less people and results in a much lower impact on the budgeted income statement.

Ultimately, the salary increase can be a function of the operating margin resulting from all the various volume, revenue, and other expense assumptions used in the budget. This is the case if the initial budgeted bottom line does not meet the targeted board levels, the two areas that are often used to bring it into balance is reduction of the proposed salary increase or FTEs.

Fringe Benefit Levels and Increases

This has become a major expense category over the years as fringe benefits have become a significant tool for recruitment and retention of staff. As was recounted in Chapter 1 in reviewing the MRI pro forma, fringe benefits can now account for as much as an additional 30% of the actual salaries paid to the staff.

As shown in Table 7–4, the largest expense item within the fringe benefit category is health insurance expenses. RHMC, like any other employer, is always

TABLE 7–4

Ridgeland Heights Medical Center
Fringe Benefits Expenses
For the Budget Year Ending December 31, 2000

	1999 Budget	1999 Projected	2000 Budget
Non-FICA benefit expenses:			
Health insurance premium:			
Employer cost	$3,200,000	$3,200,000	$3,300,000
Employee offset	(1,000,000)	(1,080,000)	(1,050,000)
Post-employment expenses			
Pension	1,000,000	980,000	1,050,000
Tax deferred annuity employer match	500,000	480,000	525,000
Life insurance	130,000	140,000	145,000
Long-term disability	100,000	110000	110,000
Short-term disability	200,000	200,000	205,000
Worker's compensation	300,000	290,000	300,000
Unemployment insurance	60,000	55,000	60,000
Tuition reimbursement	60,000	62,000	65,000
Other expenses	50,000	40,000	60,000
Total non-FICA benefit expenses	4,600,000	4,477,000	4,770,000
FICA expense	2,400,000	2,450,000	2,500,000
Total benefit expenses	$7,000,000	$6,927,000	$7,270,000

evaluating these expenses in order to minimize its overall impact on its bottom line. Over the years, it has moved its health insurance from an indemnity plan to a managed care plan. Several years ago it also started to require its employees to pay for a portion of the health insurance premiums. In the current year, this amounts to 30% of the total insurance premium. In its benchmarking analysis, RHMC has determined that its competition requires its employees to pay between 20% to 50% of the premiums.

For the upcoming budget year, the human resources department is suggesting that the budget include an expense increase of 4% for the health insurance premium based on competitive bidding of its account. No increase in the employee paid portion of the insurance premium is recommended because of competitive human resource issues in the region.

The other fringe benefit line items are basically status quo for the upcoming year. No contentious issues are on the radar screen.

Controllable Nonsalary Expense Changes

These items constitute considerably less than 50% of the total expenses for the organization because salaries and fringe benefits tend to make up over 50%, and noncontrollable nonsalary expenses can make up between 15% and 25% of the remainder. Noncontrollable nonsalary expenses are generally defined as interest and depreciation expense. Controllable nonsalary expenses therefore make up between 25% and 35% of total expenses.

Controllable nonsalary expenses are categorized into eight parts. As stated earlier in this book, RHMC uses a publishing service that specializes in analyzing trends in healthcare costs.[1] The analysis goes backward and forward three years. It is published in annual percent increases or decreases. RHMC uses the published upcoming year percentages as a guide to their budgeting. There are times when one or several administrators believe they can beat the published increases either through more aggressive negotiating skills or changing the mix of products or services currently being acquired. Table 7–5 is a summary of the methodology used by Rate Controls and employed by RHMC.

July 15—Review Gross Revenues and Contractual Adjustments and Validate Payor Mix

This is a meeting internal to the finance department and its administrators. The assumptions used by the financial analysts leading to the July 11 revenue and contractual adjustments summary, shown in Table 7–2, is reviewed with a fine tooth comb. It is imperative that all the assumptions used are validated to the greatest extent possible. While it is not possible to actually see the future, it is essential that the entire set of assumptions track from the past to the future using internal and external assessment tools.

---

[1] Rate Controls Twice Monthly Newsletter. Rate Controls Publications. 602-995-9435.

TABLE 7-5

Ridgeland Heights Medical Center
Salary and Nonsalary Expense Changes
Summary of Projected Price Increase
For the Budget Year Ending December 31, 2000

| | National Indices as of September 30, 1998 | | | | | |
| | Historical | | | Projected | | |
	1995	1996	1997	1998	1999	2000
Salaries and wages	6.1%	3.5%	2.5%	2.8%	2.8%	2.9%
Employee benefits	5.6%	1.7%	1.1%	1.3%	1.4%	1.5%
Professional fees	4.0%	3.5%	3.1%	3.2%	3.4%	3.6%
Supplies—medical/surgical	1.1%	0.6%	−2.1%	−0.5%	−0.3%	0.0%
Pharmaceuticals	4.2%	2.1%	3.4%	5.0%	5.2%	5.4%
Dietary	3.9%	3.4%	−0.9%	0.1%	0.2%	0.3%
Utilities	1.4%	4.6%	0.5%	0.3%	0.4%	0.4%
Insurance	5.0%	1.5%	4.9%	4.3%	4.3%	4.4%
Purchased services	3.5%	5.4%	3.6	3.7%	3.8%	3.8%
Other expenses	2.5%	3.3%	1.7%	1.7%	1.8%	1.9%
Plant and equipment	4.5%	2.2%	3.1%	2.6%	2.4%	2.3%
Total hospital inflation	**4.7%**	**3.5%**	**2.4%**	**2.6%**	**2.7%**	**2.8%**

Source: *Rate Controls—Trends in American Health Care.* Rate Controls Publications, Inc. 800-975-8100.

During this meeting, the finance administrators grill the analysts to determine if there are any holes in the logic of the analysis. Because these finance bosses will present the outcomes to the rest of the administration in just a few days, they want to assure themselves that the information is solid and acceptable. In the case of RHMC, both the analysts and the administrators have been together for years and so all the questions are expected and the answers are already available. Had this not been the case, there is a good possibility that some questions would need to be further researched and answered outside the meeting, but within the next 24 hours, so that it is available for the meeting on July 18, three days hence.

July 18—Review 2000 Budgeted Income Statement, Determine Price Increase Targets, and Revise Salary and Nonsalary Assumptions

This is the big meeting of the year. It is the when the executives and other administrators first see the projected budgeted bottom line. This bottom line is based on the dozens of assumptions that have been discussed and debated over the past six weeks. In summary, these assumptions include the following.

- Inpatient and outpatient volumes based on historical trends and future expectations of physician referral patterns
- Gross revenues based on the above volumes with no price increases yet proposed
- Contractual adjustments based on best guess Medicare, Medicaid, and managed care rates
- Salaries based on the number of employees and the proposed wage increase percentage
- Fringe benefits expenses based on the proposed employee health and welfare package, including the recommended medical plan and the amount of premium that the employees will be expected to pay
- Nonsalary expenses based on any changes over the current year and the projected rate of inflation for these expense items

The meeting immediately turns to the current year projected and budget year operating margin, as shown in Table 7–6. If the budget year margin amounts to the targeted 4% of net patient revenues, then the meeting is over, well short of its two-hour time limit. In the late 1990s, this is not likely to be the case. Declining reimbursement rates and generally reduced inpatient admissions resulting from utilization controls required by managed care health plans have made bottom line management much more difficult.

In fact, the cover story in the 1998 year-end issue of *Modern Healthcare* highlights the growing operating margin problem for hospitals and health systems. In addition to drastically reduced reimbursement rates from Medicare, Medicaid, and managed care, "many are grappling with losses on failed physician and HMO investments. They are also widening use of expensive medical technologies and making larger than planned expenditures on 'millennium-bug' cures. And heightened competition and soaring expectations for quality and service are pressuring the bottom line." [2]

Thus, it is likely that there will be a gap between the initial budgeted bottom line and the target at most healthcare organizations. This is true at RHMC. The initial 2000 budgeted operating margin presented by the finance administrator at this meeting is a $4,200,000 loss. Meanwhile, the hospital needs an operating margin of $3,800,000 to achieve the board mandated 4% target. This establishes a gap of $8,000,000 that needs to be closed.

This gap is large but not necessarily surprising to many of the administrators in the room. Many have sat through dozens of budget meetings in their time and seen initial bottom lines almost as bad as this. They are not highly disturbed. There is,

---

[2] Pallarito, K. (1998). Paying for Innovation—Failed Strategies Add to Hospitals' Reimbursement Losses. *Modern Healthcare*, December 21–28, p. 2.

TABLE 7-6

Ridgeland Heights Medical Center
Preliminary Budgeted Statement of Operations
For the Budget Year-to-Date Ending December 31, 2000
July 18, 1999 (in thousands)

	1998 Actual	1999 Budget	June 1999 Actual	1999 Projected	2000 Budget	Percentage Change 00B vs 99B	Percentage Change 00B vs 99P
Revenues							
Inpatient revenue	$ 74,000	$ 79,000	$ 38,500	$ 77,800	$ 84,000	6.33	7.97
Outpatient revenue	69,000	77,000	37,600	76,100	86,000	11.69	13.01
Total patient revenue	143,000	156,000	76,100	153,900	170,000	8.97	10.46
Less							
Contractual and other adjustments	(48,000)	(60,000)	(29,000)	(59,000)	(72,000)	20.00	22.03
Charity care	(2,200)	(2,700)	(1,300)	(2,500)	(3,000)	11.11	20.00
Net patient service revenue	92,800	93,300	45,800	92,400	95,000	1.82	2.81
Add							
Premium revenue	1,300	2,100	1,100	2,100	1,000	−52.38	−52.38
Investment income	5,500	5,000	3,500	6,000	5,000	0.00	−16.67[1]
Other operating income	1,200	1,200	600	1,100	1,200	0.00	9.09
Total revenue	100,800	101,600	51,000	101,600	102,200	0.59	0.59
Expenses							
Salaries	34,000	35,500	18,000	36,500	39,000	9.86	6.85[2]
Contract labor	1,500	1,400	400	800	1,200	−14.29	50.00
Fringe benefits	6,800	7,000	3,500	6,900	7,800	11.43	13.04[3]
Total salaries and benefits	42,300	43,900	21,900	44,200	48,000	9.34	8.60

Bad debts	4,400	4,400	2,400	4,400	5,000	13.64	13.64[4]
Patient care supplies	15,000	15,200	8,200	16,000	17,100	12.50	6.88[5]
Professional and management fees	3,600	3,400	1,900	3,800	4,200	23.53	10.53[6]
Purchased services	5,600	5,600	2,900	5,600	5,600	0.00	0.00
Operation of plant (including utilities)	2,500	2,700	1,300	2,600	2,800	3.70	7.69
Depreciation	10,500	11,000	5,600	10,500	11,500	4.55	9.52
Interest and financing expenses	7,600	7,400	3,700	7,400	7,200	−2.70	−2.70
Other	4,600	3,800	2,000	4,000	5,000	31.53	25.00[7]
Total expenses	96,100	97,400	49,900	98,500	106,400	9.24	8.02
Operating margin	4,700	4,200	1,100	3,100	(4,200)	−200.00	−235.48
Nonoperating income							
Gain/(loss) on investments	600	1,200	800	1,400	1,000	−16.67	−28.57
Total Nonoperating Income	600	1,200	800	1,400	1,000	−16.67	−28.57
Net income	$ 5,300	$ 5,400	$ 1,900	$ 4,500	$ (3,200)	−159.26	−171.11
4% targeted operating margin					$ 3,800		
3% targeted operating margin					$ 2,850		
2% targeted operating margin					$ 1,900		

however, a new twist this year. The twin whammies of Medicare and managed care revenue reductions are unprecedented. It will make it harder to close the budget gap this time.

Value of Price Increases

The remainder of the meeting is devoted to figuring out how to initially close the budget gap. Several techniques will be used. The first decision will be to decide how many dollars the organization will net for every 1% increase in its listed prices. Because RHMC's primary payor mix is Medicare and managed care, it would initially appear that price increases would have no impact on the bottom line. In fact, the administrators at RHMC are aware that this is not case. There are at least two reasons for this.

1. Not all managed care contracts are per diem based. There may still be a number of contracts that are based on discounts from gross charges. If so, a piece of any price increase will be passed along to the managed care plan depending on the particular level of discounts that have been negotiated.

2. There are still payors that are reimbursing RHMC on gross charges. Even if it is only a small percentage, say 10%, that can still have a positive impact on the bottom line.

In the case of RHMC, analysis performed by the finance department indicates that every 1% increase is worth an incremental 25 cents on total dollars charged. This estimate is based on payor mix assumptions, level of managed care contracts paid on a percentage of charge basis, and percentage of payors still paying full charges. Based on this estimate, it is concluded that net revenues generated from a 1% price increase is $425,000 ($170,000,000 total gross charges × 1% price increase × 25% net revenue realization).

Although the administrators now know the value of each percentage point increase, they still need some context in order to determine how much of an increase will be acceptable to their community and the managed care payors. Although very few patients still continue to pay for their healthcare out-of-pocket, there is a continuing fascination with the healthcare organization's price list. Leading the region in high charges can create a public relations problem for the organization. And in Illinois, as in many other states, RHMC is required to report to a state agency a series of specific charges as well as a group of bundled procedure charges. These items are then *published* by the responsible state agency and available to anyone who wants a copy.

Like any other good finance department, RHMC reviews the output of this report to determine the level of its charges compared to its competitors. Finance staff members report the organization's position during this phase of the budget meeting. For the latest report year available, RHMC is directly in the middle of the pack for most of its charges, fifth out of a total of nine competitor organizations. Based on this knowledge, and some anecdotal information that some of the other organizations will be raising their charges by the approximate level of healthcare inflation, the administration decides to preliminarily propose a price increase of 4%. While this will increase the gross revenues by $6.8 million ($170,000,000 pre-increase gross revenue × 4% average price increase), it will also net $1.7 million on the bottom line.

Budgeted Expense Reductions

With this 4% price increase set, the administrators are then able to determine how much additional expense needs to be cut, or if there are any other revenue sources that could be considered. From the expense side, the staffing levels are once again the first item on the list to be discussed. Although this was discussed in depth only a week ago at the July 14 meeting, now that the preliminary bottom line is in play, it is reviewed again to determine where cuts could possibly be made.

The best way to determine these cuts would be with appropriate productivity measures. RHMC is currently in the process of developing these productivity measures. There is a lot of work involved in developing, maintaining, and then tracking productivity measures. Once an organization makes the decision to do so, it is taking a step to practice better management. Productivity management is an art. It provides the administrators and department managers with information they never had before. While managers believe they know the amount of time it takes their employees to perform individual tasks, research conducted for cost accounting studies indicates that manager perception is never a good measure of actual time spent.

Productivity management techniques allow department managers to understand the following things.

- The task being performed
- Whether or not the tasks are value-added
- How long these tasks take

When all the tasks and their time frames are totaled up, the total minutes should indicate the number of staff members needed. If the organization sets its parameters between 90% and 110% of standard, then it is possible to more scientifically determine which departments are overstaffed or *understaffed*.

Table 7–7 shows a list of possible cuts that were discussed by the RHMC administrators during this meeting. The initial outcomes are provisional and dependent on the subsequent requests of the department managers. The finance staff will therefore issue departmental budgets with an aggregate total bottom line of $1,400,000. All the administrators are aware that additional decisions will need to be made after the managers return their budgets in about a month.

July 25—Issue 1999 Projected/2000 Budgeted Worksheets to Department Managers

Based on all the decisions made in the previous budget meetings, the finance department is now ready to issue the following year's budget to the department managers. This is first time that most of the managers will get an inkling of what will be expected

T A B L E 7–7

Ridgeland Heights Medical Center
"Closing the Gap" Analysis
2000 Budget
(in thousands)

Operating margin July 18th meeting		$ (4,200)
4% net price increase		1,700
Improvement in investment income		1,000
Salary expense reductions		
@$40,000 average per employee		
10 FTEs	400	
20 FTEs	800	800
30 FTEs	1,200	
40 FTEs	1,600	
50 FTEs	2,000	
Fringe benefits		
Reduce additional benefits proposed in initial budget meeting of July 14th		
	200	
	300	300
	400	
	500	
Reduce bad debt expense through better collection efforts		
	250	
	500	500
	750	
	1,000	
Reduce patient care supply expenses		
	300	
	400	
	500	500
	600	
	700	
Reduce professional and management fees		
Cut consulting fees	200	
	300	300
	400	
Reduce other expenses		500
Revised operating margin		$ 1,400

of them in the upcoming year. This submission is crucial to the levels at which the manager can operate his or her department, now and in the coming year.

The first thing that the managers will review is their staffing level. They will be concerned whether administration has already made any cuts. In addition, because RHMC is a top down budget organization, the managers are also aware that they will not be able to add any staff unless they can prove the following.

- They are not already appropriately staffed
- The additional staff member will do either of the following.
  - Improve net revenue production above the cost of the new FTE
  - Decrease other departmental costs

Of course, this is seldom the case. Instead, requests for most new FTEs are justified on the grounds of improvements in patient or physician satisfaction or a decrease in overwork.

The managers will also be interested in the other revenue and expense assumptions that were made by the administration. Revenue producing managers did have some input into the volumes, of course, but they want to know if their assumptions have been changed. In any event, the most important reason that the administration issues this preliminary budget to the managers is so that they can review every line item and determine if the finance staff made any clerical or technical errors that need to be changed. After doing error checking, studying appropriate volumes, and reviewing all other nonsalary expense items, the managers will be expected to return their budgets with any changes to their administrators by August 15.

CAPITAL BUDGET—JULY

Concurrent with the operating budget, the capital budget process continues. The finance department staff is now working overtime. They are trying to keep up with the volume of analysis materials coming into the department as well as the volumes of material going out to the department managers and the administrators during the month.

Following are the steps that need to be completed in the July capital budget process.

July 11	Submit 2000 capital budgets by department managers back to the finance staff through the electronic capital budgeting software
July 12–July 23	Review by finance staff of all capital proposals for completeness
July 24–August 6	Capital budgets reviewed by proposal reviewers—facilities management, materials management, and information systems

On July 11, the department managers are mandated to return all of their capital budget requests to the finance department with all required elements filled in.

Over the two to three weeks that the managers have to complete their portion, they are expected to contact any individual who has a need to obtain equipment within the department. So, for example, in a clinical department such as radiology, the manager should speak to the physician in charge of the clinical aspects of the department to determine if this physician is aware of any of the following things.

- New equipment that has come on the market that could
  - Improve patient outcomes
  - Provide a new revenue stream to the organization
  - Decrease costs of the operation
- Current department equipment that has become
  - Obsolete
  - No longer state-of-the-art for diagnosis or treatment
  - Harmful to the patient's care

The physician may want the manager to submit a request for updated equipment during this capital budget process. This is in fact the appropriate time to do so.

The manager will need to fill in all the blanks of the electronic capital request form for their request to be appropriately considered. Box 7–1 summarizes the required elements of the electronic capital request form. The managers have already been told that their capital proposal will be returned to them if they leave out any of these required elements.

In fact, that is exactly what the finance staff will be doing during the next project step. Between July 12 and July 23, the staff reviews all of the proposals to be sure that these elements are met. Acting in an advisory and consulting role, the finance representatives assigned to all these projects will help the managers fill in any of the

B O X   7–1

RIDGELAND HEIGHTS MEDICAL CENTER

Capital Budget Form Required Elements

1. Proposal name
2. Proposal preparer name, title, department, phone number
3. Purchase information—vendor name, manufacturer, model number
4. Description of item
5. Price of capital item
6. Classification of item
7. Executive summary—why should it be acquired?
8. Detailed summary—why should it be acquired? Explanation and justification
9. Detailed pricing details
10. Five-year pro forma profit and loss statement

elements that have been left blank. They will also advise the managers how they might be able to strengthen their proposals, where appropriate. Some managers do not write and/or justify proposals as well as others. It is RHMC's practice to attempt to level the playing field in this regard. The task of the finance staff member responsible for the capital budget is to ensure that all the proposals that will be reviewed by the administrators are complete so that the review process will be as fair as possible.

Between July 24 and August 6, the proposal reviewers get their crack at each of the proposals. These proposal reviewers are derived from three technical areas— facilities management, information systems management, and materials management. Each area is required to review every proposal to determine if any additional costs will be needed for the requested item to become operational in the organization. At RHMC, the information management department is required to review every capital item that is powered by a microchip. They are attempting to determine if the following is applicable.

- There are any nonstandard set-ups that may be required
- There are any potential Year 2000 problems lurking in the weeds
- The requested purchase requires information management expertise that may not be currently available on-site

The role of facilities management is similar. Almost every piece of requested capital equipment plugs into the wall. Most managers take that plug and the wall outlet for granted. However, each of theses additional power requirements adds up, sometimes resulting in the need for facilities management to acquire new power distribution equipment at substantial cost. It is their job to know all the volts flowing through the organization. Therefore it is absolutely necessary for them to perform their review before the evaluators see the proposals. The facilities management review may increase the cost of the proposed item. It is good to know this at the time the evaluators evaluate, not after.

Finally, materials management will ultimately have to issue the purchase order for all the approved capital items. Therefore, their review ensures that all the data elements that they require have already been included in the proposal.

REGULATORY AND LEGAL ENVIRONMENT

Still, routine and capital budgets are not the only aspects of the organization's operation that are being managed during the month of July. The administrators of the various divisions (clinical, operations, and financial) have been spending time making sure that they and their staff have been performing all of their duties in compliance with the many laws and regulations governing the operations of healthcare facilities.

Like every industry in America, healthcare is heavily regulated. Not only is the industry governed by state, federal, and local laws, it is also subject to additional regulations, formal rulings, and interpretations. In addition to being governed by several common sets of regulations, each of the various industry segments have specific rules that they need to follow.

As with all things, the highest levels of authority are laws, which are passed by legislative bodies. Healthcare laws are extensive and tend to cover a wide variety of areas within the industry. The federal laws, which must be followed, are passed by Congress and signed by the president. To properly follow the laws, providers seek guidance through regulations issued by the government agency that has the responsibility for each program. In healthcare, the appropriate federal agency is the Health Care Financing Administration (HCFA), which is charged with administering the Medicare program through the authority of the Department of Health and Human Services (HHS).

Medicare/Medicaid Fraud and Abuse

As we explored the Medicare and Medicaid programs in Chapter 5, it was evident that these are highly technical programs. The technical specifications of the programs create huge holes that are occasionally taken advantage of by unscrupulous individuals. While not dealing only with the inherently unscrupulous, the laws were designed to ensure that bad and/or crooked providers would be punished.

The framers of the Medicare and Medicaid programs were concerned that the government pay only for applicable services that should have been appropriately rendered under the law. Historically they were aware that other government programs had, over the years, been billed for goods or services not rendered or received. On occasion, the bills had been inflated above the rates that had been agreed to. Because of this, at the conclusion of the process, the Social Security Act of 1965 contained several provisions to combat this problem. They included the following.[3]

- Criminal penalties, applicable to persons convicted of committing specified fraudulent acts such as the following.
  - Filing of false claims
  - Misrepresentation of the qualification of an institution
  - Solicitation, receipt, or offering of kickbacks, bribes, or rebates
- Civil money penalties, applicable to persons determined by the Secretary of HHS to have committed the following acts.
  - Filed fraudulent claims under the programs
  - Charged beneficiaries for the services in violation of agreements entered into with the HHS Secretary
- Exclusion from the Medicare and Medicaid program participation for those providers and practitioners who are convicted of crimes involving the following
  - Health programs established under the Social Security Act or
  - Patient abuse or neglect

---

[3] Summaries of these fraud and abuse items were derived from the information in the HFMA's Fellowship Certification Preparation Manual—*Core* Examination, pp. 4-19–4-21.

There is a very special language surrounding much of these regulations. There was great concern that providers would attempt to illegally profit from the Medicare and Medicaid programs through the submission of inappropriate or bogus claims. To combat this, the Social Security Act authorizing the programs created express provisions against any individual who knowingly and willfully submits false claims to the government (in this case, the Medicare or Medicaid program).

Kickbacks, Bribes, and Rebates

In addition, the laws spend a considerable amount of time and effort in detailing efforts to prevent kickbacks, bribes, and rebates. The government was particularly concerned with the possibility that individuals would conspire with others to illegally obtain Medicare and Medicaid monies. These laws penalize individuals who knowingly and willfully solicit or receive any remuneration (including any kickback, bribe, or rebate) directly or indirectly, overtly or covertly, in cash or in kind in return for the following.

- Referring an individual to a person for the furnishing or arranging for the furnishing of any item or service for which payment may be made in whole or in part under Medicare
- Purchasing, leasing, ordering, or arranging for or recommending purchasing, leasing or ordering any good, facility, service, or item for which payment may be made in whole or in part under Medicare

If convicted of these offenses, the individual will be guilty of a felony and fined or imprisoned for not more than five years, or both.

Further, the law penalizes individuals who knowingly and willfully offer or pay any remuneration (including any kickback, bribe, or rebate) directly or indirectly, overtly or covertly, in cash or in kind to any person to induce someone to do the following.

- To refer an individual to a provider for the furnishing or arranging for the furnishing of any item or service for which payment may be made in whole or in part under Medicare
- To purchase, lease, order, or arrange for or recommend purchasing, leasing, or ordering any good, facility, service, or item for which payment may be made in whole or in part under Medicare

If convicted of these offenses, the individual will be guilty of a felony and fined or imprisoned for not more than five years, or both.

These are just a few of the many laws and regulations that providers are required to observe if they want to continue to participate in the Medicare program and stay out of jail. Other laws that are currently on the books and used by the government to enforce compliance are the following.

- Health Insurance Portability and Accountability Act of 1996, which has a number of fraud and abuse provisions built into it

- False Claims Act, which was enacted in 1863 to combat fraudulent claims billed for services to the federal government during the Civil War. This statute has been much in use by the Office of Inspector General (OIG) during the late 1990s as they have attempted to combat fraudulent healthcare claims resulting from services billed for Medicare beneficiaries.

Office of Inspector General Workplan

In fact, the OIG has been extremely busy in its attempt to eliminate healthcare fraud in both billing and nonbilling issues. It is easy to determine which areas of potential fraud and abuse they are targeting in any given year. The OIG publishes its annual work plan on its Internet Web site, *www.hhs.gov/progorg/oig*. Table 7–8 displays selected items from the OIG's 1999 work plan.

As can be seen, the OIG is involved in many different types of reviews and audits. They are focused on more than just billing and claims processing issues that were highlighted in Chapter 5. Their vision, as "guardians of the public trust" is to ensure effective and efficient Health and Human Services (HHS) programs and operations by minimizing fraud, waste, and abuse in those programs.[4] In addition to pure billing issues, they get involved in PPS rate formulation to ensure reasonableness. They also monitor utilization patterns to determine if providers are "gaming the system" in an illegal way to improve their Medicare or Medicaid reimbursement.

Other Regulatory and Business Compliance Issues

In addition to the very highly complex and punitive requirements of the Medicare fraud and abuse rules and regulations, RHMC is also responsible for following normal business compliance. Following are some examples.

1. Occupational Health and Safety Administration laws
2. All Labor Department rules and regulations
3. State Health Department rules
4. Tax or tax-exempt rules and regulations

Furthermore, as a healthcare provider, RHMC needs to comply with a whole series of supplementary rules and regulations designed specifically for the industry. Some of these follow.

1. Special state requirements pertaining to licensing as a healthcare facility
2. Private insurance requirements, usually administered by the state insurance commissioner

---

[4] Department of Health and Human Services, Office of Inspector General, Health Care Financing Administration Projects, Work Plan, Fiscal Year 1999.

T A B L E 7–8

Department of Health and Human Services
Office of the Inspector General
Fiscal Year 1999 Work Plan
Selected Areas of Review—Excluding Billing and Claims Processing

Area of Concern	Issue
Hospitals	
Hospital owned physician practices: Provider-based status	Identifying the potential vulnerabilities to Medicare arising from the proliferation of provider-based physician practices
Hospital owned physician practices: Financial impact	Reviewing the financial impact of trends in physician–hospital integration
Same-day discharge and readmission to same hospital	Examining Medicare claims for beneficiaries who discharged and subsequently readmitted on the same day to the same PPS hospital, to determine if the claims were appropriately paid
Outpatient base year costs	Conducting a series of audits of the base year costs used to develop the PPS rates for hospital outpatient services to determine if the outpatient rates are reasonable
Home Health	
Home healthcare year costs	Performing a series of audits of the base year costs used in developing PPS rates for home health agencies in order to evaluate the reasonableness of the prospective rates
Access to home health services	Assessing the effect of the Medicare home health interim payment system on beneficiary access to home health services
	Examining how home health agencies have responded to the new interim payment system and what effect this has had in beneficiary access to home health services
Utilization patterns of home health services	Determining if recent reimbursement changes to certain hospital discharges altered the use of home health services, specifically determining whether home health services have increased three days after certain inpatient discharges
	Under the BBA, Medicare pays no additional reimbursement if home health services are initiated within this three-day window

Continued.

Department of Health and Human Services *(Concluded)*

Area of Concern	Issue
Skilled Nursing Home Care	
State resident abuse data	Examining trends in nursing facility patient abuse reports to state agencies by reviewing types of reports received, investigations, and confirmations of abuse, which is one in a series of reviews to determine the quality of care in nursing homes
Resident assessments and plans of care	Determining whether quality of care concerns exist with resident assessment and plans of care and whether Medicare and Medicaid payment levels are correct
Skilled nursing facility base year costs	Performing a series of audits of the case year costs used in developing the PPS rates for skilled nursing facilities in order to evaluate the reasonableness of the rates
Physicians	
Podiatry	Assessing whether podiatry services paid by Medicare were medically necessary and met HCFA coverage policy
Reassignment of physician benefits	Evaluating the practice of allowing physicians to reassign their billing numbers to clinics
	This practice shifts the accountability and liability for billing abuses away from the physician to the clinics. Past reassignment abuses will be examined to determine specific vulnerabilities.
End Stage Renal Disease	
Medical appropriateness of tests and other services	Assessing the medical appropriateness of laboratory tests and other services ordered for ESRD patients
Drug Reimbursement	
Effect of average wholesale price discount on Medicare prescription drugs	Determining if average wholesale prices used to calculate Medicare reimbursements for prescription drugs have increased since January 1, 1998 and the effect of any such increases on Medicare savings projected in the BBA of 1997

Source: Department of Health and Human Services, Office of Inspector General, Health Care Financing Administration Projects, Work Plan, Fiscal Year 1999.

3. Special requirements by the federal government for participation in programs such as Medicare, Medicaid and Champus
   • Eligibility
   • Payment
   • Utilization review
   • Quality (which takes the form of accreditation)
   • Fraud and abuse (as represented by the OIG's work plan)

All of these areas require management and employee vigilance to meet. This book has already highlighted some of these areas and the types of techniques and methodologies that enhance the organization's financial performance, such as Medicare and Medicaid payment issues in Chapter 5 and fraud and abuse issues immediately preceding this section.

CORPORATE COMPLIANCE

Good managers expect to exceed many of the basic practices that are required in the above section. Ultimately, the organization is responsible for ensuring that there are no deviations from rules necessary to maintain licensure or accreditation. As we've seen, failure to do so can lead to fines for the organization or individuals. Furthermore, it can lead to jail time for the individual offender(s). So, these alone should be deterrent enough to ensure that neither the organization nor its employees engage in any "hanky-panky."

Yet, given all of the various rules, regulations, and interpretations that healthcare providers are required to follow, it has become an ongoing process to identify and monitor compliance. Up until the government became more diligent in its enforcement efforts in the early to mid-1990s, the providers did not devote a great deal of time, money, or energy to compliance. This started to change when the OIG began extensive Medicare cost report audits of selected academic medical centers around the nation. This brought enforcement attention to the industry at large because of the visibility of the targeted institutions. These audits resulted not only in publicity for the government's efforts, but it also wound up collecting millions of dollars in fines, which were turned back to the treasury.

That was just the beginning. Larger and better-funded government efforts followed. Most of these were billing audits, some of which were highlighted in Chapter 5. Still, the industry was now on notice; it needed to clean up its act. In 1996, the government issued a Model Laboratory Compliance Plan. This was followed in 1997 with a Model Hospital Compliance Plan. While providers did not have to follow these model plans explicitly, the mere existence of a plan at a provider's site could obviate more severe government imposed penalties if some errors were uncovered. This was important because the government was now taking the position that those seemingly unintentional errors, often clerical in nature, were being considered as fraud and abuse and were being threatened with prosecution as such.

Ridgeland Heights Medical Center, like most of its competitors and peers, always believed that it followed all the required rules and regulations. Its administrators believed they knew the rules and had systems in place to ensure compliance. Yet, this new persistence by the government to make sure the rules were followed convinced RHMC administrators that they needed to observe the rules with even more diligence and rigor.

To this end RHMC has developed a major corporate compliance policy. Its purpose is (1) to ensure that all RHMC employees are aware of and follow all the laws, regulations, and policies affecting their duties and (2) ensure that all employees recognize the organization's values and reflect such value in their actions.

While the organization and its administration always believed in "doing the right thing," this new initiative codified policies and further reinforced and established new procedures towards compliance standards. The plan states that the organization is committed to conducting its business in a manner that facilitates quality, efficiency, honesty, integrity, respect, and full compliance with applicable laws and regulations. In addition, it expresses an ongoing commitment to ensure that its affairs are conducted in accordance with both the letter and the spirit of laws and regulations and its own policies and practices. It requires its employees to maintain

BOX 7–2

RIDGELAND HEIGHTS MEDICAL CENTER

Key Compliance Plan Features

1. Designation of specific RHMC officials responsible for directing the effort to enforce compliance
2. Identification of a corporate compliance code of conduct, including an educational and training plan for dissemination of the code
3. Incorporation of standards and policies that guide RHMC employees and other third parties affiliated with the organization in regards to their conduct
4. Coordinated education and training for RHMC employees and other third parties affiliated with RHMC in regard to their conduct
5. Publication and uniform mechanisms for employees and other third parties affiliated with RHMC to raise questions and receive appropriate guidance concerning their conduct
6. Provision of a framework for specific compliance areas, such as billing and collection activities
7. Publication process for employees to report possible compliance issues and the development of a procedure for the investigation and resolution of reports of possible compliance matters
8. Formulation of corrective action plans to address any compliance problems that are identified
9. Development of a plan to monitor the organization's overall compliance efforts

standards of behavior that are both lawful and ethical. Box 7–2 sets out the key features of the compliance plan.

ACCREDITATION ISSUES

Healthcare organizations have more to worry about than just criminal and civil penalties if they fail to comply with applicable laws, regulations, and policies. Many have also chosen to participate "voluntarily" in accreditation programs. Box 7–3 shows a list of the most prominent healthcare accrediting organizations. There are significant practices that need to be followed in order to be considered in compliance with the accrediting organization's rules. There are reasons that these healthcare providers have chosen to be involved in accreditation. Following are the most important reasons.

1. Accreditation by the Joint Commission on Accreditation of Healthcare Organizations (JCAHO) automatically deems the provider eligible to participate in the Medicare and Medicaid program and able to bill for and receive reimbursement from the government payors.

2. There are marketing advantages available to organizations that have been accredited. Being able to advertise the accreditation allows the healthcare provider to imply or express a higher standard of care, if they so chose.

3. The ability to contract with managed care organizations (MCOs) is enhanced with acceptance by a reputable accrediting organization. Another way to say this, organizations that are not accredited will probably not be able to contract with any MCO to provide care to the health plan's enrollees. Because of this, it is extremely difficult to act as a healthcare provider without accreditation.

B O X 7–3

MAJOR HEALTHCARE ACCREDITING ORGANIZATIONS IN AMERICA

1. Joint Commission on Accreditation of Healthcare Organizations (JCAHO)
   a. American Hospital Association (AHA)
   b. American Medical Association (AMA)
   c. American Osteopathic Association (AOA)
   d. American Dental Association (ADA)
   e. American College of Surgeons (ACS)
2. Accreditation Association for Ambulatory Health Care (AAAHC)
3. College of American Pathologists (CAP)
4. National Committee on Quality Assurance (NCQA)—HMOs

The largest accrediting body in America is the JCAHO. It evaluates and accredits more than 18,000 healthcare organizations and programs. As can be seen in the chart in Box 7–3, the Joint Commission is an amalgam of five major healthcare provider associations. Since 1951, the JCAHO has developed professionally based standards and evaluated the compliance of healthcare organizations against these benchmarks. As is evident in Box 7–4, the Joint Commission's evaluation and accreditation services are extensive and cover the entire spectrum of healthcare provider type organizations.[5]

The Joint Commission has had its ups and downs over the years. Its biggest triumph was being deemed the accrediting body of choice by the federal government for the Medicare and Medicaid programs in 1966. However, in recent years some providers have challenged some of the Joint Commission's practices and procedures. The Joint Commission has attempted to evolve over the years, trying to lead its provider organizations into newer quality management techniques. Although the controversies may not quiet down anytime soon, the ongoing debate seems destined to strengthen overall provider quality simply by keeping it constantly on the administration's front burner.

B O X 7–4

JOINT COMMISSION ON ACCREDITATION OF HEALTHCARE ORGANIZATIONS

Evaluation and Accreditation Services

1. General, psychiatric, children's, and rehabilitation hospitals
2. Healthcare networks, including health plans, integrated delivery networks, and preferred provider organizations
3. Home care organizations, including those that provide home health services, personal care and support services, home infusion and other pharmacy services, durable medical equipment services, and hospice services
4. Nursing home and other long-term care facilities, including subacute care programs, dementia programs, and long-term care pharmacies
5. Behavioral healthcare organizations, including those that provide mental health, chemical dependency, and mental retardation/development disabilities services for patients of various ages in various organized service settings, and managed behavioral healthcare organizations
6. Ambulatory care providers, including outpatient surgery facilities, rehabilitation centers, infusion center, group practices, and others
7. Clinical laboratories

Source: Facts about the Joint Commission on Accreditation of Healthcare Organizations, www.jcaho.org/about_jc/jcinfo.htm

---

[5] Facts about the Joint Commission on Accreditation of Healthcare Organizations, www.jcaho.org/about_jc/jcinfo.htm

The other three organizations listed in Box 7–3 have the same goals. The last organization on the list, the National Committee on Quality Assurance (NCQA), does not accredit healthcare providers. Instead, it certifies health plans or MCOs that act as third-party payors to over 70 million insured enrollees. The NCQA is a private, not-for-profit organization dedicated to assessing and reporting on the quality of managed care plans.

The NCQA is relatively new. It began accrediting MCOs in 1991 in response to the need for standardized and objective information about the quality of these organizations. Since then it has expanded the range of organizations that it certifies to include managed behavior healthcare organizations, credentials verification organizations, and physician organizations.[6]

Like the JCAHO, the accreditation program is voluntary. And regardless of the motivation of the providers and health plans for participating, these accreditation programs enable the industry to properly claim a basis for quality care.

PATIENT SATISFACTION ISSUES

There is one more major issue not directly related to the finance function that can have a significant impact on the healthcare organization's bottom line. Because healthcare organizations really do care about providing very good service to their customers, over the years, many have attempted to understand the satisfaction of its patients but had not been able to effectively measure it. More recently, over the past 10 years or so, a few major national patient satisfaction firms have sprung up to provide an assessment mechanism for healthcare providers.

These organizations permit the provider to allow each patient within various service categories (such as inpatient, emergency department, or ambulatory surgery) to evaluate their satisfaction levels. More importantly, because these patient satisfaction firms have many clients, it is possible to compare each provider against a peer group and determine its own ranking. This is critical because it allows the provider to set certain goals, not only for improvement against its prior scores but also against the peer group.

At RHMC, the organization has developed criteria so the level of patient satisfaction is part of the annual incentive compensation model. By incorporating it into its incentive compensation formula, the organization believes it is "putting its money where its mouth is," making the point to its employees and its community that it takes patient satisfaction very seriously. The RHMC administration believes that its community and its physicians will notice high levels of patient satisfaction. It is believed that physicians will be more willing to refer and patients will be more willing to come to an institution that has an objective record of excellent patient service. It appears that this has been borne out over the past few years because RHMC has had a lower reduction in its admission levels than some of its competitors. Patient satisfaction ranks as one of the differentiators for this.

---

[6] National Committee for Quality Assurance—An Overview, www.ncqa.org/overview3.htm

8
CHAPTER

August

Margaret McGregor, RHMC's vice president of patient care services and nursing, was enjoying a pleasant morning, reviewing improved patient outcome scores that had just been delivered. She was aware that some of the improvement was the result of increased levels of care management provided to the patient and the physician. They were aimed at standardizing care through enhanced consumption and utilization controls. But she had a nagging feeling that something was missing. So she picked up the phone and made a call to the one person who might know the answer.

"Hi, Sam, it's Maggie. How are you this morning?" she said with a slight lilt in her voice.

"Maggie, I'm fine. It sure is a pretty morning. I was just looking out the window and wondering how we could extend this weather year round. Of course if we could then we'd be like San Diego and everybody would want to live here," Sam rhapsodized. "Anyway, I digress. What's up this morning?" he asked quizzically.

"Well I was just wondering about something," she questioned. "I was just looking over patient outcome results and they are very encouraging, but I also noticed that there is no cost data on the reports. I can't tell if these improvements cost us or saved us any money."

"You're right, Maggie," he opined. "When we initiated the care management program before you started here, we did not have a cost accounting system. Because of that, we could not produce a baseline analysis. Therefore, we can't tell how much we've improved. We can however tell you how much each patient is costing us now. We can tell you the length of stays of each patient. We can even develop analyses allowing you to compare our physicians resource consumption and costs against each other or against regional or national benchmarks and create trend lines over time."

Maggie responded, "Sam, that sounds really good. I know that would help us a lot as we try to continuously improve both our clinical outcomes and our cost base. With that kind of information, my nursing directors and their staff will be able to focus considerable efforts on those areas that require the most improvements."

"That's great," said Sam. "I'm aware that the biggest bang for the buck would be to identify utilization patterns by individual physicians, determine the averages, and try to bring those physicians that are outside of the norms back in line. The opportunities to save money for the organization while the patient satisfaction scores increase are significant."

"So, Sam, how come you didn't tell me about all this great stuff before?" asked a bewildered Maggie.

"Mags, that's a real good question. You need to understand that I've been trying to get the nursing division to accept and use this information for the last few years. They have just shown no inclination to use them. That's why I'm really pleased that you are here now. I know that you've used these kinds of data before and that you know the value of it. So I'm thrilled that you are asking for it now," Sam said excitedly.

"Yeah, yeah, yeah, Sam," said a suddenly peeved Maggie, "but next time, I expect you to come to me with something like this first, okay."

The dog days of summer. Hot days. Even hotter nights. As the temperatures soar into the triple digits, an extraordinary amount of city and suburban dwellers have gone fishin.' The workers have taken their companions, their kids, their dogs, and sometimes their gerbils and left town. They have left behind whatever work didn't get done. It's a theme at this time of year. The pace slows down to a delightful crawl. Margaritas and moonlight meet. Daytime is extended as daylight is magnified.

As hot as it is outside, it is even hotter inside the four walls of Ridgeland Heights Medical Center. August is the month that final decisions will be made on the operating and capital budgets. For the finance staff, no vacations are scheduled and no vacations are allowed. They are busy crunching numbers and providing support for both the department managers and the administrators, helping them improve some of their budget presentations late in the game. They are in an all-out blitz to ensure that all the deadlines in a month of meetings are met. And so it goes . . .

CAPITAL BUDGET—AUGUST

Now that August has arrived, the role of RHMC's administrators in the capital budget process takes center stage. Prior to this month, a lot of preliminary work has been performed. The department managers have prepared all of their capital requests with input from their medical directors, where appropriate. The finance staff has reviewed each proposal for completeness and consistency in order to allow them equal chances of success during the administrator's evaluation phase. Finally, facilities management, materials management, and information systems management examined the proposal to ensure that the proposals included any extra information that could potentially affect their areas. So, the proposals are complete, clean, and ready to be judged on their merits.

The steps that need to be completed in the August capital budget process include the following.

August 11	Detailed discussion of all proposals over $100,000 and training of all proposal evaluators
August 12	Discussion of all pool proposals with the pool evaluators
August 12–15	Evaluate proposals online
August 22–25	Various pool consensus meetings with pool evaluators
August 25	Consensus meeting for all proposals over $100,000
August 26–28	Revise ratings, if necessary, on the reviewers desktop

August 11—Detailed Discussion and Training for All Proposals over $100,000

The meeting of August 11 is highly anticipated by the administrators. This is first time that they will see the entire list of capital items being requested for acquisition in the year 2000. Prior to this, each administrator has seen only the capital requests from their division. Now they will get to see the competing items requested from all other divisions. The primary purpose of this meeting is to allow each administrator to present a verbal detailed story about the capital items being requested from their division. In effect, each administrator is given an opportunity to lobby for the items they are championing for their division. The secondary purpose of the meeting is to train each of the administrators in the use of the computer software that they will use for analysis.

In this meeting, it has already been determined that the dollar cut-off point for major project evaluation will be $100,000. This decision was made by the finance administrator within the past three weeks and only after the entire list of requested capital items was assembled. The dollar cut-off number is not fixed but can vary from year to year. It depends on the total number and dollar value of capital items being requested. Essentially, experience has shown that the evaluators can effectively review no more than 40 to 45 projects in a detailed manner. If they are asked to do more, they lose effectiveness and the objectivity of the criteria-based capital budget process is diminished.

In the case of the 2000 RHMC capital budget, the requested items were stratified into dollar categories as shown in Table 8–1. Capital items are defined as equipment or building items that do the following.

- Cost at least $2,500
- Have a useful life greater than one year

Table 8–1 shows that 194 capital items were requested in total. Accumulating the item number backwards, it is clear that in order not to exceed the 40 to 45 item limit, the 2000 capital budget cut-off should be at $100,000. This dollar limit can change each year. It is entirely dependent on the dollar value and number of requests. There can also be a finer stratification of the requests. Therefore, the stratification jumps can be whatever makes sense to the organization. Although RHMC used $25,000, other organizations might use $10,000 or even $100,000. All items under the $100,000 cut-off level will be evaluated in a somewhat different manner. These items will be grouped into six pools and evaluated separately by a small team of expert users and administrators.

During the first part of the meeting, the proposal evaluators (administrators) will be trained on how to use the software. They are advised to set aside about two hours of concurrent time so that they can perform their review in one sitting. This is necessary because they are being asked to score each proposal against all the others within each of the 10 criteria.

The methodology they are trained on works in the following way.

- The evaluators will be reminded that their review is based on the 10 strategic plan criteria. They will be refamiliarized with these criteria. Box 8–1 is a listing of the criteria.

- The evaluators are told to review each proposal in total one time before doing any scoring. This allows them to get an overall feel for the entire mix of proposals before them.

TABLE 8–1

Ridgeland Heights Medical Center
Summary of 2000 Capital Budget, by Number of Requests

Dollar Value of Requests	Number of Requests	Backward Accumulation of Requests	Total Dollar Value of Requests
$2,500–$24,999	78	194	$800,000
$25,000–$49,999	42	116	$1,400,000
$50,000–$74,999	19	74	$1,200,000
$75,000–$99,999	15	55	$1,300,000
$100,000–$124,999	18	40	$2,000,000
$125,000–$199,999	12	22	$2,400,000
$200,000–$249,999	7	10	$3,200,000
Over $250,000	3	3	$4,000,000
Total Requests	194		$16,300,000

- Then they are told to go back to review and score each proposal on just the first strategic plan criteria, in this case community health promotion.
- The key concept in the scoring, they are told, is to determine after reading all proposals which of the 40 do they consider that *best meet the criteria.* This proposal will be awarded 1,000 points on a scale of 0–1,000. The other 39 proposals will then be judged against this "best" proposal. The evaluators are strongly encouraged to give out zeroes where a proposal does not have any features that meet the criteria. So, for example, using this methodology, an evaluator may decide that one of the other proposals is only 10% as effective in meeting the community health promotion criteria. Therefore, that evaluator would then award the second proposal only 100 points for the criteria.
- After completing the scoring for all the proposals on the first criteria, they are told to go back to the second strategic plan criteria and continue the process, and so on until they finish all 10 criteria.

This system is extremely efficient and relatively fast. The use of the desktop PC and the software creates an amazingly compact process. In fact, one of the administrators has been known to complete the 40-item list, with its 10 criteria, in 45 minutes. The average time among the group is about 90 minutes. Remember, that means that each RHMC administrator spends an hour and a half a year allocating as much as $10 million. Not bad. And far superior to the previous smoke-filled backroom process.

The software enhances the process in several ways. First, each detailed proposal is just a mouse click away if the administrator needs to research any specific aspect. Particularly important in this regard are the justifications within any of the criteria that the department managers have claimed. The software summarizes these on one easy to read screen. Second, the software actually leads the administrator through the process, forcing them to complete the first strategic plan criteria before allowing them to move on to the second. This therefore enforces a discipline in the process. Lastly, the software encourages the managers to complete a screen for any additional information that they may deem important to

B O X   8–1

RIDGELAND HEIGHTS MEDICAL CENTER

Strategic Plan Criteria

1. Community health promotion
2. Facility quality
3. Image and reputation
4. Information and decision support
5. Market share

6. Operating efficiency
7. Patient/family satisfaction
8. Patient outcomes
9. Physician outcomes
10. Physician satisfaction

making their case. This screen is always available to the evaluator with a single mouse click.

The administrators are given one additional piece of information during this meeting that is critical to fully understanding the criteria-based capital budget. Although these administrators serve as evaluators for each proposal and cumulatively their scores are totaled and ranked, high to low, there is still one additional concept that significantly effects the final total.

It turns out that the 10 criteria are not evenly weighted at 10% each. Instead, this process mandates that the chief executive officer (CEO) gets to weight the 10 criteria, allowing the CEO to decide which are more important to the organization's well being and which are less important. And, at RHMC, this weighting was kept secret from the evaluators so that these same administrators would not be allowed to game the system by trying to over justify those highly weighted criteria in their own division's requests. The only two people who know this weighting are the CEO and the finance staff member assigned to inputting it into the computer.

This is all explained to the administrators before they and their colleagues begin to attempt to verbally sway each other. Now that they know what they will be evaluating over the next few days in the privacy of their own offices, each of these evaluators can better formulate their question during the second part of the meeting they are currently attending.

August 12 —Discussion of All Pool Proposals with the Pool Evaluators

There has been a lot written about the main capital budget process for all requests over $100,000. A significant amount of information is requested and then evaluated for equipment and projects above this threshold. Yet, as we saw in Table 8–1, there are many other requested projects under the threshold. The criteria-based capital budgeting process has a streamlined process for these items that does not generally involve all the administrators, yet it still meets the objective of using strategic plan criteria in making yes/no decisions.

There is a reason for the streamlined process. It follows the classic 80/20 principle of finance, which expresses that in almost every case, the top 20% of a process accounts for 80% of the value, while conversely, the bottom 80% of a process accounts for only 20% of the value. The principle works to a large extent in this case. Twenty percent of the 194 requests means 39 proposals should be reviewed. In this case if we round up to the 40 cases that just happen to meet the $100,000 threshold, we can see, again in Table 8–1 that these proposals have a dollar value of $11,600,000. This is 71.2% of the 194 cases, which is fairly close to once again proving the 80/20 principle ($11,600,000 divided by $16,300,000 = 71.2%).

The process for all requests under $100,000 divides all the items into five categories, clinical equipment, facilities construction and renovations projects, information systems, market development, and office equipment. Small specialty groups are assembled to review the requested items in their categories. Each group develops

TABLE 8–2

Ridgeland Heights Medical Center
Pool Evaluators

Pool	Evaluators
Clinical equipment	Vice president, patient care services Directors of nursing Director of clinical services
Facilities/construction	Director of facilities Manager of environmental services
Information services	Chief information officer Manager of hardware services Manager of application services
Market development	Chief strategy officer Director of external communications
Office equipment	Finance administrator Materials manager

a smaller set of criteria related to the strategic plan. They use these criteria to rate and score the requests.

The groups are made up of directors and managers with significant responsibility for the areas in question. Table 8–2 shows the representative groups responsible for pool evaluations.

At the first meeting, the finance facilitator will explain the role of each group, how the group will operate and how much money is available for funding. They will then review all of the requested proposals for the first time. The review will consist of detailed discussion of each item and how it relates to the decision criteria set by the group. If there are any questions that cannot be answered at this meeting about any of the proposals, a small additional amount of time will be set aside to get the answer. At the end of the meeting, the group is told to do the following.

- Think about what they have just discussed
- Get answers to any unanswered questions
- Return between August 22 and 25 to make final decisions on the requests

Funding Availability

The amount of money available to both the over-$100,000 items and the under-$100,000 items is determined by taking the initial total funding determined by the finance administrator and allocating it between the categories. For example, after the

TABLE 8-3

Ridgeland Heights Medical Center
2000 Proposed Capital Budget
Funding Summary

		Total Funded		
	Total Requested	Total	Criteria Based	Noncriteria Based
Main strategic	$11,600	$8,184	$3,184	$5,000
Clinical equipment	1,800	1,270	870	400
Facilities/construction	1,500	1,058	258	800
Information services	900	635	635	—
Market development	300	212	212	—
Office equipment	200	141	141	—
Total	$16,300	$11,500	$5,300	$6,200

organization decided to fund its capital at 100% of its depreciation expense, it then needs to determine the allocation between the over and under $100,000. At RHMC, they look at the dollar level of requests between the over and under $100,000 and use the percentage ratios between the two. So, again if we examine Table 8–1, RHMC will fund 71.2% of its depreciation expense for the over $100,000 requests and 28.8% for the under $100,000.

This funding limitation sets up the constraints for the organization and justifies the need for this type of capital budgeting process. Table 8–3 summarizes the differences between the capital requests and capital available by category.

First, it is obvious that some department managers will not be approved for all the capital they requested. The organization's funding level is $11,500,000. The capital requests are $16,300,000. That's a gap of $4,800,000. The organization will be able to approve only 70.5% of its requests.

Noncriteria-Based Capital Funding

A counter-intuitive concept inherent in this criteria-based capital budgeting system is the noncriteria aspect built into the process. At its heart, this concept expresses that not all capital acquisitions need to or are even able to formally meet strategic plan criteria and therefore need a safety valve for approval. In addition, there are capital items that might compete well in the main process, but because the administration as a whole agrees that these items need to be purchased no matter what, they are deemed eligible for automatic approval.

Examples of RHMC noncriteria-based capital items are Year 2000 information system upgrades and fixes and information system infrastructure upgrades to support

Year 2000 fixes. In addition, the administration has determined that it is in the organization's best interest to approve the construction of a new emergency department and renovation of one of their medical/surgical nursing units. These items alone amount to $4,800,000 in capital. This amount is therefore deducted from the total amount available to be funded; thereby reducing the amounts available for those criteria-based projects that need to compete against each other.

August 12–15—Evaluate Proposals Online

Finally between August 12 and 15, the administrators (proposal evaluators) get their opportunity to score each of the proposals against all the proposals using the 10 strategic plan criteria. This is done on the evaluator's PC, which is attached to a local area network (LAN) so that all the scoring is linked and aggregated by the software. This will result in a streamlined and efficient outcome at the end of the process. They will follow the rules set down at the meeting of August 11. They are given three days in which to find a two-hour time block to get it done. The finance division has two staff members available during these three days to come over to any evaluator's office in the event of a question or problem with the concepts or the software. At RHMC, over these three days, no problems are encountered.

August 22–25—Various Pool Consensus Meetings with Pool Evaluators

Between August 22 and 25 the pool evaluators will get together again to make final recommendations on their category requests. If there are no controversies, they will be done. If however, no consensus has been reached, each of the groups will get one more chance to settle on their recommended lists over the following week. In essence, these meetings are held to give any of the pool evaluators one more chance to lobby for their own proposal or champion any other. These meeting are usually short and conclusive.

August 25—Consensus Meeting for All Proposals Over $100,000

This is the day that many of the administrators have been waiting for. It is when they will learn if the capital requested by their division has made the cut of the criteria-based capital budgeting system. All of the previous process has been very important, but it was also a prelude to this. The power of the criteria-based capital budget now becomes evident.

At this meeting, a list for the 2000 recommended and nonrecommended capital items will be presented. It is the culmination of the administrator's rating and the CEO's weighting of the 10 strategic plan criteria. The initial output from the licensed software is called the weighted value score (WVS). It is literally the administrators' judged priority ratings multiplied by the CEO's priority weighting. This output, when arrayed from the highest WVS to the lowest, is a clear indication of which requested capital items meet the administrator's concept of strategic plan importance.

But this array is not the final list of recommended projects. The final step required to produce the best outcome is to divide each of the WVSs by their cost. This produces a benefit to cost ratio that can then be ranked. The higher the result the more likely that the capital request will be approved. This simple mathematical equation allows the administration to put the requested capital expenditures into context. For example, there could be a request for an item that had a high WVS but also had high cost. The result could easily move it down the list, lower than an item with a lower WVS but a much lower cost.

These rankings allow the administration to make rational decisions using objective criteria and techniques, something that was not available before at RHMC. The rankings are machine generated from their own consensus inputs. Still, they are not required to use it, all or in part, if they so choose. As a group, they can decide not to fund a machine-recommended item in favor of one that did not initially make the cut. An administrator may try to lobby for a project that missed the cut. However, the odds are stacked against a change because everyone went through the process and if a substitution is made, one of the other recommended projects will have to be cut.

It is a zero-sum game. The funding is set and will not be increased. So, when the software ranked the projects, it drew the cutoff point above the funding limit. Replacement requires substitution. Because of this, the arguments are eliminated in the meeting. Everyone has participated and is aware of the process. They understand that they have met criteria and it is completely defensible to the losers.

RHMC, in fact, experienced an intended consequence of the process that was very positive for the organization. During last year's capital budget, the organization's chief operating officer (COO) requested a CT scanner costing $800,000. Based on the final WVS and benefit cost ratio, this project did not make the cut. Still, the COO felt strongly that this was an important project and needed to be funded. This was based on the fact that the request was initiated by the medical director for the radiology service, a very powerful and politically connected individual.

In the past, based on the requester and the project champion, this argument would have prevailed over the strategic plan importance. However, because of the new process, the COO decided to go back to the radiologist and explain the situation, the objectivity of the process, and the desire of the group not to override the criteria outcome. Lo and behold, the radiologist backed off on his request and decided to come back the following year with a request for an even more enhanced scanner. This was a major success for this year's process. Next year will take care of itself.

As the meeting progresses, the finance administrator can make changes to any of the inputs online and real time to the software program. Because the results are being projected up on a screen in the front of the room, the results of revised assumptions can be analyzed and reviewed immediately. The software reoptimizes the results instantaneously. This also enhances the value of the process, where the assembled brain trust can pursue their desired results.

At the end of this meeting, the capital budget will have been set based on established funding levels and strategic plan criteria or else there may be a need to bring back certain additional information on some of the projects, if so desired. If this is so, there will be the need for the administrators to perform one more set of evaluations to finalize their ratings. If this is not necessary, the 2000 capital budget is done.

August 26–28—Revise Ratings, if Necessary, on the Reviewer's Desktop

These next three days will be necessary only if there were any kind of dispute at the August 25 meeting involving any administrator's pet projects, or if any additional information is requested during the meeting. It is really used as a fail-safe device, allowing the capital budget to have extra time built into the process. Although the capital budget software allows the administrators to immediately see the results of any changes to the funding levels, it is possible that they need some additional data in order to make an informed decision. If this is so, that information will be transmitted electronically into the networked software for all the administrators to see and react to online by possibly changing their evaluation scoring.

If this is done, the group will meet again early next month to perform one final review of the capital budget requests in order to finalize it.

OPERATING BUDGET

While the finance staff is hard at work on the capital budget, the beginning of August is a time when they are able to take a breather on the operating budget. The department managers and their bosses, the administrators, are doing almost all of the work this month. They are reviewing the operating budgets that have been in their hands since July 25. The main role of the finance staff during this time is to be available to answer any questions that the managers have. They also continue to hold small formal classes on how the managers can best do their budgets. Still for the most part, in August, the finance staff is devoting most of their time to the capital budget.

August 15 ——Department Managers Need to Return Their Operating Budget Worksheets to Their Vice Presidents

By August 15, the managers have had the operating budget worksheets in their hands for three weeks. They were expected to review the full time equivalent employees (FTEs) and salary levels, the volume assumptions, and the nonsalary line items to determine if there were any clerical or technical errors made by the finance staff in preparing their budget. If there were any errors of this sort, they are expected to make a note of it on the budget so that it can be corrected when it is returned to finance.

After the error check is complete, the managers have an opportunity to request additional resources for the department. This is problematic. Healthcare in the late 1990s is an industry under considerable financial pressure. Because of the reimbursement limitations, additional resources are not easily granted. The best way to ensure that a request for additional staff is approved is to prove that net revenues will exceed the cost of the position. Proof is the problem. It's easy for a manager to say that additional volume and revenues will accumulate if another staff member is added. It is much harder to prove because for the most part this is tantamount to telling the future.

In Chapter 1, the validity of volume assumptions was discussed at length in the MRI pro forma section. The administrators, who have dozens of years of cumulative experience, have heard all kinds of stories from managers about how this added FTE or that added FTE will allow the managers to earn significant additional revenue for the organization. But it doesn't always happen, and then the organization will have lost money on the assumption. The addition of the MRI service was an example of the organization taking a chance on proven medical technology where they thought that there was a good chance of meeting the pro forma volumes.

Similarly, revenue-producing department managers are currently deciding where they too may have an opportunity to expand their department's services. For example, the cardiology department manager may decide that there is an opportunity to expand the CT scan service. They know there is an absolute capacity level to their one and only CT scanner. They also know that they are currently open for two full shifts, from 6:30 in the morning until 10:30 at night. Finally, there is currently a two-week waiting list for outpatient testing. Because of these facts, the department manager decides that it would be appropriate to request a second CT scanner as well as 3 additional FTEs to run the new machine. Once again, because of the magnitude of this purchase, a pro forma analysis is prepared to determine if the net revenues will exceed the additional expenses, including the staffing, the additional fringe benefits, the supplies, and the depreciation on the new equipment.

Smaller projects involving revenue-producing departments will need similar analyses. For example, the physical therapy department may have been built to accommodate a far greater volume of patients than is currently being serviced. However, if RHMC just recruited a new orthopedic surgeon, it may be presumed that the need for additional therapies will commence soon. In this case, the request for a new physical therapist in the department will almost certainly be accepted.

But, it may not be as easy if the physical therapy manager can show no particular event that would increase revenues. Still, the manager believes that additional staff will bring additional people to the organization for service. This is the "if we build it, they will come" theory of management. It almost never works and will be rejected out of hand by the RHMC administrator. If, however, this manager had done her homework, and written a marketing plan that included specific actions that would be taken to recruit physicians, health plans, and individual patients, there is a better chance that the extra FTE(s) would be accepted.

Still, if it is difficult for a revenue department manager to add new staff, it is even harder to do so for a nonrevenue manager. Nonrevenue-producing departments find it very difficult to justify additional staff as a result of additional workload because it is always so hard to prove. Later in this chapter we will look at cost analysis and decision making. In this section, there will be a discussion on how to measure workload. This is an important discussion and, if performed correctly, can truly help to justify additional staff.

Still, the most likely method for a nonrevenue-producing manager to justify additional staff is to claim *cost-reduction* in other areas of their department. Yet it is usually rejected because it almost never is verifiable. Like the volumes argument used by the revenue-producing managers, the proof is elusive. Because this argument will usually fail, the nonrevenue manager does not have many good remaining justifications for additional staff.

Nonsalary expenses are the other line items that the managers will review for accuracy. They will determine whether the supplies, purchased services, and all other services reflect the current year's reality and the upcoming budget year projection. They will do this using some financial analysis techniques but mostly it will be determined by gut feel. Because they know what they are spending this year using the financial reports provided by finance, the managers can speculate on next year's expenses. It is easy for many managers to recognize if any of their large expense items have been lost through clerical errors. If these nonsalary expenses appear correct, then they are ready to accept the budget and move it onto their administrator for further review.

August 18–28—Review of the Proposed Operating Budget by the Divisional Vice Presidents and then Return to Finance

During this 10-day period, each administrator will receive a budget package that has been reviewed and accepted by each of his or her department managers. Each administrator's role is to aggregate all these department budgets and determine how the total volumes, revenues, and expenses equate to the current year's budget and the current year's projection and how they relate to the original following year's budget proposed at the July 18 meeting.

Their role is to understand the budget assumption of each one of their departments. They will be required to present and defend any request that deviates from

---

B O X 8–2

DEPARTMENT MANAGER ACTIONS THAT DECREASE THE BUDGETED BOTTOM LINES

1. Volume reductions
2. Gross revenue reductions due to the following.
    a. Price decreases (to conform with market forces)
3. Expense increases characterized by the following.
    a. FTE increases
    b. Salary increases above the organization's established averages
    c. Supply cost increases caused by additional consumption above the current averages

the July 18 budget, particularly if they reduce the bottom line. Box 8–2 are some of the kinds of actions that could reduce the budgeted bottom line.

Administrators also need to be prepared to speak up at the upcoming September 9 administrative budget meeting if the budgeted bottom line has once again failed to meet the board's established targets. They need to bring contingency plans and expense items to "give up," when, as is almost certain, additional expenses will need to be cut.

The administrators also understand that their role is fraught with peril. They need to walk a fine line between supporting the perceived needs of their managers, whose job it is to run the day-to-day operations of the departments, and supporting the board goals, which mandate specific bottom line requirements. They will use their experience and training attempting to achieve these goals.

BUDGET VARIANCE ANALYSIS

While managers, directors, and the vice presidents are performing all this work in order to present the best budgeted bottom line for the upcoming year, the current year is taking place. During the year, the administration constantly monitors not only its actual financial results but also how those results compare to this current year's budget. That really is the whole point of the budget. The budget is a plan that has been developed by management and approved by the board. It is meant to be followed. Deviations from the budgeted results need to be explained in order to understand why these variances occurred.

Accounting and finance track and report budget variances diligently. In general, budget variances are not inherently bad or good. They are just deviations from the expected. Yet, budget variances are a concept that many managers have a hard time accepting.

Budgets are not effective without appropriate feedback mechanisms. Feedback allows the managers to review the variance between their actual operational results, including volume, revenues, and expenses against their expected (budgeted) results. All budget variances should be explainable. The concept of *explainable variances* should not be foreign to clinical managers, many of whom have a scientific background and should understand the concept of deviation from the norm. An explainable variance is a variance that resulted from a specific event that was different from the expected event.

For example, let's say that a water main on the second floor of RHMC broke in the month of August. The resulting flooding caused water damage to six rooms on the first floor. Ignoring any potential insurance claim, the cost to fix the damage was $10,000 and was charged to the facilities department. The manager of the department is disturbed because this $10,000 charge has put him over budget by $9,000 for the month. He is concerned that he will be singled out for criticism when the monthly financial statement is distributed because of the negative budget expense variance.

This should not be the case and it is not so at RHMC. The administrators understand the concept of explainable variances. As long as the managers can appropriately explain significant negative or positive variances, they will not be maligned or disparaged. In the above case, the administrator will be reminded of the reason for the overage when they review the monthly variance analysis report that is required to be completed by all managers. Box 8–3 is a copy of the report used at RHMC.

This variance report allows the manager to record reasons for positive or negative differences of net revenues, salary expenses, and/or nonsalary expenses. The purpose of the report is to require the managers to research and discuss their variances with their administrators. It allows both individuals to know their businesses better. In addition, the finance administrator uses these reports to explain the vari-

B O X   8–3

MONTHLY VARIANCE ANALYSIS REPORT

MONTHLY DEPARTMENTAL "KNOW YOUR BUSINESS" REPORT

Use this form to provide information if your actual operating margin for the MONTH was ± 10% of budget.

DEPARTMENT_____

COST CENTER #_____   MONTH_____

OPERATING MARGIN VARIANCE____% $_____

In the space below, identify the major factors contributing to the variance.

ACCOUNT	AMOUNT ($'s)	AMT (%)	EXPLANATION OF VARIANCE
		Net Revenue	
		Salary Expenses	
		Nonsalary Expenses	

THIS FORM IS DUE TO YOUR VICE PRESIDENT NO LATER THAN THE LAST BUSINESS DAY OF EACH MONTH, FOR THE PREVIOUS MONTH'S PROFIT AND LOSS STATEMENTS.

ances to the finance committee. It is the best way to get and maintain a complete record of the activities that deviate from the financial performance expected when the budget was developed in the previous years.

Budget Variance Parameters

A key element of the variance report is the parameters set by the organization that triggers the need for an explanation. The organization's culture has a great deal to do with the parameter levels. For example, RHMC uses a ± 10% level. This means that it does not question revenue and expense variances that fall within the 90% to 110% range around the budget. Other organizations may be tighter or looser with the parameter range.

Regardless of the range, it is important for the organization to enforce the variance analysis. This allows administrators to maintain an understanding of the financial record of its departments. Departments with consistent problems maintaining positive variances to their budgeted margins need to be monitored closely. If necessary, the organization needs to consider replacing any manager who does not contribute positively to budgeted organizational results.

Flexible Budgeting

Flexible budgeting is another aspect related to budgeting and budget variance reporting. A flexible budget is a budget that is adjusted for changes in volume. The budget used by RHMC is not a flexible budget, it is a static budget. Static budgets "are not adjusted or altered, regardless of changes in volume or other conditions during the budget period."[1] That is why RHMC department managers use the variance report in Box 8–3 to explain if their variances are the result of volume variance and whether it is positive or negative to the original budget.

An organization that uses a flexible budget will already flex the budget column in the monthly departmental financial report to factor out any volume variances. The flexible budget is "based on a knowledge of how revenue and costs should behave over a range of activities."[2] Because RHMC does not use a flexible budget, it will not be discussed in detail. However, there are many healthcare organizations that use flexible budgeting rather than static budgeting. It is a cultural preference that can be changed depending on the preference of the CEO, COO, or CFO.

COST ACCOUNTING AND ANALYSIS

Cost accounting in healthcare has had an interesting and rich existence since 1966, when the Medicare and Medicaid programs were created. Prior to these programs,

---

[1] This is the definition used in the legendary textbook: Horngren, C.T., Foster, G. (1987). *Cost Accounting—A Managerial Emphasis*. 6th ed. Prentice Hall: Englewood Cliffs, NJ, p. 181.
[2] Ibid.

the healthcare industry was smaller and less sophisticated. There was a perception at that time that because of the more charitable nature of the industry, accurate costing of the organization's activity was unnecessary and unwarranted. Many not-for-profit organizations did not care as much about their bottom lines. Often, they had donors who agreed to fund any bottom line losses at the end of each year. These losses were usually moderate and reflected a time when less dramatic care was furnished to patients. A hospital's mission then was more convalescent, less intensive.

The advent of Medicare made healthcare into a big industry. All of a sudden, money flowed freely. With this came the need for better accounting of the organization's revenues and costs. In fact, the Social Security Act that brought Medicare into existence mandated the annual filing of a Medicare Cost Report for each organization treating Medicare patients. As reported in some detail earlier in Chapter 4, the MCR mandated a cost accounting methodology for the industry called the ratio of cost-to-charges (RCC). The RCC was developed by allocating the organization's indirect (or overhead) costs to the revenue-producing cost centers based on a step-down methodology. Because of the relative ease of this methodology, much of the industry accepted this as their own cost accounting system. Unfortunately, the RCC system is not totally accurate for developing or determining the actual cost of doing business at the unit of service level.

The RCC costing method is faulty because it does not meet the general requirements needed for a good cost accounting methodology. *Cost accounting* is a financial management technique that requires costs to be separated into meaningful categories allowing for its identification. These relevant cost components are as follows.

- *Direct costs*—costs that are directly attributable to the operating or revenue-producing department in question
- *Indirect costs*—also called overhead costs, these are costs that are not directly attributable to operating departments
- *Variable costs*—costs that vary (increase of decrease) with changes in volume
- *Fixed costs*—costs that do not vary with increases or decreases in volume

The RCC and step-down methods of cost accounting do not do a reliable job of separating the components in a relatively accurate way. In fact, while these methods purport to at least separate the direct from the indirect component, they

- Do not do so at the unit of service level.
- Do not even attempt to separate the variable from the fixed component.

So, if a healthcare organization wants to "know" the cost of producing any of its services, it will need to adopt different and better techniques to do so. Box 8–4 elaborates on why the organization would want to have a good idea of the component parts of its costs at the unit of service level. Each of the objectives is important in their own right. The cumulative effect of the objectives makes it an organizational imperative to be able to perform reasonably accurate cost accounting.

BOX 8–4

OBJECTIVES OF A COST ACCOUNTING SYSTEM

Cost Accounting Separates Costs into Meaningful Categories Allowing Managers to do the Following.

1. Measure the effects of changes in intensity and case-mix
2. Evaluate and measure performance against a plan
3. Acquire the information required to manage resources efficiently
4. Identify those costs that can be converted from fixed to variable
5. Identify inefficient functions and demonstrate the nature of the problem, such as price, volume, or practice.

There Is no Such Thing as "True" Cost!

While reviewing established cost accounting techniques, it is important to discuss some reasons why there is no "true" cost in cost accounting. There are many people, including administrators, department managers, and physicians who believe that the cost accounting figures presented by the finance staff are an accurate and objective portrayal of cost components. The problem is that this is just not true. Developing costs at the unit of service level involve *assumptions*. In any finance or accounting concept, the very first time an assumption is used, complete accuracy is lost. The very best that can be said of cost accounting is that it is representative of the cost picture.

To understand why unit cost can never be completely true or accurate, let's look at the example of a reasonably common test done at a hospital, a CT of the abdomen. This is a digital diagnostic test ordered by physicians to rule out or determine whether a medical problem exists in the patient's abdomen. As we'll see, there will be assumptions used to determine the direct and the indirect (overhead) costs at the unit level. In order to ascertain costs at the unit level, the financial analyst has to first determine the direct costs. In the case of a CT of the abdomen, costs of staffing and nonsalaries have to be determined.

For staffing, at least three ways are utilized to determine unit costs.

1. Time and motion studies
2. Department manager time studies
3. Department manager perceptions

In all three of these methods, several assumptions are used. The biggest *assumption* is the amount of time that it takes each employee to perform each of the various jobs within the department. Table 8–4 shows an example of the tests performed in the CT scanning department and the technician time that has been determined to be required to perform each test.

T A B L E 8–4

CT Scanning Department
List of Tests Performed

Test	Technician Time
CT of the head	30 minutes
CT of the chest	45 minutes
CT of the abdomen	30 minutes
CT of the pelvis	45 minutes
CT of the spine	60 minutes

To develop what is called *microcosting* within each department, it is important to have a list of all the services performed. The direct departmental costs will then be split between staffing and nonstaffing costs. All of these direct costs will then be segregated into their various component parts. In the case of staffing at RHMC, this will be done through the use of *time logs* kept by the staff and reviewed by the department manager over the course of a four-week period. In the case of supply costs, actual invoices will be used wherever possible.

Table 8–5 is a summary of the direct cost inputs for the CT of the abdomen. The direct costs for the test are assembled and split between variable and fixed components. In this case, there were no direct fixed costs, just direct variable costs. A computer model is then used to *allocate* all of the direct departmental costs across all the tests.

The allocation of the direct staffing costs will include several additional costs components not already included in the time log such as fringe benefits and nonproductive time. In fact, nonproductive time doubles or triples the actual direct cost of performing tests. Nonproductive time is often categorized as *stand-by time,* which is when the technician is standing around, waiting for the next patient to present himself or herself for treatment. Other nonproductive time includes paid breaks and holidays, sick, and vacation time. All of these costs are included in the CT scanning department (also known as a cost center), and they all need to be allocated back to the individual tests.

After the computer model completes its direct cost allocations at the unit level, it allocates indirect costs to revenue-producing departments through a statistical methodology based on usage. Table 8–6 shows the most common allocation basis for the list of indirect cost centers. This allocation scheme deposits these indirect costs into the revenue producing departments awaiting a mechanism to further allocate the costs down to the unit of service or procedure level. Costs will be assigned at the procedure level through an allocation based either on departmental revenues or volumes.

Furthermore, one final assumption is used to determine unit costs. The 80/20 rule is used to determine the number of service/procedure codes to study. In this

TABLE 8–5

Development of Procedure Level Unit Costs
CT of the Abdomen

Inputs			
Direct variable costs		**Average Test Time**	
Labor costs	**Pay Rate**	**(in minutes)**	**Total Cost**
Senior radiology technician	17.90	30	8.95
Nonlabor costs	**Unit Cost**	**Quantity**	**Total Cost**
Film	1.59	11	17.49
Contrast media	40.44	1	40.44
	Total Departmental Cost	**Annual Tests Performed**	
Other			
Equipment depreciation	200,000	5,000	40.00
Equipment service contract	50,000	5,000	10.00
(on the CT scanning machine)			
Total direct variable cost inputs			**106.88**

case, the 80/20 rule theorizes that 80% of the departmental costs will be used by only 20% of the departmental tests performed. As previously reported in Chapter 7, this rule applies to many resource-based subjects. Therefore, the RHMC department manager needs only to analyze the top 20% of the tests in the department, not 100%, in order to feel confident in the costing outcomes. A computer matrix will allocate the unstudied procedures based on gross charges.

After all the allocations are done, the computerized cost accounting system provides a detailed analysis of the unit cost for each test. It allocates all the costs between fixed and variable, direct and indirect because each of these components acts differently in the course of departmental business. Table 8–7 represents the output of the cost allocation process for CT of the abdomen. It is interesting to note that the variable salary output is $31.67 versus the input costs of $8.95. The difference represents those stand-by and nonproductive costs mentioned earlier. In this case, the fully allocated salary is 3.5 times the direct salary. That alone should raise some questions about the productivity level in the department.

It is also interesting to note that total costs at $249.55 are 87.8% greater than direct costs at $132.91. This means that the indirect cost mark-up for CT of the

TABLE 8–6

Ridgeland Heights Medical Center
Development of Indirect Department Cost
Statistical Basis

Department	Statistical Basis
Building depreciation	Departmental square feet
Employee benefits	FTEs
Human resources	FTEs
Information services	Total expenses
Plant operations	Departmental square feet
Environmental services (housekeeping)	Departmental square feet
Cafeteria	FTEs
Administration	Total expenses
Financial services management	Total expenses
Materials management	Supply expenses
Laundry and Linen	Laundry pounds
Patient accounting	Inpatient and outpatient units of service
Medical records	Inpatient and outpatient units of service
Planning and marketing	Total revenues
Medical staff	Total revenues
Central transportation	Adult admissions
Food services	Adult patient days
Community services	Total revenues
All other overheads	Total expenses
Bad debts	Total revenues

abdomen is 87.8%. This is another area that the managers and administrators can review for cost savings opportunities. It may mean that the overhead costs are too high.

In summary, it is now obvious that a considerable number of assumptions are used to develop cost accounting standards at the procedure or unit level. Thus, while cost accounting is very useful to understanding an organization's cost components within the various revenue-producing procedures performed, the costs that are developed are not "true" or "accurate." They are reasonable and are consistently applied.

RHMC uses these cost accounting standards to produce a number of reports and analyses that aid in the understanding of departmental financial performance. They are used to determine which departments are making or losing money (winners and losers). Because the costs are developed at the procedure level, winners and losers can be aggregated in many different ways.

- Diagnostic related groups
- ICD-9-CM clinical diagnostic codes

TABLE 8–7

Development of Procedure Level Unit Costs
CT Scan of the Abdomen

	Outputs		
Direct Costs		**Indirect Costs**	
Fixed costs:		Fixed portion	$63.21
Salaries	$0.16		
Nonsalaries	2.17		
Total fixed costs	2.33		
Variable costs		Variable portion	41.16
Salaries	31.67		
Nonsalaries	46.42		
Equipment service contracts	12.49		
Total variable costs	90.58		
Equipment depreciation	40.00	Equipment depreciation	8.93
Building depreciation	0	Building depreciation	3.34
Total direct expenses	$132.91	Total indirect expenses	116.64
		Total direct expenses	132.91
		CT of the abdomen total unit costs	$249.55

- Nursing and ancillary departments
- Charge code
- Physicians
- Payor
- Patient
- Service area
- Zip code
- Age
- Sex

Cost accounting leads to decision making. If used properly, it becomes an important tool in the administration's management arsenal. Winners can be rewarded and enhanced. Losers can be disbanded. Loss leaders can be established and endured because they were developed by intent. Cost accounting is an art that acts like a science. In this case, the artist can paint with a broad brush.

AUGUST FINANCE COMMITTEE SPECIAL AGENDA ITEMS

Review Next Year's Budget Assumptions

At the August finance committee, the finance administrator will present an abbreviated list of budget assumptions that the administration will be formally presented at the October meeting. It is still too early to present a preliminary budgeted profit and loss statement, but this list allows the administration to introduce some of its preliminary thinking on the upcoming year. By doing so, the administration is able to gauge the mood and thinking of the finance committee. If there is some apparent disagreement in the direction being taken, it permits the administration to change its focus over the next few weeks prior to the October meeting.

Table 8–8 is the budget assumptions presented to the finance committee at the August meeting. The assumptions are strictly volume related because no revenue or expense assumptions are ready. The assumptions include an abbreviated explanation for the volume changes. This helps management to begin its discussion with these board members about the direction they believe the organization is heading.

Annual Materials Management/Inventory Level Review

Once a year, RHMC management presents a report to the finance committee on the status of the organization's materials management goals and accomplishments. The features of this report highlight the various efforts taken and achieved by the department in the areas of the purchasing and receiving and central sterile supply, processing, and distribution. The report is presented in the following format order.

- Supply expenses per day trends
- Revenue enhancements
- Expense reductions
- Operational efficiencies

A summarized version of the report is presented to the finance committee. It contains the gist of the important concepts needing to be communicated and understood by the finance committee to further their governance role. The finance committee usually needs to take no action on the information it receives as long as the report does not contain information showing some problems with the inventory levels or the supply expense per adjusted patient day.

T A B L E 8-8

Ridgeland Heights Medical Center 2000 Budget Assumptions
August, 1999

The 2000 budget is being prepared at this time to be presented for approval in October. The information below summarizes the volume assumptions being considered for this budget. The variances are based on the explanations noted at the bottom of the page.

	1998 Actual	1999 Budget	1999 Projected	2000 Budget	Percent Variance 00 Budget vs. 99 Projected
Acute care					
Adult admissions	8,100	8,760	9,023	9,787	8.47
Average length of stay	3.89	4.05	4.05	4.20	3.72
Adult patient days	31,500	35,496	36,561	41,131	12.50
Skilled nursing facility					
Number of admissions	800	840	850	900	5.88
Average length of stay	11.00	10.00	9.50	8.30	−12.63
Patient days	8,800	8,400	8,075	7,470	−7.49
Newborns					
Admissions	1,950	2,145	2,165	2,382	10.00
Average length of stay	2.00	2.00	2.00	2.00	0.00
Patient days	3,900	4,290	4,330	4,763	10.00
Total inpatients					
Admissions	10,850	11,745	12,038	13,069	8.56
Average length of stay	4.07	4.10	4.07	4.08	0.39
Patient days	44,200	48,186	48,966	53,364	8.98
Outpatient visits	167,150	181,000	194,400	210,000	8.02

Explanations for Variances:

1. Maternity admissions increase 10% due to newly expanded unit and recruitment of four obstetricians.

2. Psychiatric admissions increase 20% due to addition of several new psychiatrists on staff.

3. Medical/Surgical admission increase 4% due to additional affiliation of several primary care physicians.

4. Outpatient visits increase 8% based on prior year trends and continued emphasis on physician and consumer marketing.

9

C H A P T E R

September

"Damn it, Barnes, you've screwed me up again," screamed Frank Jacobs to Sam Barnes over a telephone that was bristling with static and a high level of distortion.

Sam Barnes had but a moment to react. It was early in the morning and he had not yet had his first cup of coffee. Recognizing the voice on the other end of the phone as one of his usual complainers, Sam responded, "Oh come on, Frank, what did I do *now?*"

"Listen, Barnes, you can't fool me. I know that you were personally responsible for signing that managed care contract that cheated me out of a whole lot of revenue," said Dr. Jacobs, one of the leading orthopedic surgeons on the Ridgeland Heights Medical Center staff.

"Now, Frank, really, you and I have talked about this before. You know that although I did sign that agreement, I did not do it unilaterally. This contract was discussed with the board of the IPA (independent practice association) as well as an advisory group of your colleagues on our PHO (physician hospital organization). They all felt that it was in the best interest of the hospital and all the physicians in the IPA to sign this contract rather than lose all the business generated by it," replied Barnes with his usual candor.

"Horsepuckey, Barnes," retorted Jacobs with more than his usual candor. "I just know that the hospital will benefit from this contract a lot more than the doctors. You are fully conflicted in your role of lead negotiator for the hospital and the IPA."

Sam Barnes was getting steamed, but he decided to keep his cool. "Frank, I'm really sorry that you feel like that, but it just isn't true. I know that you were around here when the PHO was formed 10 years ago so that the hospital and physicians who chose to join the IPA, like yourself, could jointly present themselves in a united way to the managed care companies. In fact over those 10 years, we have jointly contracted with over 50 managed care companies. Your representatives on the IPA monitor these negotiations. Frank, I'm not out to get you. It's in the best interest of the hospital to get you the best deal that can be made."

"Barnes, you're full of it," said Jacobs, not so diplomatically. "The rates you are negotiating are killing my office income. I can hardly afford to keep my whole staff together and still maintain my lifestyle anymore. I know that you are driving the rates down every time you accept a lower reimbursement."

"No, Frank, I'm not!" said Sam adamantly. "I know you believe that but our acceptance of the lower rates are not causing the rates to plummet. This is an industry-wide phenomenon. The payment structure has changed over the last several years and we are not immune. In fact, you should be thanking me rather than harassing me. We've actually held the line a lot longer than many of the PHOs around the area. I'm sorry your income is going down. But I also know that you do need to look at the management of your office practice. It's probably the best way you have right now to try to maintain your income. There are many ways you can economize without hurting your quality of care and patient satisfaction."

"Barnes, thanks for the advice, but I'll pass. Your advice on behalf of my business is already killing me. I'll figure out what's in my best interest by myself," blurted Dr. Jacobs as he slammed down the phone.

———

The first part of September. Always an interesting time of year in the northern region of the United States. Almost ideal weather conditions predominate. Cool Canadian air wafting down out of the north mixing with the warm breezes traveling up from the Gulf of Mexico. The best time of the year to live in this part of the country. Temperatures in the high 70s during the day, the low 60s at night.

But with Labor Day fast approaching, the end of the unofficial summer season is near. The roadways around the densely populated region are already beginning to get more congested. The grocery stores and shopping malls are getting busier while the swimming pools are getting ready to close. It is a season of melancholy for many. The end of summer means the distant winter season is not too far away. It's time for many to put away their toys and return to the real working world.

Of course, at the RHMC finance offices, real work never went away. The summer was one of their two busy seasons with budget preparation dominating the effort. Other tasks also needed to be done. For instance, this month the chief executive officer (CEO) requested additional financial analysis of the physician practices owned by the organization. There was a concern that these practices were not contributing to the overall bottom line of the organization and were operating negative to budget. The multifaceted analysis was designed to highlight the financial condition of the practices as well as the impacts that the practices have on the hospital's bottom line. The finance department was prepared to provide the CEO with a detailed analysis by the end of the month.

OPERATING BUDGET

Meanwhile, September is the month that the heavy technical work performed by the finance staff on the operating budget is completed. Subsequent work will be more clerical in nature. There is only this one additional short stretch for the finance staff to stimulate their enthusiasm. The efforts in September are as follows.

September 9	Validate or adjust budget assumptions and semi-final budget approval by the administrators
September 17	Final review and approval of the operating budget and review the human resources committee package
September 30–October 14	Prepare first draft through final copy of the 2000 budget for the finance committee

Right around the Labor Day weekend, the work needed to be performed by the finance staff on the operating budget revs up again. After the vice presidents complete their operating budget review on August 28, they are returned to the finance division for processing. The finance staff has only 11 days to "crunch" the volumes, revenues, and expenses submitted by the department managers into an understandable set of reports. At the September 9 meeting, the administrators will validate or adjust the department manager submitted assumptions. Therefore they need the best descriptions and summaries of the submitted financial data to make the best budgeting decisions for the organization.

In order for the finance staff to provide the best summary of the data, they will once again perform significant analyses at the detailed department line item level. This is done to determine whether the manager-requested changes make sense in the overall scheme and scope of the operating budget. The manager's job during August was to do the following.

- Review the full time equivalent employees (FTES) and salary levels
- Review the volume assumptions and the nonsalary line items for any clerical or technical errors made by the finance staff in preparing their budget
- Request any additional resources for their department, whether staffing or nonsalary

The finance staff's job is to review the manager's changes for objectivity and purpose. If a mistake was made, this is the time to correct it. It is imperative that any mistakes get corrected before final decisions are made. They are much more difficult to correct, from a political standpoint, after final administrative approval is granted. Because this is the version that will ultimately go to the finance committee, no CEO or chief financial officer will want to make any changes and admit to a mistake if at all possible.

An even worse time to find a mistake is after the budget is approved by the board of directors. The approved board budget is the formal direction of the healthcare organization and cannot be changed administratively. Going back to the board for subsequent approval is the only way to change the current year's budget. No administrator wants to take a weak story back to the board. Therefore, common or small mistakes will need to be absorbed by the responsible divisions. It is to everyone's advantage to catch any errors at this point in the process.

The outcome of this work by the finance staff will be a presentation to the executive and administrative staff on the upcoming year's budgeted profit and loss statement. This is done at the September 9 meeting.

September 9—Validate or Adjust Budget Assumptions and Semifinal Budget Approval by the Administrators

Another big meeting date for the finance and nonfinance administrators. Once again, there will be trepidation as each enters the room to learn the financial fate of the upcoming year. How much money will we still have to cut? How many employees will need to be eliminated in order to balance the budget? Who will remain to take care of the patients, the facility, and electronic backbone of the computerized medicine now being practiced?

This particular budget meeting is often the hardest one of the year. This is where most of the final decisions will be made. It becomes all the more difficult when the department managers request a great deal of expense increases without any offsetting net revenues. During this particular budget process, 10 additional FTEs were requested in the areas of facilities management, information services, planning, and marketing.

In addition, the clinical services division requested two additional FTEs for their rapidly growing MRI and CT scanning departments. Diagnostic services, particularly high-tech imaging services, is an extremely fast growing segment of the organization's business. The physicians are fully aware of the value of these diagnostic devices. Thus, the diagnostic imaging manager is planning to add a late afternoon and evening shift for both services and needs a technician in each area. These two FTEs will be approved because the incremental revenue far outpaces the expenses of the additional staff and supplies.

The other positions are more problematic and not as automatic. In fact, the only other two positions that are approved at this meeting belong to the information services department. They are granted two additional network specialists who are responsible for maintaining the local area network (LAN) and the devices attached to the LAN. This means that they are the installation and troubleshooting team for over 1,000 personal computers, 300 local printers, and all the network hardware and system software. As RHMC places more pieces of software on the network, the problems multiply, and more attention is required by the information services staff. Because these problems are visible to the administrators, it is easier for the information services administrator to get approval for these new jobs.

At this meeting, the finance administrator presents the modified *preliminary budgeted statement of operations* based on (1) the changes suggested at the July 18 meeting and (2) changes requested by the department managers (Table 9–1). In both

TABLE 9-1

Ridgeland Heights Medical Center
Preliminary Budgeted Statement of Operations
For the Budget Year-to-Date Ending December 31, 1999
Including 4% price increase
September 9, 1999
(in thousands)

	1998 Actual	1999 Budget	1999 Projected	7/18/99 2000 Budget	Admin 9/9/99 2000 Budget	Managers 9/9/99 2000 Budget	Percentage Change 00B vs 99B	00B vs 99P
Revenues								
Inpatient revenue	74,000	79,000	77,800	$84,000	87,360	87,360	10.58	12.29
Outpatient revenue	69,000	77,000	76,100	86,000	89,440	89,440	16.16	17.53
Total patient revenue	143,000	156,000	153,900	170,000	176,800	176,800	13.33	14.88
Less:								
Contractual and other adjustments	(48,000)	(60,000)	(59,000)	(72,000)	(77,100)	(77,100)	28.50	30.68
Charity care	(2,200)	(2,700)	(2,500)	(3,000)	(3,000)	(3,000)	11.11	20.00
Net patient service revenue	92,800	93,300	92,400	95,000	96,700	96,700	3.64	4.65
Add:								
Premuim revenue	1,300	2,100	2,100	1,000	1,000	1,000	-52.38	-52.38
Investment income	5,500	5,000	6,000	5,000	6,000	6,000	20.00	0.00
Other operating income	1,200	1,200	1,100	1,200	1,200	1,200	0.00	9.09
Total revenue	100,800	101,600	101,600	102,200	104,900	104,900	3.25	3.25

Expenses							
Salaries	34,000	35,500	36,500	39,000	38,200	38,600	7.61	4.66
Contract labor	1,500	1,400	800	1,200	1,200	1,200	−14.29	50.00
Fringe benefits	6,800	7,000	6,900	7,800	7,500	7,600	7.14	8.70
Total salaries and benefits	42,300	43,900	44,200	48,000	46,900	47,400	6.83	6.11
Bad debts	4,400	4,400	4400	5,000	4,500	4,500	2.27	2.27
Patient care supplies	15,000	15,200	16,000	17,100	16,600	16,900	9.21	3.75
Professional and management fees	3,600	3,400	3,800	4,200	3,900	4,000	14.71	2.63
Purchased services	5,600	5,600	5,600	5,600	5,600	5,600	0.00	0.00
Operation of plant (including utilities)	2,500	2,700	2,600	2,800	2,800	2,800	3.70	7.69
Depreciation	10,500	11,000	10,500	11,500	11,500	11,500	4.55	9.52
Interest and financing expenses	7,600	7,400	7,400	7,200	7,200	7,200	−2.70	−2.70
Other	4,600	3,800	4,000	5,000	4,500	4,700	18.42	12.50
Total expenses	96,100	97,400	98,500	106,400	103,500	104,600	6.26	5.08
Operation margin	4,700	4,200	3,100	(4,200)	1,400	300	−66.67	−54.84
Nonoperating income								
Gain/(loss) on investments	600	1,200	1,400	1,000	1,000	1,000	−16.67	−28.57
Total nonoperating income	600	1,200	1,400	1,000	1,000	1,000	−16.67	−28.57
Net income	5,300	5,400	4,500	$(3,200)	$2,400	$ 1,300	−55.56	−46.67
4% targeted operating margin				$ 3,800	$ 3,868	$ 3,868		
3% targeted operating margin				$ 2,850	$ 2,901	$ 2,901		
2% targeted operating margin				$ 1,900	$ 1,934	$ 1,934		

cases, the changes include a 4% price increase and suggested improvements in investment income. There are two issues surrounding the investment income change.

1. RHMC reports its investment income "above the operating margin line" in its GAAP audited financial statement. Therefore, any improvements to its investment income will help to improve the operating margin target. However reporting the investment income above the line is somewhat controversial. In many organizations, increases or decreases to investment income will not be considered appropriate changes to the operating margin.

2. Still, in its attempt to improve its investment income, RHMC will need to change its investment strategy to invest in somewhat riskier positions. Because "past results do not guarantee future outcomes," this is one of the bigger gambles in the budget package. In fact, it is possible that the finance committee, the investment committee or the board of directors will reject this recommendation as too radical.

Some other expense changes involve *reducing* the following.

- Some additional fringe benefit increases initially proposed by the human resources administrator
- Bad debt expenses through better collection efforts
- Patient care supply expenses
- Consulting fees

According to the budget compiled by the finance staff, the budgeted operating margin, after all requested changes are processed would be $300,000, or 0.3%. This is still considerably below the original 4.0% mandated by the board. Therefore, the administrators must now do the job they are paid to do, which is to make final determinations on how to achieve the budgeted target.

To aid in this effort, the finance staff once again presents the "closing the gap" analysis from the July meeting (Table 7–7). The administrators are reminded of the cost reduction opportunities that they already used and the levels at which they used them. They need to decide if they want to make further cuts in any of these line items or if they have any additional ideas. The finance administrator also reminds them that the radiology manager brought the only revenue enhancements above and beyond the original budgeted volume targets. Because there is very little additional net revenue being proposed, expense reductions are the only remaining areas that can be used to reach the budget targets.

After some discussion, the administrators agree to make a further series of cuts to the proposed 2000 budget (Table 9–2). The biggest reductions come from staffing. Instead of the original cut of 20 FTEs proposed at the July 18 meeting, they agree on a total cut of 38 FTEs. It is interesting to note that although the administrators have agreed to cut these 38 FTEs, the overall FTE count will decrease by only 17.2 because the department managers had already requested an additional 20.8 FTEs in

TABLE 9–2

Ridgeland Heights Medical Center
Final "Closing the Gap" Analysis
2000 Budget

Operating Margin July 18th Meeting	**$ (4,200)**
4% Net price increase	1,700
Improvement in investment income	1,000
Salary Expense Reductions	
38 FTEs @ $40,000 average per employee	1,520
Fringe Benefits	
Reduce additional benefits proposed in initial budget meeting of July 14th	500
Reduce bad debt expense through better collection efforts	1,000
Reduce patient care supply expenses	500
Reduce Professional and Management Fees	
Cut consulting fees	400
Reduce other expenses	500
Final set of changes since July 18th budgeted income statement	7,120
Revised operating margin	**$ 2,920**

July. So the impacts of the 38 cuts is not as severe as originally proposed. It is also agreed that these FTEs will not be cut proportionately or "across the board" as often happens. Instead, for this budget cycle, the revenue producing departments will absorb a cut of only 25%, while the nonrevenue areas will disproportionately take 75% of the cut. It is the responsibility of the finance staff to develop the formula for this before the September 17 meeting.

One additional and extraordinary decision was made at this meeting. As all the administrators struggled to determine any other places to cut the expenses to meet the 4% operating margin target, the CEO decided that no additional cut should be made beyond the 3% level. He reasoned that there were exceptional changes imposed by the Medicare Balanced Budget Act reductions coupled with increasing intransigence on the part of managed care companies to negotiate reimbursement rates in good faith. He further decided that RHMC could not absorb the full brunt of these changes in one year. Therefore he was willing to support a measure at the finance committee and board level to change the 4% operating margin target to 3% for the upcoming year. He fully reserved the right to move this target level back up to 4% for the 2001 budget year depending on circumstances.

With these changes, the budget was essentially completed. The finance staff still needed to crunch the numbers one more time to make sure all the changes did, in fact, add up to the 3% operating margin. They would have eight days in which to do so and also to recommend the number of staff members that needed to cut by division.

September 17—Final Review and Approval of the Operating Budget and Review the Human Resources Committee Package

At the September 17 meeting, the administrators will be presented with the final version of the 2000 operating budget. Table 9–3 represents this final budget. Through a series of columns, it also shows the progression of changes made to bring it home. This version, without the intermediate columns will be presented to the finance committee for approval at their October meeting.

The administrators are also presented with the finance-produced list of FTE cuts by division. It is the responsibility of the division heads to determine how they will implement the cuts required by the list. There are a number of techniques they will employ to make these determinations. Some of them are as follows.

- Eliminate all vacant positions (#1 answer of all time)
- Cut the level of overtime
- Replace FTEs with part time employees
- Replace part time employees with "as needed" employees (known as PRNs)
- Eliminate currently filled positions

These are hard decisions to make, but always necessary. The vice presidents are also responsible for deciding which of the departments within their division need to make the cuts. Fairness is not always involved at this point. The cuts may be made proportionate or disproportionate. But they must be made because there will be no budget dollars available to support these positions in the new year.

This meeting will also be used to present the human resources committee package prepared by the finance staff with the assistance of the human resources staff that will be going to the board. It includes a narrative of the human resources decisions that are being proposed by the administration, such as the actual, projected, and budgeted staffing levels by dollars and FTEs; details of the fringe benefits package; and a discussion of the wage and salary levels. These include minimum and maximum pay scales across various job classifications and the going market rate pay scales around the region. This allows the entire administrative staff to see what the board will see and gain any additional understanding of the subject at this time.

September 18–October 14—Prepare First Draft Through Final Copy of the 2000 Budget for the Finance Committee

Over the next four-week period, the finance staff will be heavily involved in preparing, and the finance administrators will be heavily occupied in reviewing the budget reports for the human resources committee, the finance committee, and the board of directors meetings. These reports are between 16 and 30 pages in length and contain varying degrees of detailed information. Preparing and reconciling the various schedules between volumes, revenues, staffing levels (FTEs), and staffing dollars are very tense and intense chores. It takes an individual with a high level of commitment, organization, and perfectionism to lead this effort. RHMC is fortunate to have an Accounting Director with such drive and skill to do so.

The budget drafts will be prepared on schedule so that effective review can be performed. As the dates of presentation get closer and closer and the draft copies get cleaner and cleaner, the final implications of the budget packages are revealed.

Operating Budget System of the Near Future

In subsequent years, it is expected that much of this paper pushing between the department managers and the finance staff during the budget process will be eliminated by the use of computers and networks. While the steps in the process may not change, a lot of the manual steps performed by the finance staff can actually be done through the work that is already required to be performed by the department managers and the vice presidents. There is a considerable amount of work that typically flows back and forth between the finance department and the department managers in a manual mode. There are ways to improve this process.

Computers are already capable of streamlining this budget process. RHMC plans to install this specialized budgeting software in the near future. The organization will be able to use this software to enhance its budget process because it has already invested in the construction of a computerized LAN. By going to the expense of installing the computer infrastructure (wiring, cabling wall outlets, and the various computer closets needed for coordination), all the personal computers at the organization are hooked up to a common computer (known as a server). Because of this linkage, all the PCs can "talk" to each other without needing to access any outside communications service, such as the phone company. Following are some of the functions available to the organization and its staff because of the LAN linkage.

- An internal electronic mail system (e-mail)
- An external e-mail with a firewall to maintain overall system security
- The Internet with the firewall attached
- A common calendar program, which enables any eligible staff member to request a meeting with one or many other staff members electronically
- The heavily developed financial and clinical decision support system and data warehouse available to all management staff
- The networked capital budgeting system, which has been thoroughly discussed in the previous three chapters

The near future will bring electronic capabilities to the operation budget. These new capabilities will allow the finance staff and the department managers to conduct

Ridgeland Heights Medical Center
Preliminary Budgeted Statement of Operations
For the Budget Year-to-Date Ending December 31, 2000
Including 4% Price Increase
September 17, 1999
(in thousands)

	1999 Budget	1999 Projected	7/18/99 2000 Budget	Admin 9/9/99 2000 Budget	Managers 9/9/99 2000 Budget	9/17/99 2000 Budget	Percentage Change	
							00B vs 99B	00B vs 99P
Revenues								
Inpatient revenue	79,000	77,800	$ 84,000	$87,360	87,360	87,360	10.58	12.29
Outpatient revenue	77,000	76,100	86,000	89,440	89,440	89,440	16.16	17.53
Total patient revenue	156,000	153,900	170,000	176,800	176,800	176,800	13.33	14.88
Less:								
Contractual and other adjustments	(60,000)	(59,000)	(72,000)	(77,100)	(77,100)	(77,100)	28.50	30.68
Charity care	(2,700)	(2,500)	(3,000)	(3,000)	(3,000)	(3,000)	11.11	20.00
Net patient service revenue	93,300	92,400	95,000	96,700	96,700	96,700	3.64	4.65
Add:								
Premuim revenue	2,100	2,100	1,000	1,000	1,000	1,000	−52.38	−52.38
Investment income	5,000	6,000	5,000	6,000	6,000	6,000	20.00	0.00
Other operating income	1,200	1,100	1,200	1,200	1,200	1,200	0.00	9.09
Total revenue	101,600	101,600	102,200	104,900	104,900	104,900	3.25	3.25

Expenses								
Salaries	35,500	36,500	39,000	38,200	38,600	37,480	5.58	2.68
Contract labor	1,400	800	1,200	1,200	1,200	1,200	−14.29	50.00
Fringe benefits	7,000	6900	7,800	7,500	7,600	7,300	4.29	5.80
Total salaries and benefits	43,900	44,200	48,000	46,900	47,400	45,980	4.74	4.03
Bad debts	4,400	4,400	5,000	4,500	4,500	4,000	−9.09	−9.09
Patient care supplies	15,200	16,000	17,100	16,600	16,900	16,600	9.21	3.75
Professional and management fees	3,400	3,800	4,200	3,900	4,000	3,800	11.76	0.00
Purchased services	5,600	5,600	5,600	5,600	5,600	5,600	0.00	0.00
Operation of plant (including utilities)	2,700	2,600	2,800	2,800	2,800	2,800	3.70	7.69
Depreciation	11,000	10,500	11,500	11,500	11,500	11,500	4.55	9.52
Interest and financing expenses	7,400	7400	7,200	7,200	7,200	7,200	−2.70	−2.70
Other	3,800	4,000	5,000	4,500	4,700	4,500	18.42	12.50
Total expenses	97,400	98,500	106,400	103,500	104,600	101,980	4.70	3.53
Operation margin	4,200	3,100	(4,200)	1,400	300	2,920	−30.48	−5.81
Nonoperating income								
Gain/(loss) on investments	1,200	1,400	1,000	1,000	1,000	1,000	−16.67	−28.57
Total nonoperating income	1,200	1,400	1,000	1,000	1,000	1,000	−16.67	−28.57
Net income	5,400	4,500	$ (3,200)	$ 2,400	$ 1,300	$ 3,920	−27.41	−12.89
4% targeted operating margin			$ 3,800	$ 3,868	$ 3,868	$ 3,868		
3% targeted operating margin			$ 2,850	$ 2,901	$ 2,901	$ 2,901		
2% targeted operating margin			$ 1,900	$ 1,934	$ 1,934	$ 1,934		

their business online. In a nutshell, the finance staff will be able to send the budget out electronically over the LAN (also known as "the network") instead of on paper. The managers will then be able to perform their analysis online and send back their changes over the wires. Because the changes are already in a digital format, the finance staff will no longer have to reenter the data. Instead they can devote their efforts to analysis of the changes. This is a much better use of the analyst's time and energy.

CAPITAL BUDGET—SEPTEMBER

September 4—Meeting to Discuss Results of Main Strategic Capital Budget Evaluations and Final Administrative Approval of 2000 Capital Budget

This meeting is necessary only if the administrators were unable to come to any final decisions during the meeting on August 25. If there were still open issues present at the end of that meeting and additional evaluation scoring was performed over the past week, then the administrators will use this meeting to finalize the budget. This approval is required because the finance staff needs to budget depreciation expense on the operating budget and to do so, it needs to know the capital assets that will be acquired in the upcoming year.

In this particular year, the RHMC administrators were able to complete their review and come to a consensus at the prior meeting. This is due in large part to the new process and software used by the organization to produce a much more efficient and effective outcome. Because of the early conclusion, the finance staff is able to determine the depreciation expense for the operating budget in record time.

CASH BUDGET

Once a year, at the conclusion of the capital and operating budget phases, the finance department staff prepares a cash budget. This is a necessary step that allows the organization to determine how to optimize the value of the cash being generated by its operations. Consider all the following facts. Excess cash can be used in the following ways.

- Kept in an interest bearing checking account at a rate equal to 350 basis points below the prime lending rate. In this case, RHMC could perhaps receive 5% interest income on its excess cash (100 basis points is equal to 1%)
- Invested on a short-term basis (defined as 12 to 18 months) for approximately 5.5% to 6% in a set of very low risk intermediate term bonds
- Invested in a moderate risk, longer-term basis in a mix of fixed instruments (bonds) and equities (stocks). A moderate risk portfolio would consist of a 65%/35% mix of stocks and bonds. The previous 10-year average return on this investment mix has been 11.3% annually based on analysis performed by the organization's investment consultants

If the board has an appetite for a moderate risk strategy that offers a greater than average return on their investments, it becomes imperative to invest the maximum amount of excess cash in the higher earning alternative. To do so, however, the organization has to have a very clear understanding of its stream of receipts and disbursements, preferably on a weekly basis. This allows them to remove the optimum amount of cash from the checking account so that it can be invested in the longer term, higher earning assets.

At the conclusion of the annual budget process, the finance staff prepares a 52-week cash budget that attempts to forecast the receipts and disbursements represented by the income statement revenues and expenses. Table 9–4 shows an eight-week set of the 2000 cash budget prepared by the finance staff. The most problematic line in this budget is labeled "patient cash" receipts. It is the most difficult line to forecast because of the problem with the industry's third-party payors (Medicare, Medicaid, managed care plans). Many of the third-party payors, particularly the non-government-based managed care plans have varying definitions of "clean claims." These are claims that should be paid within a narrowly defined time period. However, many of the major healthcare provider segments have had their share of trouble collecting promptly on these clean claims. This makes it difficult to prepare a reasonable cash budget.

Still, it is achievable assuming that the cash receipts are collected evenly throughout the year. The method that RHMC uses to budget receipts takes several steps.

1. The finance staff spreads the annual budgeted net revenue across the 12 monthly time periods based on days in the month (e.g., January is allocated 31/365th of the net revenue, February is allocated 29/365, etc.).

2. The staff splits the months into seven-day weeks and applies a proportionate amount of the monthly receipts to each week.

3. The weeks are reviewed to detect any anomalies, such as whether a holiday falls within the week. Those weeks are adjusted accordingly.

The caveat to the budgeting of cash receipts is that a change in the accounts receivable can wreak havoc on the forecast. The initial cash budget should prophesy the collection of 100% of the budgeted net revenues. If this does not happen, the cash budget could fail, leading to the following problems.

- A shortfall to pay the required disbursements, such as payroll and trade vendor payables
- A need to borrow funds at a rate higher than is being earned by the invested funds

It is important to remember that a budget, whether operating, capital or cash is nothing more than a forecast based on a set of assumptions for future activities. Because the cash budget can have so much potential negative impact if the forecasts are not reasonable, it is imperative to update these budgets on a weekly basis.[1] This

---

[1] Note: Forecasts can never be "accurate" because it is not possible to accurately foretell the future.

allows close monitoring of the actual cash balances, which leads to a better ability to move the cash into its most appropriate asset category.

The RHMC board has requested that the administration maximize its investment income, wherever possible, without resorting to a risky investment strategy. One of the ways this can be accomplished is by keeping its checking account balances as close to zero as possible without going into an overdraft position ("going negative"). Table 9–4 shows a $4,000,000 actual opening balance for the week ending December 17. Eight weeks later, the projected balance is still $3,997,200.

Given this information, it appears that if the organization wants to maintain a balance closer to zero, it could transfer, let's say, $3,000,000 out of the checking account and into its stock portfolio. That would still leave it with a $1,000,000 cash cushion in its checking account. Unfortunately RHMC would overdraft its checking account if it transferred the $3,000,000 according to this weekly forecast because the forecast for the week ending January 14 shows an ending balance of $2,734,500. If the $3,000,000 had been transferred prior to that date, the ending balance would have therefore been a negative $265,500. Not good!

The moral of the story is that cash balances fluctuate with normal organizational activities and organizations need to look at the *lowest* weekly cash balances when forecasting checking account balances if they do not want to overdraft. The organization should also negotiate a line of credit, at favorable interest rates, with its bank to cover a situation where there could be an overdraft. In this case, the finance administrator would not be as concerned about a short-term overdraft. In short, cash budgeting can have great value to an organization if there is a desire to maximize cash assets, comfort in the forecasting, and availability of overdraft protection or a line of credit.

PHYSICIAN PRACTICE MANAGEMENT

General Concepts

Physician practice is a major segment of the healthcare industry. As we saw in Chapter 1, physician practices accounts for more than $200 billion a year encompassing 20% of the industry's financial outlays. Although they literally make up "only" 20% of the industry, the impact of physicians, and their office practice on the process of healthcare is enormous.

In all the important ways, physicians impact most of the healthcare costs generated in this country. Not only do they personally control the $200 billion of their own pure office revenues, they also have a great deal of control over the expenses generated in the $350 billion hospital segment of the industry. It is important to note that most clinical hospital expenses are originated by physician orders. Thus, the costs of every hospital inpatient case are the result of the type and quantity of diagnostic tests, therapies, drugs, and supplies ordered by the physicians. Still, the manner in which physicians manage their own office practice is often an indicator of how frugal or profligate they will be in managing the resources of other healthcare organizations with which they are affiliated.

TABLE 9-4

Ridgeland Heights Medical Center
2000 Cash Budget
Selected Weeks

	Actual December 13–17	Actual December 20–24	Actual December 27–31	Actual January 3–7	Forecast January 10–14	Forecast January 17–21	Forecast January 24–28	Forecast January 31–4
Cash Receipts								
Patient receipts	2,400,000	1,400,000	2,100,000	2,100,000	2,109,000	2,109,000	2,109,000	2,109,000
Other operating receipts	30,000	40,000	30,000	40,000	35,000	35,000	35,000	35,000
Miscellaneous items	5,000	3,000	8,000	3,000	—	—	—	—
Total Receipts	2,435,000	1,443,000	2,138,000	2,143,000	2,144,000	2,144,000	2,144,000	2,144,000
Cash disbursements								
Trade vendors payable	1,100,000	1,150,000	1,800,000	1,500,000	1,025,000	1,025,000	1,025,000	1,025,000
Self insured healthcare payments	—	60,000	—	170,000	—	—	—	80,000
Debt payments	—	—	—	—	—	—	—	—
Miscellaneous items	5,000	5,000	4,000	5,000	—	—	—	—
Total accounts payable and other	5,000	65,000	4,000	175,000	—	—	—	80,000
Transfers to payroll	850,000	250,000	800,000	260,000	841,500	268,500	841,500	268,500
Payroll taxes	450,000	40,000	—	500,000	444,000	43,400	444,000	43,400
Other payroll transfers	100,000	2,000	100,000	2,000	105,000	—	105,000	—
Total payroll disbursements	1,400,000	292,000	900,000	762,000	1,390,500	311,900	1,390,500	311,900
Total cash disbursements	2,505,000	1,507,000	2,704,000	2,437,000	2,415,500	1,336,900	2,415,500	1,416,900
Net activities	(70,000)	(64,000)	(566,000)	(294,000)	(271,500)	807,100	(271,500)	727,100
Cash balance—beginning	4,000,000	3,930,000	3,866,000	3,300,000	3,006,000	2,734,500	3,541,600	3,270,100
Cash balance—ending	3,930,000	3,866,000	3,300,000	3,006,000	2,734,500	3,541,600	3,270,100	3,997,200

229

There is an art to physician practice management (PPM). And there are many variables to running a successful office practice. One of the biggest variables is the *size* of the practice. Physician practices can range in size from a solo practitioner's office to a building housing a 400-physician multispecialty clinic. Regardless of size, there are still a number of basic financial characteristics that all physician office practices must adhere to. Box 9–1 illustrates the basic ways that a physician office practice can optimize its financial condition.

Unfortunately over the last several years, it has become obvious to many physicians and physician groups that they are no longer capable of optimizing their own financial condition. The rapid rise of managed care plans dealt a crippling blow to many of the old physician back offices. Managed care plans mandated dozens of new requirements, some for billing but mostly for referrals. Primary care physicians (PCPs) that signed up with managed care plans are required to get preapproval for all treatment modalities that take place outside of the physician's office. This has caused an avalanche of paperwork unknown in prior eras.

Specialists are not immune to this phenomenon. First, they are the recipients of referrals requested by the PCP and processed by the health plan. Therefore, the specialist's staff has to be sure that each managed care patient that is being treated by the specialist has the required approvals for payment. This is an onerous task; health plans do not always process their approvals in a timely manner, yet the patients have a need to be seen promptly creating a potential conflict between the physician and his or her patient. Second, they too need to request referrals back to the PCP if they want to perform additional tests or treatments on the patient beyond the original referral.

There are other medical practice issues that physicians have to deal with in the current era.

BOX 9–1

METHODS USED TO OPTIMIZE FINANCIAL CONDITION OF PHYSICIAN OFFICE PRACTICE

Revenue Enhancement

- Improve documentation in order to bill for and support higher reimbursement procedures
- Improve patient throughput
- Retain ancillary revenues in the office setting

Expense Reduction

- Trim the payroll through the use of benchmarks and levels of support staff
- Cut office space costs—consider timesharing
- Reduce malpractice premiums
- Hold down supply costs through reduced usage and less costly items

1. Fraud and abuse, particularly related to Medicare rules and regulations under the Stark II laws, as characterized by the following.
   - Billing issues
   - Documentation issues
   - Corporate structure of the practice
2. Cash flow, due to the long length of time that it takes some health plans to pay capitation premium and other insurance claims
3. The need for capital to fund the acquisition of efficiency producing and revenue enhancing information technology
4. Consumers who are demanding new tests, treatments, and drugs caused by the influence of print ads, televisions ads, and the omnipresence of the Internet
5. If it is a small practice (a less than five-physician group), the need for capital to continue to compete for managed care contracts against the much larger groups that are being courted by the large consolidated managed healthcare plans

Into the breach to straighten out these problem rode the physician practice management companies (PPMCs). These companies had many corporate structures. There are for-profit and not-for-profit hospital-based, equity-based, and academic medical center-based PPMCs. Their mandate was to operate the physician office practice in a more professional, businesslike manner. It was their conviction that many solo and multispecialty practice settings operated with little financial focus, or ability to manage these issues.

Therefore these PPMCs sold physician practices, both solo and multispecialty, on their ability to optimize revenue enhancement and cost reduction strategies. They became popular in the early to mid 1990s as a vehicle to improve the financial condition within the physician office setting.

Wall Street became enchanted with the PPMCs in the early 1990s. They enjoyed exceptional growth in the equity-based market. As shown in Figure 9–1 the market capitalization for PPMCs increased from just under $1 billion in 1993 to $12 billion three years later. At the same time the number of publicly traded PPMCs increased from 3 in 1990 to 27 in 1996, an explosion in a nascent industry as can be seen in Figure 9–2.

In 1997, it appeared that there was no limit to this industry's size. Doctors were selling themselves to PPMCs by the thousands. The PPMCs targeted medium- and large-sized groups for acquisition. The PPMCs were on a roll. Although they had not yet proved that they could improve the financial condition of the physicians' practices, they were able to acquire many vulnerable groups because of a hard-to-refuse come-on that was, "Come be a part of us and we will make you very rich through the increase in our stock price." Because equity- or stock-based companies always sell at a premium to their underlying value, equity-based PPMCs could offer physicians stock in the PPMC that was 10, 15, 20,

F I G U R E   9–1

Equity Based PPMC Market Capitalization 1993–1997

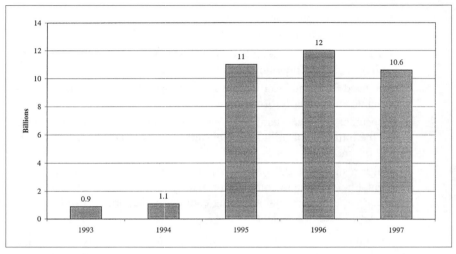

Source: The Advisory Board.

F I G U R E   9–2

Number of Publicly Traded PPMCs for Selected Years Between 1990–1997

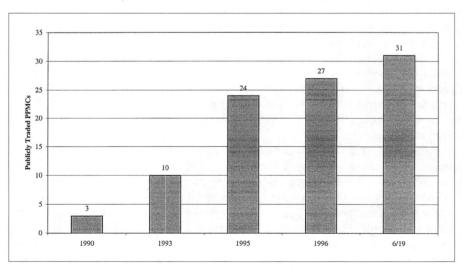

Source: The Advisory Board.

maybe 30 times the value of the practice. It made some physicians in the early adopter practices multimillionaires.

The come-ons were relentless. Every independent physician or physician group was talking about their future in relation to the PPMCs. They were hoping to be courted by, making the initial overtures to, or talking about rejecting the PPMCs if extended an offer because of cultural differences or the simple desire to stay independent. The equity-based PPMCs grew exponentially, fueled more by their tremendous acquisition binge than by improved earnings based on practice improvements.

Meanwhile, this phenomenon did not go unnoticed by the hospital and health systems side of the industry. They were worried. There are historical linkages between hospitals and their affiliated doctors. In most not-for-profit hospital/health system settings, the physicians maintain independent status while gaining the privilege to use the hospital for those specific services for which they were granted credentials. Hospitals have a financial interest in granting these credentials. After all, it is these privileged physicians who refer patients to the hospital for inpatient and outpatient services. Physicians can get privileged in any of the following categories, each of which confers different rights and responsibilities. Box 9–2 is a listing of the categories of the RHMC medical staff and some of the privileges afforded to them. These categories create the linkages between the healthcare organization and the individual medical staff members.

Anything that disrupts these linkages is viewed as an obstacle by the hospitals. Thus, the hospitals attempted to counter the trends of "their" physicians selling or aligning themselves with equity-based PPMCs. One of the steps that many hospitals/health systems took was to organize the equivalent of their own PPMC. Often called management services organizations (MSOs), they would offer to purchase the physicians' practice or manage the physicians' practice while the physician(s) retain control.

It was extremely important to the hospitals that they maintain the linkages, particularly in the era of expanding managed care. They knew that being able to strike a bargain on managed care contracts was enhanced when a single negotiator could speak for the hospital and physician providers. It provided a small amount of leverage against the health plans in contrast to the hospitals and physicians coming to the contract table separately. In addition, *single signature contracting* keeps hospitals and their physicians on the "same side," allowing both entities to maintain contracts with the same MCOs. It was therefore in the interest of RHMC to do its best to create a strong affiliation with its many primary care and multispecialty physicians on its staff.

RHMC did this in two ways.

First, it encouraged its affiliated (credentialed) physicians to form an independent practice association (IPA). This gave the physicians a legal base from which to negotiate as a single unit with the managed care companies. Any physician who became a member of the IPA gave the IPA the authority to negotiate rates for him or her and the practice. So long as the IPA board approved a deal, the individual physicians in the IPA had to accept it.

B O X   9–2

RIDGELAND HEIGHTS MEDICAL CENTER

Categories of Medical Staff

Provisional Staff—newly appointed to the staff—this is essentially a one-year probation period.

Courtesy Staff—Physicians whose practices are exclusively office-based but who seek membership to use hospital services or specialists or participate in hospital-based MCOs. They will be credentialed but not privileged to admit or treat patients within the inpatient or outpatient hospital setting. (Some hospitals may allow a limited number of patient admissions.)

Associate Staff—Three-year term after completion of provisional status. It is available to staff members who have done the following.

1. Demonstrated an increasing need for the hospital facilities through satisfaction of their respective utilization criteria
2. Have shown an active interest in the affairs of the hospital
3. Whose professional work has demonstrated qualities of maturity and responsibility to indicate that they are likely to become eligible for promotion to active staff

Consulting Staff—Physicians whose work is not primarily at this hospital but are exceptionally qualified and experienced in their specialties. Their appointment to the consulting staff shall be determined by their potential for contributing service both to the hospital and to the community. They shall not have admitting privileges, shall be exempt from all utilization criteria policies, and shall not have the right to vote or hold office.

Active Staff—Physicians who have completed associate staff and have satisfied organizational bylaw requirements that qualify them to conduct the business of the medical staff. They are entitled to admit patients to the hospital, vote on all members, and hold elective office.

Second, while RHMC had no control over the IPA (which was 100% physician owned and operated), it was now able to work with the IPA to develop a 50/50 owned physician hospital organization (PHO). This allowed the unified physician organization and the hospital to negotiate deals with health plans.

Management Services Organizations

Meanwhile, RHMC took one additional giant step. Like other healthcare organizations in the country, they set up a MSO to do the following.

- Provide back office services to independent physicians who felt the need to outsource these efforts

- Provide the management services for PCPs who were employed by the healthcare organization

The rationale for the MSO's formation was to allow RHMC to have some control over the patient referral pattern within its primary and secondary service areas. Employed physicians refer 100% of their nonoffice-based clinical services back to RHMC. It also provided RHMC with a growing physician practice, giving it some additional leverage with the managed care companies.

The MSO was another operating company within the overall RHMC corporate structure. Its creation was costly to RHMC. It set up a back office operation that consisted of billers and collectors, physician office managers, and administrative personnel. These individuals were responsible for operating the physician's offices, from hiring all the office personnel including the nurses, to procuring the supplies, and making the office facility meet very high standards. The point of the MSO was to allow the physicians to concentrate on the clinical issues pertaining to their patients and not worry about the office management.

One of the biggest features of most MSOs was its responsibility to negotiate all the managed care contracts. In the case of the RHMC MSO, this was not applicable because every member of the MSO was also a member of the IPA. Thus, the IPA through the PHO was providing the negotiating muscle for the MSO.

There were several areas in which the MSO was particularly effective. These included the management of the office staff, including the hiring, firing, supervising and reviewing of the nursing and clerical staff. A key responsibility of the clerical staff was to process the PCP's referral for any other medical or surgical service. This could include referrals to specialist physicians, hospitals, and/or home health agencies.

Making referrals for other medical and surgical services encompassed some difficulty in the late 1990s in America. The most important piece of information that the physician's clerical staff needs to know is the patient's insurance carrier and plan. This allows the clerk to determine the exact benefits applicable to the patient. This also allows the PCP to know which specialist physician or hospital the patient could be referred to. This is possible because each and every insurance plan has a different provider panel attached to it. Insurance companies will allow only a contracted PCP to refer to other physicians in the panel associated with the insurance plan being paid for by the individual employers.

Billing and Collection Issues

Another service that the MSO provides is billing and collecting. There are very specific rules and regulations that need to be followed by physician billers and billing services. Some of the rules and regulations are the result of laws written for the Medicare and Medicaid programs. Other rules are the results of contractual stipulations agreed to between the organization and all the managed care companies with which it has decided to do business. The rules involve all phases of the operation. Below are some of the main rules that need to be followed.

- Determination of patient third-party status—capitation or fee-for-service
- Amount of the copay that needs to be collected from the patient
- Second opinion
- Referrals
- Preauthorization of services
- Coordination of benefits
- Fraud and abuse regulations

It is extremely difficult to perform all the required steps properly and not run afoul of the contract stipulations or the law. It is akin to trying to juggle a set of rare china dishes without letting any of them fall and break. Proper identification of the patient during the check-in period is critical to the success of the billing process. Determining the third-party payor's requirements then becomes essential to the speedy billing and collection of the account if it is a fee-for-service type contract. If the patient is capitated, no bill for collection will be sent, to either the payor or the patient.

The rapid increase in the managed care volume in many physician offices set off a rush by some physicians to acquire the tools to manage these additional new requirements. As mentioned earlier in this chapter, there was a great need to acquire state-of-the-art information technology that enhances the ability to bill and collect patient accounts from Medicare, Medicaid, and managed care payors in a highly efficient manner. Some of these information systems included "edits" within the programming to identify and flag gaps in information required to be submitted with bills based on the payor. This was very useful to the billers. It avoided the need for them to manually review every bill against a payor's contract.

But, there was one enormous downside to the acquisition of these new information technology billing and collecting tools. They are very expensive. The cost of the systems vary depending on the size of the practice, the number of patients that are treated, the number of members that are capitated, and the number of physician sites that are being connected. There are several information system vendors that cater to the physician office practice market and their products come in a variety of shapes and sizes.

Some of the very popular features and functions of a PPM billing and collecting system are as follows.

- Electronic charting
- Voice recognition
- Optical imaging
- Office scheduling
- Managed care[2]

---

[2] Worley, R., Ciotti, V. (1997). Selecting Practice Management Information Systems. *MGM Journal*, May/June, p. 55.

These features and functions will aid the physician and his or her office staff in optimizing their billing and collections. It should also help in clinical practice. However, given the current healthcare reimbursement climate, the problem is deciding what mechanism to use to finance the acquisition of these systems. Many practices in the 1990s turned to PPMCs for help.

Patient Throughput

One of the most important concepts in PPM involves patient throughput. Patient throughput is defined as the number of patients that a physician can see in defined time period, usually stated in hours or days. Stated another way, patient throughput concerns the amount of time that a physician spends treating his or her patients.

This is more easily explained using the following example.

Let's say that a physician currently treats, on average, 21 patients a day over a standard seven-hour day. That means the physician is treating three patients per hour (21 patients divided by seven hours). Put another way, the physician is seeing, on average, one patient every 20 minutes. There are two important concepts inherent in this example.

- In regards to the physician seeing a patient every 20 minutes, it is critical to understand all of the work that the physician needs to perform during this time period. First and foremost, the physician needs to "put hands on" the patient. When a patient enters a doctor's office, what they want is for the physician to physically poke and prod them. This gives the patient comfort that the physician is doing his or her job. It is this spending of time that is the physician's most valuable commodity.

   But, because of the nature of 21st century practice, the physician needs to perform many more functions than just sitting with the patient while making a diagnosis and devising a treatment plan. Box 9-3 describes the steps that a physician might take with a patient during an office visit.

- Now, consider the patient. Did he or she think that 20 minutes was enough time for the care rendered? Did they want more? Did they think that the physician was able to do an effective job in that time period? The answer to most of these questions is NO! Patients are demanding and often aware that the physician is on a short time schedule. It's always been this way, hasn't it? Well, of course physicians have always had calendars. The biggest difference is that back then in the Marcus Welby 1950s and 1960s, physicians often booked patients into 30- and 45-minute time slots. Nowadays, the 20-minute time slot described above is *too long!*

   These days most PCPs (this era's Marcus Welby) schedule four patients an hour. This is of course one patient every 15 minutes. In fact, there are some physicians who book patients every 10 or 12 minutes apart (five or six patients per hour) in order to maximize their revenues.

Improving patient throughput in a physician's office was a sure-fire way for the PPMC to increase the physician's revenue, as long as there was a pent-up

BOX 9–3

STEPS TAKEN BY PHYSICIANS DURING AN OFFICE VISIT

- Examine the patient!
- Fully document all the relevant signs and symptoms of the patient in order to allow the physician coder and biller to accurately produce a bill that will stand up to scrutiny by a federal government or managed care auditor.
- Review the patient's chart from prior periods to ascertain if any previous illness or injury is connected to the current medical problem, and if so, review the previous treatment patterns for success or failure.
- Create any referral notes and paperwork that may be needed so that the patient can move on to a higher level of care, if warranted.
- Write up any prescription that the patient may need.
- Explain to the patient any particular instructions that need to be given for home care.

---

demand for the physician's services. It was one of the first things looked at by a PPMC that was performing due diligence in the event of a practice acquisition. PPMCs could immediately ascertain if the practice had throughput of 2.0, 2.5, 3.0, and so on of patients per hour. It was easy math to determine immediate improvements.

The equation seems too easy—like pushing the speed-up button on the assembly line in order to produce more cars, thus generating more revenues. Unfortunately, in the late 1990s, the theory rarely could be turned into practice. The main reason is that most physicians who have been in practice for a few years have developed a practice pattern with which they are comfortable. Altering this pattern is akin to changing a successful baseball player's batting style or a golfer's swing. Yes, it's possible, but only after a lot of hard work and effort. And they have to want to change!

The method used by most PPMCs was to develop physician incentive compensation arrangement. These arrangements provided the physician with financial incentives for meeting productivity goals. Thus, a physician might be able to earn between 10% and 50% over his or her base compensation for producing patient throughput in various levels above an agreed upon standard. For example, over the course of a year, the physician and the PPMC may have agreed on a base salary of $110,000 with a stipulation that the physician would see 6,174 patients (28 patients per day $\times$ 4.5 days per week $\times$ 49 weeks). However if the physician sees two more patients per day, on average, the physician could earn 15% of his or her base salary and if they see four more patients per day, the incentive could rise to 30% of the base salary. This is just one physician compensation method that may have been attempted to raise physician throughput. There are dozens more, some very esoteric. Many books, articles and seminars around the country concentrate on these methods and should be referred to for advanced discussion in this area.

Although PPMCs emerged because of the rise of managed care and the reduction to physician's incomes, when push came to shove, many physicians chose not to alter their practice patterns even with the carrot of the incentive compensation being waved in front of them. Thus, the physicians did not increase their incomes because there were little, if any, improvements in patient throughput and the PPMCs did not generate the kinds of revenues that they expected.

The concept of improving patient throughput as a driver to physician financial success and lack of success with it became a beacon in the industry. Physicians began to rebel against throughput guidelines. Other physicians who had not yet signed on with PPMCs as employees, but might have been considering it, stopped. In effect in 1997 and 1998, the PPMCs ran out of physician practices to acquire. Through 1993 to 1996, the only thing fueling the PPMCs growth was physician practice acquisition, not bottom line improvements. Thus, when the acquisitions dried up, so did a good part of the industry.

Equity-Based Physician Practice Management Companies

Take the case of the two largest equity-based PPMCs, MedPartners and PhyCor. In 1995, MedPartners was trading at a stock price of $17. By 1996, it highest stock price was $32. Yet in late 1998, its price, which had been tumbling since late 1997, hit a low of just under $2 a share. Similarly, PhyCor was trading at just over $3 a share in early 1992. Throughout 1993, 1994, and 1995, it experienced a steadily rising stock price until it hit its peak in late 1996 with a stock price of $40 a share. However, subsequent to that date, it suffered a precipitous drop in its stock price, back down to $4 a share.

PPMCs fell out of such favor that MedPartners abandoned its commitment to its physician practices in November 1998 in favor of pharmacy benefit management and therapeutic services. In its own news release dated November 11, 1998, Mac Crawford, the company's president and chief executive officer said that "we believe that it is in the best interest of our shareholders and our affiliated physicians to divest our PPM operations because it allows MedPartners to exit an industry that is viewed unfavorably by the investment community as presently configured."

Thus was the meteoric rise and subsequent fall of the equity-based PPMCs. Yet the future is not yet told for this segment of the industry. Consider that there are still many physicians under contract to several other smaller PPMCs. In addition, the underlying issues that gave rise to the PPMCs still exist. Managed care is still dominant in many parts of the country. Physician earnings are still impacted by managed care rates and there is still opportunity for expense reductions and revenue enhancements in physician office practices. In fact, "to achieve continued success, PPMCs must be prepared to show how they will boost physician incomes, save physicians' time, manage capitation, reduce malpractice exposure and enhance care."[3]

In addition, a new type of PPMC is emerging to fill some of the gap left by the failure of some of the previously bigger players. These new companies are termed

---

[3] Peters, J. (1998). Rough Waters Ahead—Its Time for PPMs to Slow Down and Get Their Bearings. *Modern Physician,* May, p. 47.

"outsourcing firms." They typically have shorter term and incentive-based contracts with physicians. The main advantage of outsourcing is that it has none of the constraints common to the other type of PPM agreements (i.e., it allows doctors to keep control of their practices). The outsourcing firms focus on handling billing services, payor contracts, or other administrative services. And this could still be a heavy growth business because according to a survey released in December 1997 by the National CPA Healthcare Advisers Association, 72% of physician practices still do not outsource.[4]

Hospital Owned PPMCs

Still, not all PPMCs are alike. Even with the turmoil in the equity-based PPMC industry, there are still segments of the industry that have not been as heavily tarnished. "Good PPMCs—defined mostly as single-specialty and hospital-based PPMCs—are suffering from a backlash caused by a few companies problems, but they will survive any industry shakeout because they still provide the money and management skills most physicians lack."[5] In fact, hospital owned PPMCs continue to operate into the new millennium with a renewed purpose and greater financial returns.

Like many of the equity-based PPMCs, those sponsored by hospitals did not produce very good financial results during the mid to late 1990s. In fact, according to the Center for Healthcare Industry Performance Studies, hospitals were more likely to lose money on physician practice acquisitions than equity-based PPMCs. This was the conclusion of a survey conducted between 1994 and 1996 representing over 1,200 physicians and 460 practice acquisitions.[6] There tended to be a number of reasons for this conclusion. Hospitals tend to pay higher salaries to employed physicians than do other firms that may offer equity (stock) as an added inducement. They do this because they believe there are opportunities to raise practice revenues or decrease costs to make the practice more profitable. Also, there are substantial opportunities for additional revenues as employed physicians may legally make appropriate referrals back to the hospitals.

The higher practice losses did not deter many hospitals that had the opportunity to establish PPMCs. As stated earlier in the chapter, these hospital owned PPMCs met the criteria that included the following.

- Keeping control of some of the organization's best doctors rather than losing them to an outside influence
- In some cases, establishing new practices in undeserved parts of the service area, thereby generating new referral revenues

---

[4] Cook, B. (1998). A New Contender—Outsourcing Firms Fight for Physicians' Business. *Modern Physician,* May, p. 44.

[5] Cook, B. (1998). Judgment Day—MedPartners' Pullout Raises Questions About the Future of PPMs. *Modern Physician,* December, p. 2.

[6] Cleverly, W.O., Knott, P.J., Dye, C.F. (1998). *The 1997–1998 Physician Practice Acquisition Resource Book.* The Center for Healthcare Industry Performance Studies (CHIPS): Columbus, Ohio.

Still, hospital organizations did not go out of their way to create physician practice losses in the PPMC. Most of them had every intention of making these business segments profitable. Many of the losses experienced by the hospital-based PPMCs could be construed as start-up losses over the first few years of their existence. In fact, steep investment costs and pressures to pay higher physician salaries led many hospital owned physician practices into the red. But a 1996 survey by the MGMA predicts that the combination of time and experience may soon pay off.[7]

The decreasing losses reported for hospital owned PPMCs is the situation that is being experienced at RHMC. When they entered the PPMC business in the mid 1990s, they expected to lose money in the early years of the practices, and they budgeted to do so. Although practice acquisition was a major thrust of their plan, in their market, they were not many physician practices that wanted to be acquired. They turned instead to developing their own physician practices, hiring relatively young PCPs who agreed to be employed. RHMC then acquired office space for these physicians in those parts of the service area that RHMC wanted to seed.

The biggest problem with new physician practices is that they take a long time to mature. Depending on the area, it could take from three to five years for a practice to mature (i.e., bring in enough revenue to offset the total practice costs, which includes the physician's salary). Developing a volume and revenue base involves becoming known in the community and applying for certification by the several managed care plans that provide medical insurance coverage in the area. This allows the physician to be included in the managed care plan's pamphlet of eligible providers, thus allowing a managed care member to access the physician. This cycle could take a year or longer.

The start-up costs during this cycle tend to be high. The two largest costs are 1) the salary of the physician who will be sitting around waiting for the next patient to come through the door and 2) the office rent, a fixed cost that needs to be amortized by patient volumes. Almost all the other costs are variable and thus more easily absorbed in a low volume environment. Still, while these losses are real, they can be somewhat offset by the volume of patients who are referred to the hospital for required testing, when appropriate.

RHMC has developed a monthly board report that provides a summary financial review of the physician practices. It includes the profit or loss on the office practice itself as well as the incremental revenues generated by the hospital on the services provided through referrals by the office practices. Table 9–5 shows an example of this report. While the finance committee of the board continues to be dissatisfied with the direct losses generated by the physician practices, they are well aware of their value in extending the healthcare organization's reach out into the deepest reaches of the service area. In addition, their dissatisfaction is somewhat ameliorated by the last line on the report that shows an overall positive physician financial contribution to the overall organization.

---

[7] Tschida, M. (1998). Fade to Black—Hospital-Owned Physician Practices May Soon Begin to Pay Off. *Modern Physician,* February, p. 18.

TABLE 9-5

Ridgeland Heights Medical Center
Physician Development Key Success Factor
For the Month and Year Ended September 30, 1999

	Month						Year to Date				
	Prior Yr.	Actual	Budget	Percent Prior Yr.	Variance Budget		Prior Yr.	Actual	Budget	Percent Prior Yr.	Variance Budget
Employed physicians											
Total no. of capitated lives	360	380	370	5.6	2.7		2,000	2,400	2,200	20.0	9.1
Office visits—new patients	1,820	1,870	1,900	2.7	−1.6		4,000	4,100	4,200	2.5	−2.4
Office visits—established patients	2,180	2,250	2,270	3.2	−0.9		18,000	22,000	22,000	22.2	0.0
Office visits—total							22,000	26,100	26,200	18.6	−0.4
Patient satisfaction rating (scale = 1–5)	4.57	4.75	4.8	3.9	−1.0		4.65	4.78	4.8	2.8	−0.4
Accounts receivable											
A/R balance (in thousands)							350	450	0	28.6	N/A
Days net revenues in A/R							42.0	41.0	40.0	−2.4	2.5
Total hospital activity											
Patient days	180	200	190	11.1	5.3		2,000	2,100	2,200	5.0	−4.5
Inpatient admissions	32	35	36	9.4	−2.8		380	400	420	5.3	−4.8
Outpatient services	310	330	350	6.5	−5.7		3,000	3,400	3,600	13.3	−5.6
Physician practice operating margins	(190)	(150)	(140)	−21.1	7.1		(2,400)	(2,000)	(1,800)	−16.7	11.1
Total gross revenues (in thousands)	450	520	490	15.6	6.1		5,000	6,000	5,800	20.0	3.4
Total net revenues (in thousands)	265	320	300	20.8	6.7		3,000	3,600	3,500	20.0	2.9
Incremental contribution margin (in thousands) (net revenues minus incremental expenses)	160	180	200	12.5	−10.0		1,800	2,100	2,300	16.7	−8.7
Total physician contribution to the corporation (in thousands)	(30)	30	60	−200.0	−50.0		(600)	100	500	116.7	−80.0

In addition, the board is aware that the direct losses suffered by the physician practices are slowly decreasing. Over the few years that the practices have been in existence, the practice managers have quickly learned the reasons for the losses and have taken steps to improve the problems. RHMC's problems are very similar to those described in a November/December 1998 article in *Medical Group Management (MGM) Journal* on the subject. In summary, the factors contributing to the practice losses include the following.

- Reduced physician productivity (throughput)
- Decreased collection rates
- Expansion problems
- Managed care contract negotiation issues
- Centralization of ancillary department revenues
- New costs such as computer and facility upgrades
- Occupancy issues
- Level of physician compensation[8]

RHMC management and staff assigned to the physician practice have made significant improvements in many of these areas as the direct losses experienced by the organization are moving towards breakeven. This also tends to be the case in other hospital owned physician practices around the country. The RHMC finance committee and board continue to support the efforts in regard to their hospital owned PPMC but continue to demand improvement.

In summary, the rise of PPMCs in the country has wrought some interesting and everlasting changes to the healthcare industry. Physicians are the dominant group of healthcare practitioners in the country by virtue of their education, experience, and licensure. Only they can prescribe medical testing, order inpatient hospital admissions, order drugs and medical supplies, and prescribe all other medical/surgical type referrals. The 1990s have brought upheaval to established physician practices, particularly the dramatic oversight function by managed care companies. This story is far from over. It is likely that the physicians, as a group, will attempt to reexert the control they have historically enjoyed as leaders of the healthcare community.

---

[8] Bohlmann, R.C. (1998). Hospital-Affiliated Practices Reduce 'Red Ink.' *MGM Journal,* November/December, p. 30.

10

CHAPTER

October

It was 7:30 in the morning. Josephine Morton, RHMC's vice president of information services and chief information officer (CIO), had just arrived at her office. She had a big day ahead of her and she was trying to brace herself for it. As she was heading for her first cup of coffee of the morning, she ran into Sam Barnes, whose office was just down the hall.

"Hey Jo, slow down," said Sam as Morton literally ran into Sam.

"Oh, sorry Sam, I've got a lot on my mind today," she uttered. "We're rolling out the final phase of the electronic nurse charting system. I'm on my way to a nursing floor right now to see how it's working in action."

"Final phase, today. Jo, that's fantastic. I thought we'd never get there," offered the always optimistic Sam.

"Yeah," said Jo, "I'll tell you, this has been a heck of a year. Between working through the Y2K problem and replacing our complete information system during the past several months, I think the organization owes me about two months of sleep."

"I know how you feel, Jo. I often feel that way during certain phases of the budget process. Still, I know that the job you've been through is quite a bit bigger and longer than the annual budget."

"Sam, speaking of the budget, between the main hospital computer replacement and the Y2K project, we've spent even more money than the very large budget that was approved by the board," asked a suddenly worried CIO. "How are going to handle that?"

"That's a good question, Jo," responded Sam. "I've thought a lot about how to present the final dollar amounts to the board. First of all, we've been keeping them informed all along. Whenever there was a break between the budget and the actual expenses, we've let them know and asked for subsequent approval. They haven't always been happy but they usually understand why there have been budget variances, particularly capital budget breaks. You know Jo, most of our finance committee members are CEOs and they have faced these issues first hand at their own companies."

"Well I know I've prepared some analysis for you and the finance committee, Sam," stated Jo. "So that's good to hear."

"I'll tell you Jo, the toughest part of the increased budget that we needed to explain was the tremendous cost of upgrading the computer infrastructure. It was hard to describe the need to spend several million dollars to replace all the wires behind the walls and build dozens of computer closets to help in controlling the flood of digital data as it flows across those wires. The way we were able to make them understand it was to explain how we send and receive e-mail across the local area network that you are setting up."

"That's a good way to do it Sam," said Jo. "I'm glad to hear that the finance committee has accepted these budget changes. I've gotta go now. I need to get to that nursing floor to see the new system in action."

"Okay, Jo, but let me ask you to try and not have any more budget breaks. It gets harder and harder to deal with them," replied Sam.

October dawned gorgeous, as usual. The leading edge of the trees that populated the remaining forests of northern Illinois was beginning the turn from bright green to flaming orange and red. The temperatures reaching in the high 60s at noon and mid 40s at night was, likewise, perfect. The brisk autumn air invigorated the region. Productivity was very high, which was useful because October is traditionally a month when hospital beds fill up with various illnesses and injuries.

At RHMC, October is always a transitional month because of the proposed budget presentation to the finance committee and the board of directors in the middle and late part of the month. At the beginning of the month, the anxiety begins to build as the dates approach. The finance staff was working constantly to clean up the presentation package, giving particular care to explain any discrepancies that emerge. These discrepancies must be evaluated and clarified. At RHMC, because of the process employed over the previous five months that systematically weeds out anomalies, there are rarely any discrepancies that cause the finance staff to recommend a change in the budget before presentation to the finance committee.

At the same time, the finance staff is making heavy use of their computers to perform the budget work. The computer technology enhances the staff's performance in generating, calculating, and evaluating the operating and capital budgets. In fact, the finance staff would need to double or triple in size if the computers ceased to exist.

INFORMATION SYSTEMS IMPLICATIONS TO HEALTHCARE FINANCIAL MANAGEMENT

Throughout this book, it has been shown that much of the process and practice performed by the finance staff is facilitated by the use of information technology (IT). In fact, each of the staff members essentially has a computer keyboard attached to the end of their arms. Just as a carpenter has his hammer, the finance and accounting staff have their spreadsheet programs. While the accounting profession was invented in 1492 when an Italian named Pacioli invented double-entry bookkeeping using a quill pen, the current practice is somewhat more advanced. In the late 1990s, pen quills are too slow to keep up with the pace of change in the healthcare industry.

While it may be obvious that all industries have adopted IT as a cost reduction, labor saving tool, the uses for IT in healthcare have a distinctly patient-oriented focus. General ledger and payroll programs are the most basic pieces of software in any industry and thus are not at issue here. They work the same in healthcare as in any other industry. It is the other programs that provide the value in healthcare and healthcare finance.

The essential function of information systems management is *to get the right information to the right user at the right time to support effective decision making.* The improvements contemplated for healthcare IT are generally predicated around improved patient care and involve moving previously unavailable information to the clinical practitioner at the patient point of service. The practitioner might be a physician, a nurse, a physical therapist, or a dietician. It could also be a massage therapist, an acupuncturist, a pharmacist or a psychologist. In every case, the need to know what happened to the patient prior to the current visit is critical to the most effective and *cost-efficient* care.

Healthcare IT functions are extensive. There are critical needs in areas such as clinical operation, financial operations and analysis, facility management and planning, and marketing development. Yet the healthcare industry has been behind the curve in IT spending. Figure 10–1 is a representative chart of IT spending within healthcare and other industries. This failure to invest in IT has hurt the industry by holding it back from making some of the major productivity strides achieved in other industries. For example, the auto industry is a leader in automated production processes and the banking industry, which specializing in the movement of money in both global and local marketplaces, could not exist without major advances in IT. After all, the proliferation of automated teller machines allowed banks to reduce their labor costs while improving services to the customers who needed more than basic services.

So, healthcare is late to the IT table. But it is starting to close the gap in IT spending in the very late 1990s. Many healthcare chief executive officers (CEOs) and their boards are gaining a greater understanding of the organizational needs and capabilities of IT. They have accepted the need to move beyond the 2.0% to 2.5% average spending on IT. Figure 10–2 provides an indication of the types of costs that need to be expended. Each of these items has its own expense history. For example, over the past few years the cost of computer hardware has

Traditional IT Spending
Estimated IT spending as a percentage of operating costs

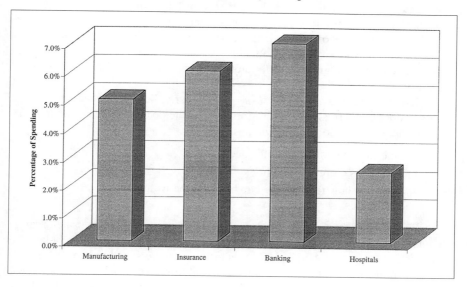

Potential IT Spending in Healthcare

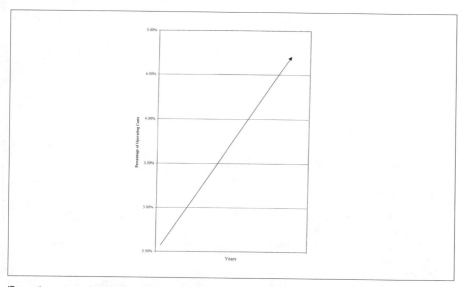

IT operating costs consist of hardware, software, telecommunications, depreciation, personnel, and other.

plummeted. Computer users now have hardware that is thousands of times faster with the ability to store and hold much greater amounts of data than just a few decades ago. On the other hand, the cost of IT personnel has increased much quicker than the rate of normal inflation as a result of the demand for personnel who can write the programs and fix any of the glitches that arise in the course of operations.

RHMC, like most of its industry counterparts, has researched its future IT needs. It does this formally through a formal IT strategic plan, updated annually. The goal of the plan is to do the following.

- Determine the organization's needs
- Review its current capabilities
- Ascertain how to close the gap between the its needs and current capabilities

The IT plan starts with a review of the strategic initiatives that the organization is attempting to achieve, in accordance with the main strategic plan. The strategic initiatives that the IT plan needs to focus on are stated in Box 10–1.

Each of these four strategic organizational initiatives need to be aligned with specific IT needs that are not currently being addressed. At RHMC this led to the determination that there should be a concentration of five key areas.

1. Build IT systems and processes to strengthen the customer support capabilities. In this case customers are defined as patients and physicians.
2. Build systems to support enhanced clinical process management and data access.
3. Integrate data and reporting to support enhanced decision making.
4. Build the IT infrastructure and delivery capabilities.
5. Become Year 2000 compliant.

B O X   10–1

RIDGELAND HEIGHTS MEDICAL CENTER

Strategic Initiatives

- Providing superior healthcare to all clients of the system and improving the health status of the community
- Integrating physicians into the health delivery system and expanding the primary care physician network
- Managing healthcare delivery across the continuum
- Reducing cost per unit of healthcare service by increasing utilization and efficiencies

Y2K IMPLEMENTATION

Although each of these areas is significant in its own right, the last item, to become Year 2000 compliant, superseded all the others beginning in mid 1997. As most everyone knows by now, the Y2K problem could potentially impact almost any electromechanical system that employs a microchip (the computer's brain). This is not limited to only computers. In hospitals and other healthcare facilities, some of the medical devices attached to patient's bodies such as heart monitors and IV pumps use microchips.

Still, as with any industry, there are critical areas that cause the greatest concern. For example, while healthcare organizations worry about patient devices, the airline industry worries about planes falling out of the sky at 12:01AM, January 1, 2000. Thus, the concerns are widespread. These concerns overshadowed most other IT planning in the two years preceding the millennium. At RHMC this meant the establishment of an expansive committee of staff and managers with responsibility for systems that could be affected by the millennium bug. This committee was headed by the organization's CIO. The committee was charged with finding and fixing every potential glitch before it could affect operations at the turn of the century.

This committee received a great deal of visibility because of its focus. Additionally, the finance committee and board were greatly concerned about limiting any potential damage before the fact. Beginning in early 1998, the CIO reported on the progress of the committee's efforts at every finance committee meeting. A report was developed to assist in the reporting. It became the standard summary for all Y2K issues. Table 10–1 is a copy of the report that was delivered at the October 1999 finance committee, just 70 days before the fateful date.

The report was developed in a logical way starting with the awareness of this potentially grave problem. It moved on down to project organization and planning and the resources that needed to be expended in order to become compliant. It moved onto the actual process of determining compliance, such as performing an inventory of all potential Y2K items in the general categories of software applications, biomedical and diagnostic devices, general purpose computers, IT and building infrastructure and control systems, and readiness of its trading partners. After identification of the inventory, the task force evaluated the importance of the item and the risk of failure. The task force then tested every item for compliance, even if the manufacturer certified it as Y2K compliant. If the item was deemed noncompliant, the task force decided whether to renovate, replace, or retire it depending on need and use.

Throughout this process, the procedures were relatively straightforward. The real problems began after the decisions were made on all of the items that the task force can see and touch. For example, many items that were the responsibility of the trading partners couldn't be tested, yet they may be crucial to the continued operation of the organization, such as receipts of funds from its third-party vendors. To deal with these issues, contingency plans were drawn up in the event they come to pass. Finally, a crisis management plan had been prepared and a team had been assembled to fight any IT fires beginning 12:01 AM, January 1, 2000.

Ridgeland Heights Medical Center
Year 2000 Compliance Report as of September 30, 1999

Task	Status	Target Date
Task Awareness		
1. Top leadership is aware and committed	Done	
2. Y2K compliance program is enterprise-wide and includes computer hardware and software, medical equipment, infrastructure/control systems, and trading partners	Done	
3. All staff have been informed of potential problems and actions	Done	
Project Organization and Planning		
1. One senior leader has overall Y2K responsibility	Done	
2. Y2K committee has overall Y2K responsibility	Done	
3. A formal project plan is in place	Done	
4. A legal review has been conducted on Y2K plan	Done	
Resources		
1. Resources required to identify, correct, test, and implement changes have been identified including personnel, office space, test environment, tools, contractors	95%	11/30/99
2. A preliminary Y2K budget has been approved by senior management	Done	
3. Users are aware of their required participation in Y2K	90%	12/15/99
Inventory/Compliance Letters		
1. An inventory of all equipment/systems has been completed for the following.		
• Software application	Done	
• Biomedical and diagnostic equipment	Done	
• General purpose computers/infrastructure/control systems	Done	
• Trading partners	Done	
2. Compliance letters have been obtained from all hardware and software vendors and all service providers for those same four areas	90%	11/30/99
Evaluation/Risk Assessment		
1. Vendor responses have been evaluated (1,100 vendors)	85%	11/15/99
2. Y2K risk has been assessed, and reported compliant items have been prioritized for testing/certification (920 vendors)	80%	11/30/99
3. Y2K risk has been assessed and noncompliant items have been prioritized for compliance management (180)	Done	
Testing/Certification		
1. Test plans have been established for compliance within the four categories	90%	
2. Testing environment including methods and tools are in place		
3. Compliant items have been tested and labeled for the four categories	Done	
Compliance Management		
1. Decision to renovate, replace, or retire noncompliant items have been made	92%	
2. Budget and other resource requirements have been reassessed and committed by senior management	Done	
3. Updates and replacement items have been purchased	88%	12/31/99
4. Testing environment including methods and tools are in place	Done	
5. A detailed implementation plan has been established	Done	
6. Documentation has been updated	92%	12/31/99
7. Testing is complete	90%	12/31/99
Implementation		
1. Necessary hardware, software, and equipment changes are in production environment	Done	
2. New operational procedures are in place	Done	
3. Back-up procedures are in place	Done	
Contingency Planning		
1. Contingency plans have been established for each item	Done	
2. Review of business interruption insurance coverage has been completed	Done	
3. Disaster recovery team is prepared to deal with system failures	Done	
Crisis Management		
1. Internal and external communication plans have been established	95%	12/15/99
2. Crisis management plan has been developed	Done	

The board is relatively pleased to see the significant progress that has been made in most areas. In addition, in performing their fiduciary responsibility, the finance committee retained the services of their auditing firm to review the progress at a detailed level with the CIO. Still, even with all this planning, no one is absolutely sure of the impacts on January 1, 2000. Because of this, most of the RHMC management team and clinical staff are expected to be in the facility at that time. The New Year's Eve party of the millennium for these people will take place in the organization's cafeteria at about 9:00 in the evening.

INFORMATION TECHNOLOGY STRATEGIC PLAN INITIATIVES

Although the Y2K project has absorbed a great deal of RHMC's personnel and capital resources for the previous two years, many of the other needs that were identified during the IT strategic plan still need to be accomplished. Interestingly, the Y2K project significantly supports the plan requirements in most areas. Let's look again at the other four IT strategic plan initiatives.

1. Build IT systems and processes to strengthen the customer support capabilities. In this case customers are defined as patients and physicians.
2. Build systems to support enhanced clinical process management and data access.
3. Integrate data and reporting to support enhanced decision making.
4. Build the IT infrastructure and delivery capabilities.

Because RHMC's current computer system is not Y2K compliant, the Y2K project allowed the organization to start fresh, revamping an IT infrastructure and delivery capability that will help strengthen customer support capabilities and enhance clinical process management and data access. The third IT strategic initiative—integrating data and reporting to support enhanced decision making—is an IT feature that, to a great extent, does not fully exist at RHMC and thus will be postponed until after the crucial Y2K fixes are completed.

Selection of a New Healthcare Information System

The opportunities to improve all the other features and functions were enormous. So, in mid 1997, the RHMC administration decided to enlist the aid of a computer consultant who would help them select the best possible system for their needs. They chose to interview a few consulting candidates in order to select the consultant who was the best fit for their culture and needs. They were aware that consultants who help in IT selection processes can be very expensive if allowed to perform extensive and unnecessary services. Instead, they chose a consultant to assist them with a narrow scope of work:[1]

---

[1] Berger, S., Ciotti, V.G. (1993). HIS Consultants: When They Are Necessary, and Why? *Healthcare Financial Management,* June, p. 45.

1. Creating the initial list of suitable vendors for RHMC's size
2. Helping to prepare the request for price quotation (RPQ), a 20-page document that asks the vendor for a defined set of information and allows the consultant and organization to gain an understanding of those IT vendors being queried without creating an unmanageable and virtually useful set of information[2]
3. Summarizing the information contained in the RPQs returned by the vendors
4. Facilitating a focused yet streamlined selection process (The staff of RHMC performed much of the analysis work related to the software applications with which they would be involved, such as evaluating the features, functions, and ease of use and applying objective scoring criteria to determine the selection.)

After extensive negotiations, RHMC and the selected vendor got down to the always troublesome implementation stage. In this stage, there were some very severe time constraints because the organization was backed up against an unmovable date, December 31, 1999, after which the Y2K bug would bite their current system. Because of the time it took to select a system, negotiate the contract, and perform significant upgrades to their IT infrastructure, the organization had only nine months to perform their complete implementation plan if they were to be done by April 1, 1999. It was important that the system be installed no later than that date because of the following reasons.

1. There was a possibility that some Year 2000 glitches could occur early in 1999.
2. There was a need to build in some time cushion just in case the system was not installed in a timely fashion.
3. No installation specialist/programmer/analyst may have been available from the software company to complete the implementation.
4. Preregistration of obstetrics patients (nine months in the future) would not have been available under the old systems.

If the major reason for acquiring and installing the new system was to overcome the Y2K problem, the secondary reason was to upgrade the organization's IT capabilities as expressed by the strategic plan. Therefore, as each department manager reviewed the features and functions of the available computer vendors, they kept in mind their departmental needs as well as their wants (the "wish list").

Features and Functions of the Selected Information Technology System

The features and functions that were ultimately chosen reflect many of the areas of focus in the IT strategic plan. Each of the four major initiatives (customer, clinical,

---

[2] Gibson, R.P., Berger, S., Ciotti, V.G. (1992). Selecting an Information System Without an RFP. *Healthcare Financial Management,* June, p. 48.

decision making, and IT infrastructure) were extensively reviewed. The "gap analysis" revealed particularly significant needs in the clinical and infrastructure areas.

The baseline system that was to be replaced included the following major areas.

- Financial (general ledger, accounts payable, payroll)
- Patient management (patient registration, accounts receivable)
- Clinical (order entry and results reporting for tests and treatments)
- Physician support (practice management, clinical information access, managed care support)
- Home health agency support (billing, coding, clinical charting)
- SNF support (registration, billing, coding)

The additional features and functions that RHMC would be gaining with its new system acquisition included the following.

- Patient integration (integrated scheduling and registration, enterprise-wide master patient index)
- Physician support (integrated clinical and administrative information access)
- Clinical data integration (nurse charting, clinical point-of-care applications, clinical data repository, clinical outcome measurement systems, electronic medical record implementation, disease management, encounter reporting)

Additionally, all of these clinical and financial upgrades requires significant improvements to the IT infrastructure.

- Local area network upgrade (wiring, data closets, integration hardware)
- Additional staff support (more full time equivalent employees [FTEs] in applications and hardware support, and network engineering)
- Additional capability for multiple, complex project execution

Much of what RHMC planned was consistent with various surveys that had been taken during the late 1990s. In general, for a majority of integrated delivery systems and hospitals, upgrading the IT infrastructure and patient-focused information were the priorities. In descending order, healthcare IT directors considered the following items as most important in fulfilling their organization's mission.

1. Upgrading the IT infrastructure
2. Integrating systems in a multivendor environment
3. Reengineering to a patient-centered computing environment
4. Migrating to client server systems
5. Implementing an Internet strategy
6. Developing an Intranet

7. Implementing mobile access for caregivers

8. Outsourcing IT services[3]

Financial Implications to RHMC

The scope of work described above is extremely costly. In fact, it easily exceeds the 2.0% to 2.5% of average organizational spending on IT mentioned earlier in the chapter. Table 10–2 shows the extent of the spending by RHMC over the three-year period between 1997 and 1999. It would appear to be an extraordinary amount of money for an organization of its size. Yet, it was absolutely necessary, and RHMC was far from unique. One survey notes that integrated delivery systems expect to spend an average of $5 million just to fix their Y2K problems. This does not include the cost of upgrading their systems to enhance features and functionality. Other estimates put the cost of Y2K fixes for integrated delivery systems at $10 million to $20 million. Some may be spending more.

Knowing how to count the cost of Y2K fixes as compared to other upgrades is difficult. At RHMC, there are a number of ways that IT costs, capital and operation, are counted. For example, back in Chapter 3, Table 3–5 was a representation of RHMC's five-year capital budget, which included $3,000,000 in 1998 and $5,000,000 in 1999 for IT. In Chapter 8, Table 8–3 showed the final 1999 capital budget, which was prepared six months after the strategic plan. It shows only $635,000 funded for IT. Yet in Table 10–2, the total amount spent for Y2K, as represented in just the conversion of the main healthcare information system from a noncompliant system to a compliant system at RHMC is reported as $13,150,000.

Each of these reports are correct in their own right and in their own reported time period. The earlier strategic financial plan capital budget did attempt to include all the known capital costs associated with the Y2K problem and all other upgrades. It turned out that even just six months earlier, the known costs were severely understated. When the 2000 capital budget was prepared and approved, the revised 1999 capital had already been approved and requisitioned. No additional funds were therefore required in the 2000 budget. In fact, so much money had been approved and requisitioned for 1999 that there was very little IT capital equipment left to request in 2000.

In addition, it is important to note that IT costs for Y2K and other issues are not only limited to capital expenditures. The operating costs of labor and supplies count, too. There are extra costs for consultants to perform evaluation and risk assessments, replacement labor when the clinical personnel are being trained on the newly installed Y2K compliant system, and the cost of redesigning all of the organization's printed forms.

All of the extra IT capital costs that were determined to be needed in 1999, particularly the Y2K costs, were funded out of equity. RHMC's board decided that the current year should not bear the brunt of this once-in-a-millennium problem.

---

[3] 1997 Healthcare Information and Management Systems Society (HIMSS)/Hewlett-Packard Leadership Survey.

[4] Elliott, J. (1998). Y2K Tops List of Priorities. *Healthcare Informatics,* September, p. 17.

TABLE 10–2

Ridgeland Heights Medical Center
Information Technology Capital Expenses for Computer Installation
1997–1999

Application Software (Financial/Operational)	
General ledger	
Accounts payable	
Payroll/personnel	
Medical records abstracting	
Medical records coding	
Enterprise medical records	
Patient accounting/billing/collections	
Patient registration	
Automated scheduling	
Data repository	
Subtotal financial/operational software	$ 720,000
Application Software (Clinical)	
Order entry and results reporting	
Radiology	
Pharmacy	
Automated nurse charting	
Subtotal clinical software	330,000
Hardware	
Computer servers	
Network	
Peripherals:	
PCs (800 units)	
Laser printers (200 units)	
Miscellaneous	
Subtotal hardware	3,300,000
Network Infrastructure	
Architect and engineering fees	
Network closets/cabling/electrical/outlets	
Expansion of computer room	
Renovations for additional classrooms	
Subtotal network Infrastructure	4,850,000
Other Hardware and Software Costs	
Interface engine	
Interface programming (12 systems)	
Conversions (8 systems)	
Subtotal other hardware and software costs	550,000
Vendor Implementation Fees	
Implementation fees to vendors (13 systems)	
Travel expenses for implementation and training	
Subtotal vendor implementation fees	1,800,000
Implementation Fees for RHMC	
Information technology staff*	
Consultants	
Implementation team*	
User training*	
Subtotal RHMC implementation fees	1,600,000
Total Health Information System Implementation Costs	$ 13,150,000

*Cost transferred to IT system conversion budget to represent the time spent by RHMC staff working on the new computer system implementation.

Therefore, the administration did not have to limit capital acquisitions in non-IT areas and was able to prepare a relatively normal capital budget.

How Improvements to Clinical Systems Benefits RHMC's Financial Outcomes

The biggest benefits that RHMC expects to obtain from its upgraded information system are in the clinical services area. New software modules for nursing and ancillary department staff are expected to generate service and patient satisfaction improvements. The modules are expected to automate some of the clinicians documentation, freeing up more time for clinical analysis. The clinicians who would being using the system in the ordinary course of the day include the following.

- Physicians
- Nurses
- Physical therapists
- Speech therapists
- Occupational therapists
- Cardiac services personnel, such as cardiac catherization, cardiac rehabilitation, and other cardiology
- Respiratory therapists
- Pharmacists
- Pastoral care
- Dieticians

Basically any clinician who currently is required to document the service or education component of the patient's encounter would be able to perform this documentation online. The benefits of this online documentation (or "charting" as it is more commonly known as) are significant. They include all of the following.

- Because the clinician can document online from any computer, they will no longer have to spend time locating the patient's paper chart. This is a time saver.
- The computers will be located at several areas around the inpatient floors, in the patient's room and in every outpatient setting. This will allow not only input capabilities, but it will also allow the clinician to review previous clinical notes as far back as has been input into the computer.
- Clinicians will also be able to review and trend items like laboratory results across various time periods, such as years. This is not effectively possible with paper charts unless very special requests are made and the analysis can never be done timely. This new ability will enhance the clinician's ability to make quicker and more accurate diagnoses.
- Computer terminals will be located not only in patient areas, but there will also be terminals installed in the physician lounges and for those

physicians associated with the hospital, connections can be made to terminals in their offices. This will allow physicians to check the progress of their patients online and in real time for lab, radiology, or cardiology results and/or nurses notes. Because of the increased resources and speed of the analysis, the physician will be able to prescribe treatment plans or drugs sooner. This should allow the patient to recover quicker, a plus for the patient, the patient's insurance company, and the healthcare organization that is reimbursed on case rates or low per diems.

- Online documentation improves legibility.
- Patient satisfaction should improve as they realize the benefits of the increased speed of treatment and recovery from their illness or trauma.
- Clinical documentation is always better the sooner it is recorded. The location of the terminals at the bedside, in the physician lounges, and in the physicians' offices should shorten the time frame to recording the documentation. Swifter documentation leads to better documentation, which leads to better clinical analysis. This ultimately leads to better coding and reimbursement!
- Quality of care should increase because nursing and other clinical personnel will be spending less time on administrative/clerical matters and more time at the patient's bedside, administering care.

In summary, the value of clinical systems is still virtually untapped. But at RHMC and many other healthcare organizations, the use of computers for documenting, analyzing, diagnosing, and researching the patient's condition is at the starting line. It should revolutionize the practice of medical care.

IMPACT OF THE INTERNET

Healthcare IT offers greater promise in the future than has been experienced in the past. There are opportunities for unprecedented progress in patient care applications that could that should have very positive implications on financial performance of healthcare organizations. In addition, there are nonfinance applications that can have very positive benefits for the healthcare organization. For example, two years ago, RHMC developed a Web site for community access to information about RHMC's patient services with hot links to dozens of consumer, clinical, and professional health-related Web sites. The RHMC Web site enjoys over 100 hits a day, creating a closer bond with consumers in its community.

In addition, RHMC has planned some major Internet applications for the next two years.

- Allow physicians Internet access from the physician's lounge and medical library for medical research. This is a burgeoning area of interest for physicians and allows them to find the types of information that can aid them in physician diagnoses and treatment issues. Further in the future, the physician will have this access at the patient's bedside and in the outpatient treatment areas.

- Provide selected key users (managers and directors) access to the World Wide Web to research new revenue-generating ideas and regulatory issues. It has already been shown to be a big asset in reducing the time spent in these areas and has enhanced the managers' abilities to keep more current in leading edge changes in their areas of expertise.

- Create an Intranet so that departments or divisions like human resources and nursing can save money and increase access to policy and procedure manuals. Intranets work like normal Web browsers but without using an external modem. Instead, using a big computer server and the organization's local area network, manuals of information can now be accessed in an easy-to-use manner. Staff looking for information can easily access it using the FIND key without having to slog through books of several thousand pages.

In summary, the uses for IT in healthcare have only just begun to have a dramatic impact on patient care and finances. The future for technology in healthcare is limitless. RHMC, like most other healthcare organizations, is running as fast as it can in order not to be left behind.

BUDGET PRESENTATION TO THE BOARD FINANCE COMMITTEE

After all the work of the previous five months, RHMC's administration will present its proposed millennium budget to the finance committee of the board for approval. Upon approval by the finance committee, it will be sent to the full board of directors for final approval. This is usually a formality as the full board has generally ceded the responsibility of detailed review and debate to the finance committee. Still, there is an occasional controversy that may occur, perhaps related to the level of budgeted capital expenditures in relation to net incomes.

For example, the administration may have proposed spending more money for capital acquisition and replacements than is available from cash inflows as shown in Table 10–3. It's possible that the finance committee could decide to approve this scenario because it has been presented as a one-time problem. This problem could be the result of a major shift or reduction in third-party reimbursements, such as the Medicare Balanced Budget Act or the incursion of managed care into the organization's region. Yet the full board may be unsympathetic to the argument that allows the administration to dip into its "rainy day" funds. It could therefore decide not to approve the upcoming budget and instead return it to the administration with instructions to rethink the cash flow results so that there is no cash flow loss (i.e., reduced planned capital spending).

In this case, RHMC's board has already discussed this issue and decided that if there were a proposed cash flow loss because of Y2K issues and dramatic changes in the reimbursement systems, they would allow it. So the presentation by

TABLE 10–3

Ridgeland Heights Medical Center
Cash Inflows and Outflows
Based on 2000 Budget

	1999 Projected	2000 Budget
Cash Inflows		
Operating margin	$ 3,100	$ 2,920
Add back: depreciation	10,500	11,500
Cash inflows	13,600	14,420
Cash Outflows		
Capital expenditures	10,000	11,500
Principle payments on outstanding debt	3,500	3,600
Cash outflows	13,500	15,100
Net cash inflows/(outflows)	$ 100	$ (680)

TABLE 10–4

Ridgeland Heights Medical Center
2000 Proposed Budget
Table of Contents

administration proceeds. At RHMC, there is 23-page document that is presented over a two-hour time frame. It is important to note that this document was sent out to the finance committee members one week before the meeting so that the members could review it in detail before the actual meeting. Table 10–4 is a representation of the table of contents. The presentation includes chart, graphs, tables, and variance analyses that are used to enhance the committee's understanding of the budget.

There is an interesting feature to the structure of this budget. Several of the budget document pages are designed to look exactly like several of the pages presented to the finance committee in their monthly financial statements. This is a great time saver to the finance staff. In prior years, the finance staff had to scurry around throughout the year to extrapolate budgeted volumes, or ratio analysis data that had not been specifically reported during the budget process. So several years ago, the RHMC finance administrator redesigned both the monthly financial statement and the annual budget report to align the outputs. All parties were pleased with the outcome of the alignment. It resulted in the elimination of many obsolete analyses and the inclusion of pages that matched the monthly financial report, such as the ratio analysis/key success factors (page 5) and key volume assumptions and gross revenue percentages (page 6).

The CEO's memorandum to the board is designed to put the entire budget into perspective from the individual with the primary organizational responsibility for success or failure. In effect this final budget product is the financial representation of the CEO's goal and vision for the organization. Therefore this memo is a personal message from the CEO to the board responsible for approving the vision. For the Year 2000 budget, the CEO's vision and the board's vision are somewhat at odds because the operating margin does not meet the board's 4% target. In this case, the CEOs memo becomes an essential tool for formally describing the reasons for the divergence. Box 10–2 shows how personal and direct this memo can get.

Following the CEO's memorandum is the final proposed statement of revenues and expenses, shown in Table 10–5. We have already seen the development of these budgeted revenues and expenses. But the board gets to see only this final version. Ratio analysis (page 5) and key volume assumptions (page 6) are then provided to place the budgeted bottom lines into context. In addition, there are explanation of variances provided as represented by the analysis of revenues and contractual allowances (page 7), salary expense and FTE summary (page 8), salaries reconciliation (page 9), employee benefits (page 10), and interest expenses (the debt issues, page 11). There are also graphs that show selected financial and statistical trend results over the previous five or six years.

Table 10–6 places much of the expected financial results in context for the finance committee and the board. It begins with the ratios that directly relate to the organization's strategic financial plan that allows the board members to review the trends in these areas. It continues with accounts receivable information, moves towards staffing information, and ends with other pertinent patient information reflecting financial outcomes. This page is set up to mimic the information presented in the financial statements every month.

In the Key Volumes Assumptions (Table 10–7), the analysis of inpatient volumes begins with admissions. This is a big change from prior years when revenues were based on per diem (or per day) reimbursement. It meant that the healthcare organization was paid for each day of stay as well as all the additional diagnostic and

B O X   10–2

THE CEO'S MEMORANDUM TO THE BOARD

October 16, 1999

To: Members of the Finance Committee
From: Richard M. Samuelson, President and Chief Executive Officer
Subject: 2000 Budget

The 2000 Budget is noteworthy for the organization. The federal government's 1997 Balanced Budget Act is beginning its third full year, producing severe consequences for the industry at large and Ridgeland Heights Medical Center in particular. Payment reductions from managed care are also accelerating, but the demand for service from patients and medical staff continues unabated. Our predicament is a national and local issue as well and was anticipated to occur several years ago during discussions of prior strategic financial plans. The fact that the "sky did not fall" previously is a reflection of the growth in outpatient revenues and our ability to delay the impact of managed care market rates (thereby generating favorable variances in contractual allowances).

The question today is, "How should management and the board evaluate our budget?" Clearly, the most significant trend is the sharp rise in the percentage of contractual allowances, which causes net revenues to remain relatively flat. Management suggests the board consider the following viewpoints.

1. The most important consideration is that we provide quality patient care and that service shortfalls are not attributed to budget considerations. The human resources committee specifically concluded that quality should not be compromised to maintain short-term margin targets. However, on a long-term basis, both quality and financial targets must be achieved. Our ability to absorb short-term declines in operating margins is a recognized asset that the committee was willing to deploy.

2. In spite of the decline in operating margins, our historical cash flow has generated a strong balance sheet including $130 million of cash and investments through September 1999. In 2000, we will generate a negative cash flow as a result of projected capital expenditures exceeding our operating margin plus depreciation expenses. This one-time reduction needs to be absorbed as we restructure our services to further maximize our financial position.

3. Although the 2000 budgets are submitted for approval, ideas to improve actual hospital results are being developed, including the following.

Continued.

THE CEO'S MEMORANDUM TO THE BOARD *(concluded)*

Existing Program Enhancement or Elimination and New Program Development.

- Analysis is being done regarding home health and skilled nursing to determine if they will continue to have a positive contribution margin. If not, other opportunities may be considered.
- Development of cardiac surgery and other new programs has not been included. These projects will have short-term negative impacts as they ramp up.

Cost Reduction Efforts are Ongoing.

- We are exploring merging some of our outpatient clinical programs, such as home healthcare, to improve overall financial results.
- Further staff reductions may arise from a new management engineering program. The strategic financial plan anticipated the need for staffing cuts.
- Efforts to further the effective use of clinical pathways and to develop "best practices" are necessary. This requires focused physician leadership intended to improve product standardization and utilization management.

4. Putting into context the risk areas imbedded within the budget is important.
   - Inpatient or outpatient volumes may not be achievable.
   - Managed care contracts, which historically have been favorable, may be at or below budget in 2000.
   - Budgeted salary reductions will be difficult and have been elusive to achieve in the past.
   - Pharmaceutical prices and use may be problematic.
   - Realized gains may decline as a result of market conditions.

In conclusion, the lack of revenue growth, in spite of volume and price increases, is the critical problem that exposes the risks identified. This requires that management remain focused on the successful execution of the strategic plan to develop new or improved clinical programs, medical staff size and capability, and cost-reduction efforts. The growth of our employed physician staff and the acquisition of new MSO clients is critical to decreasing the losses associated with this business segment. It is also essential to generating new business for the hospital. The era of declining margins makes it imperative that we maximize the returns from our core business and our investments.

---

therapeutic services it rendered during these inpatient stays. This was particularly important through 1983 when most third-party insurers paid full published charges and Medicare paid their own computed actual cost for each day of stay in the hospital. Skilled nursing facilities and physician practices were treated similarly. Since then, Medicare changed its inpatient reimbursement methodology and no longer relies on per diem costs. The Prospective Payment System (PPS) pays the organization on a per case basis. Therefore for Medicare revenue, admission is now the statistic that determines net revenues, not patient days.

T A B L E 10-5

Ridgeland Heights Medical Center
Preliminary Budgeted Statement of Operations
For the Budget Year-to-Date Ending December 31, 2000 (in thousands)

	1998 Actual	1999 Budget	1999 Projected	2000 Budget	Percentage Change 00B vs 99B	Percentage Change 00B vs 99P
Revenues						
Inpatient revenue	73,000	79,000	77,800	87,360	10.58	12.29
Outpatient revenue	72,000	77,000	76,100	89,440	16.16	17.53
Total patient revenue	145,000	156,000	153,900	176,800	13.33	14.88
Less						
Contractual and other adjustments	(49,000)	(60,000)	(59,000)	(77,100)	28.50	30.68
Charity care	(2,600)	(2,700)	(2,500)	(3,000)	11.11	20.00
Net patient service revenue	93,400	93,300	92,400	96,700	3.64	4.65
Add						
Premium revenue	2,100	2,100	2,100	1,000	-52.38	-52.38
Investment income	6,400	5,000	6,000	6,000	20.00	0.00
Other operating income	1,200	1,200	1,100	1,200	0.00	9.09
Total revenue	103,100	101,600	101,600	104,900	3.25	3.25
Expenses						
Salaries	36,000	35,500	36,500	37,480	5.58	2.68
Contract labor	1,000	1,400	800	1,200	-14.29	50.00
Fringe benefits	7,000	7,000	6,900	7,300	4.29	5.80
Total salaries and benefits	44,000	43,900	44,200	45,980	4.74	4.03
Bad debts	4,600	4,400	4,400	4,000	-9.09	-9.09
Patient care supplies	15,500	15,200	16,000	16,600	9.21	3.75
Professional and management fees	3,600	3,400	3,800	3,800	11.76	0.00
Purchased services	5,400	5,600	5,600	5,600	0.00	0.00
Operation of plant (including utilities)	2,600	2,700	2,600	2,800	3.70	7.69
Depreciation	11,000	11,000	10,500	11,500	4.55	9.52
Interest and financing expenses	7,400	7,400	7,400	7,200	-2.70	-2.70
Other	3,800	3,800	4,000	4,500	18.42	12.50
Total expenses	97,900	97,400	98,500	101,980	4.70	3.53
Operation margin	5,200	4,200	3,100	2,920	-30.48	-5.81
Nonoperating Income						
Gain/(loss) on investments	1,200	1,200	1,400	1,000	-16.67	-28.57
Total nonoperating income	1,200	1,200	1,400	1,000	-16.67	-28.57
Net income	6,400	5,400	4,500	3,920	-27.41	-12.89

Ridgeland Heights Medical Center
Ratio Analysis/Key Success Factors
2000 Proposed Budget

	1998 Actual	1999 Budget	1999 Projected	2000 Budget	Favorable/Unfavorable 2000 B vs. 1999 P Amount	Favorable/Unfavorable 2000 B vs. 1999 P Percent
Strategic Financial Plan						
Operating margin	0.0%	4.1%	3.1%	2.8%	-0.3%	-8.8%
Total margin	0.0%	5.3%	4.4%	3.7%	-0.7%	-15.6%
Current ratio	1.27	1.33	1.35	1.28	(0.07)	-5.2%
Cushion ratio	12.19	12.20	12.20	12.13	(0.08)	-0.6%
Days cash on hand	525.87	510.12	501.98	485.50	(16.48)	-3.3%
Average age of plant	6.55	7.24	7.35	7.85	0.50	6.8%
Capital expenses as a percentage of expenses	18.8%	18.9%	18.2%	18.3%	0.00	0.9%
Debt service coverage	2.28	2.16	2.04	2.04	0.00	0.1%
Debt/capitalization	64.6%	62.2%	62.5%	61.8%	(0.01)	-1.1%
Return on equity	7.66%	7.10%	6.80%	6.50%	(0.003)	-4.4%
Return on assets	2.43%	2.10%	1.99%	1.90%	(0.00)	-4.5%
Accounts Receivable Information						
Inpatient AR days	59.3	60.1	59.6	58	(1.60)	-2.7%
Outpatient AR days	65.1	66.5	65.4	64	(1.40)	-2.1%
Bad debt expense	$4,600,000	$4,400,000	$4,400,000	$4,000,000	$(400,000)	-9.1%
Net write-offs	$4,000,000	$4,300,000	$4,700,000	$4,600,000	$(100,000)	-2.1%
Allowance for doubtful accounts (ADA)	$5,800,000	$5,900,000	$5,600,000	$5,000,000	$(600,000)	-10.7%
(Also known as reserve for bad debts)						
ADA as a percentage of AR	26.4%	26.8%	25.5%	22.7%	(0.03)	-10.7
Staffing Information						
Total FTEs	980.0	1023.1	1026.0	1005.9	(20.10)	-2.0%
Salaries, benefits & contract labor as a	4.10	4.17	4.13	4.00	(0.13)	-0.6%
percentage of net revenues & premium revenues	45.8%	47.1%	47.8%	47.5%	(0.00)	-0.6%
Other Patient Information						
Medicare case mix index	1.32	1.33	1.34	1.34	—	0.0%
All-payor case mix index	0.91	1.02	1.04	1.05	0.01	1.0%
Cost per adjusted patient Day	$ 1,122	$ 1,024	$ 1,017	$ 944	$ (73)	-7.1%
Cost per adjusted admission	$ 4,774	$ 4,200	$ 4,136	$ 3,856	(281)	-6.8%
I/P managed care contractual adj. %	26.0%	29.0%	28.0%	32.0%	0.04	14.3%
O/P managed care contractual adj. %	20.0%	24.0%	22.0%	26.0%	0.04	18.2%

TABLE 10-7

Ridgeland Heights Medical Center
2000 Proposed Budget
Key Volume Assumptions and Gross Revenue Percentage

	1998 Actual	1999 Budget	1999 Projected	2000 Budget	Favorable/Unfavorable 2000 B vs. 1999 P Amount	Percent
Admissions						
Adult	8,100	8,760	9,023	9,787	764	8.5
Newborn	1,950	2,145	2,165	2,382	217	10.0
Skilled nursing	800	840	850	900	50	5.9
Total admissions	10,850	11,745	12,038	13,069	1,031	8.6
Average Length of Stay						
Adult	3.89	4.05	4.05	4.20	0.15	3.7
Newborn	2.00	2.00	2.00	2.00	—	0.0
Skilled nursing	3.89	4.05	4.05	4.20	0.15	3.7
Newborn	2.00	2.00	2.00	2.00	—	0.0
Skilled nursing	11.00	10.00	9.50	8.30	(1.20)	-12.6
Total length of stay	4.07	4.10	4.07	4.08	0.01	0.2
Patient Days						
Adult	31,500	35,496	36,561	41,131	4,570	12.5
Newborn	3,900	4,290	4,330	4,763	433	10.0
Skilled nursing	8,800	8,400	8,075	7,470	(605)	-7.5
Total patient days	44,200	48,186	48,966	53,364	4,398	9.0
Outpatient Services and Visits						
Emergency visits	19,000	20,000	20,200	21,816	1,616	8.0
Outpatient surgery	4,500	5,000	5,200	5,616	416	8.0
Same day surgery	3,700	4,000	4,500	4,860	360	8.0
Observation patients	1,950	2,000	1,890	2,041	151	8.0
Home health services	26,000	30,000	27,000	25,000	(2,000)	-7.4
All other outpatients	112,000	120,000	124,000	133,920	9,920	8.0
Total O/P services and visits	167,150	181,000	182,790	193,253	10,463	5.7
Gross Patient Revenue Percentage by Payor						
Medicare	40.0%	39.0%	38.0%	37.5%	(0.005)	-1.3
Medicaid	4.0%	5.0%	6.0%	6.0%	—	0.0
Managed care (HMO/PPO)	26.0%	28.0%	30.0%	31.5%	0.015	5.0
All others	30.0%	28.0%	26.0%	25.0%	(0.010)	-3.8
	100.0%	100.0%	100.0%	100.0%	—	—

Although many managed care companies have recently adopted per diem reimbursement as their basis for their reimbursement to hospitals, their per diem is based on negotiations with the provider, not on a cost basis. And because managed care companies have extremely stringent utilization controls, which restrict the number of days that patients can stay in the hospital, the number of days is limited. Hence, the organization earns little, if any margin from this per diem reimbursement. Therefore, while patient days are still an important statistic for determining variable costs and operating capacity, it no longer occupies the primary slot at the top of the key volumes assumptions page.

The analysis of revenues and contractual allowances (Table 10–8) is very useful in explaining levels of changes between the years. In particular, it allows the reviewers to see how contractual adjustment changes can positively or negatively impact net revenues. In addition, it breaks down the gross and net revenues into units (per case, per day) that are more easily understandable from the standpoint of financial analysis. It highlights the fact that gross revenue increases do not translate into positive net revenue results, especially in an era of declining reimbursements, like the late 1990s/early 21st century.

The remaining analyses represent expense issues, both salary and nonsalary. There is usually little discussion on most of these items, except for staffing levels and its resulting impact on salary expenses. The analyses usually are able to pinpoint the issues that are driving the staffing expenses. For example page 8 of the budget package (Table 10–9) clearly summarizes the changes in FTEs, which as we've seen in Table 7–3 of Chapter 7 has the most impact on staffing expenses. In the case of RHMC, it is clear from Table 10–9 that staffing has fluctuated as the administration has attempted to rightsize the staff through productivity and volume changes throughout the years.

Meanwhile, page 9 of the budget package (Box 10–3) provides a reconciliation and explanation of how the salaries increased or decreased between the current year's projected and upcoming budget year's salaries. The largest change is in the area of FTE increases or decreases, as it is again in this budget. Any policy or practice change proposed in the budget that has financial implications needs to be addressed in this reconciliation. Finally, the merit rate increases have a carry-over effect from the current year and an impact from the budget year. This last type of change would be similar if the healthcare organization was unionized and knew its upcoming year's negotiated wage changes.

Pages 10 (employee benefits) and 11 (financial effect of debt issues) of the finance committee budget package are summaries of specific expense items. Pages 12 to 16 present an overall summary of the capital budget as well as a listing of all recommended capital items costing $25,000 or more. This detail is presented in order to keep the finance committee informed of items and because they want to see them. The committee believes that being able to review the requested items at this dollar level is consistent with their governance and approval function. RHMC's management is pleased to present the information because it allows them to show the committee how these purchases support the organization's strategic plans.

TABLE 10-8

Ridgeland Heights Medical Center
2000 Proposed Budget
Analysis of Revenue and Contractual Allowances

	1998 Actual	1999 Budget	1999 Projected	2000 Budget	Favorable/Unfavorable 2000 B vs. 1999 P	
					Amount	Percent
Inpatients						
Gross Revenue Per Case						
Medicare	10,977	11,300	11,105	11,570	465	4.2
Non-Medicare	5,228	5,065	5,250	5,370	120	2.3
Total gross revenue per case	6,728	6,726	6,463	6,685	222	3.4
Gross Revenue Per Day						
Medicare	1,505	1,502	1,478	1,506	28	1.9
Non-Medicare	1,740	1,725	1,700	1,730	30	1.8
Total gross revenue per day	1,652	1,639	1,589	1,637	48	3.0
Net Revenue Per Case						
Medicare	4,900	4,770	4,700	4,550	(150)	-3.2
Non-Medicare	4,550	4,200	4,090	3,880	(210)	-5.1
Total net revenue per case	4,648	4,290	4,145	3,996	(149)	-3.6
Net Revenue Per Day						
Medicare	880	850	820	790	(30)	-3.7
Non-Medicare	1,400	1,330	1,300	1,365	65	5.0
Total net revenue per day	1,141	1,046	1,019	979	(40)	-4.0
Contractual and Other Adjustments						
Inpatient Contractual Adjustment as a % of Inpatient Gross Revenue						
Medicare	56.7%	58.9%	57.9%	61.0%	0.03	5.4
Non-Medicare	33.0%	38.0%	35.6%	41.2%	0.06	15.7
Total inpatient contractual %	41.1%	45.3%	44.2%	48.9%	0.05	10.6
Outpatient Contractual Adjustment as a % of Outpatient Gross Revnue						
Medicare	52.3%	61.3%	59.8%	68.4%	0.09	14.4
Non-Medicare	15.0%	23.4%	22.6%	30.0%	0.07	32.7
Total outpatient contractual %	26.4%	33.5%	31.6%	38.0%	0.06	20.3
Bad Debts and Charity Care as a % of Total Gross Revenues						
Bad debts	2.99%	2.82%	2.86%	2.26%	(0.01)	-20.9
Charity and other free care	1.69%	1.73%	1.63%	1.70%	0.00	3.8

T A B L E 10–9

Ridgeland Heights Medical Center
2000 Proposed Budget
Staffing Expenses and FTE Analysis

	1999 Budget	1999 Projected	2000 Budget	Favorable/Unfavorable 2000 B vs. 1999 P Amount	Percent
Salary expenses	$35,500,000	$36,500,000	$39,000,000	$2,500,000	6.8
Total FTEs	1023.1	1026.0	1005.9	(20.10)	−2.0
FTEs per adjusted patient days	4.17	4.13	4.00	(0.13)	−3.1
Salaries, wages, and fringe benefits as a percentage of net patient service revenue	47.05%	47.84%	47.55%	−0.29%	−0.6
Nonsalary fringe benefit expenses	$7,000,000	$6,927,000	$7,270,000	$343,000	5.0

Page 17 (Table 10–3) is a short worksheet presentation of the organization's cash budget for the upcoming year. It is the presentation that was already discussed earlier in this chapter in regard to the finance committee's willingness or unwillingness to approve net cash outflows. In this case, management's recommendation is accepted and for the short term (i.e., the year 2000), the proposed negative annual cash flow is accepted after further discussion. However, the board members challenge the administrators to attempt to beat the approved operating and capital budget. They would still like to see no negative cash flow if this can be accomplished.

The administrators accept the challenge but offer no guarantees. As with any budget or any projection, the ability to predict or foretell the future, whether in the assumptions already made or the assumption not yet known, is questionable and problematic. By far, the budget assumption with the highest degree of uncertainty involves the managed care contractual adjustments. If none of the major managed care companies propose any substantial changes for the year 2000 (which is unlikely), the administration has a good chance of beating the budget.

The updated strategic financial plan information presented on pages 18 and 19 simply revise the information presented seven months earlier. This update maintains the discipline of periodically monitoring the previous assumptions, summarizing the actual results, explaining the material variances, and reporting the current projections. The explanation of variances allows the finance committee members to gain a better understanding of the reasons for positive or negative differences.

Finally, the last four pages of the package present five-year trends of certain financial and statistical information in graph form. If one picture is worth a thousand words, then these four graphs become invaluable tools in explaining the overall trends in the inputs that drive the budget dollars and the outputs from which they are

BOX 10–3

RIDGELAND HEIGHTS MEDICAL CENTER

2000 Proposed Budget
Salary Reconciliation

Total full time equivalents were budgeted at 1023.1 in 1999. The 2000 proposal of 1005.9 in as a net decrease of 20.1 below the currently projected FTEs of 1026.0.

RHMC's salary expense is projected to be $35,500,000 in 1999 and $37,480,000 in 2000 which is an increase of $1,980,000 or 2.7%. The net increase is a result of the following changes.

1999 Ridgeland Heights Projected Salaries	$36,500,000
Salary Revisions	
Net decreases of 20.1 FTEs in 2000 (1026.0 projected − 1005.9 budgeted = 20.1 FTEs)	(824,100)
Increase due to staffing mix and rate changes	124,500
Wage Adjustments	
1999 carry over impact of merit increases ($\frac{1}{2}$ of 4.0% increase)	730,000
2000 merit increase ($\frac{1}{2}$ of 4.0%)	749,600
2000 wage contingency	200,000
2000 Proposed Budget—Ridgeland Heights Medical Center	$37,480,000

derived. Page 20 graphs the overall admissions of the organization, page 21 plots the patient days and outpatient visits, while page 22 trends total expenses on the first Y-axis and expenses per adjusted admission (which is very similar to expense per adjusted discharge) on the second Y-axis.

Page 23 (Figure 10–3) shows the trend of gross revenues, total net revenues, and total expenses. This particular chart is a very useful way to conclude the budget because in a single picture, it is easy to see the relationships between these three items and whether or not they are trending in a similar manner. If they are not, it appropriately requires the administration to explain the reasons why. In this particular case, RHMC's trend lines move in the same direction with approximately the same slope each year. It is an accurate representation of the organization's actual financial results over the previous four years as well as the results projected for the upcoming year.

OCTOBER FINANCE COMMITTEE SPECIAL AGENDA ITEMS

During the October finance committee, one of the other special agenda items included the half-yearly report on the management letter comments made by the auditors in April. However, because the auditors did not report on any internal control

F I G U R E   10–3

Ridgeland Heights Medical Center
2000 Budget
Financial Trends for the Years 1996 through 2000

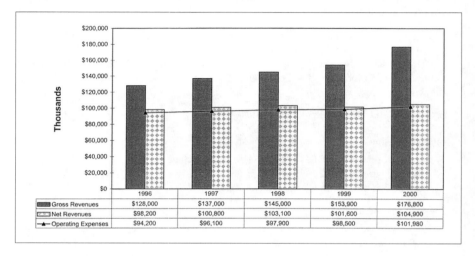

	1996	1997	1998	1999	2000
Gross Revenues	$128,000	$137,000	$145,000	$153,900	$176,800
Net Revenues	$98,200	$100,800	$103,100	$101,600	$104,900
Operating Expenses	$94,200	$96,100	$97,900	$98,500	$101,980

deficiencies in April, there are no updates that need to be given by management. Instead, as has already been reported, the finance committee continues to be extremely interested in the progress towards Y2K compliance. Thus they will review the progress report shown in Table 10–1 earlier in this chapter. The Y2K progress report is the equivalent of an internal control's status report. After all, Y2K compliance, or the lack thereof, of can have serious consequences to the ability of the organization to be a going concern.

In summary, the October finance committee will be dominated by the discussion and approval of the 2000 budget and the implementation progress on the Y2K compliance issues.

November

Rick Samuelson was pensive. He couldn't help but feel that a great upheaval was looming. But he was having some trouble getting a clear picture in his mind of just what it might be. Just them Sam Barnes popped his head into the CEO's office.

"Hey, Rick, what's going on?" asked Sam in an uncharacteristically jovial voice.

"Oh, hi Sam, come on in," said Samuelson, who had been lost in thought and was a little startled by the greeting.

"Rick, I was just reviewing some of our investment results from last month and thought you'd want to hear about it."

"Sam, I do," said Rick. "But first I'd like to share a couple of things I've just been thinking about and see what you think."

"Sure, I'd love to hear it," said the ever agreeable Sam.

"Well, Sam, you know that I've been the CEO of Ridgeland Heights for a long time. And it sure seems to be getting tougher every day. This place has so much to offer to the community. It's a place of healing. We really make people better. And we have such good people working for us. They are so committed to their jobs. But it's just getting harder and harder to maintain the high level of quality and patient satisfaction that every patient has come to expect from us."

Sam was all ears and more than happy to agree. "Rick, I know what you mean. The payors have been taking a bite out of us for the last few years and we are really feeling it now. The budget we just completed and got approved last month had the lowest operating margin in the last 10 years. In fact, thanks to you writing your memorandum to the finance committee, they were willing to allow us to work on a lower margin target than ever before."

"That's true, Sam." Rick was on a roll now. "And I've been thinking a lot about that. This past June you and I had a talk about the deteriorating margin and I remember what you said. You mentioned that there were three things we could do to improve the bottom line. It was the usual things—increase revenues through increased inpatient and outpatient volumes, reduce costs through specific cost analysis and perform process improvements. But I was concerned about the reaction from our core constituents—the doctors, the staff, and the community. I was afraid that they wouldn't understand the fundamental changes taking place in the financing of healthcare and that they would see us as a villain in this drama."

Sam was sympathetic. "I know that, Rick. But it sounds like maybe you've had a change of heart," Sam said hopefully.

"Yeah, I think that would be true," said Rick emphatically. " While we continue to strive for increased volumes, these are certainly not assured. So I want us to make a concerted and rational effort to reduce our costs. I know that you've been telling me about some techniques that seem to be working at some other providers around the country. I'd like us to put some of them into place right here!"

"Well, Rick, I think that's great." Sam was suddenly excited. "I'm really looking forward to working on that. We can get started right away. The sooner we begin, the sooner we'll be able to see some positive results. And you are right. We really need to do this because even though our budget calls for that low level of profitability, even that is not assured. As you know, since we put that budget to bed we've been hit with some enormous discount requests from some of the managed care companies with which we do the most business. And there are rumblings from Medicare for payment reductions in excess of the original Balanced Budget Act. So I'm totally supportive of these initiatives."

"Well then, what are you waiting for?" said the suddenly impatient CEO. "Stop your yapping and get started."

The ghosts and goblins of Halloween have hardly dissipated when the month of November begins. Autumn has truly fallen upon the region, with the skies remaining increasingly gray throughout the day and the nights getting increasingly colder. Residents of the northern climes are preparing for the equivalent of the big winter hibernation as they begin the preparations to hunker down against the expected turn in the weather.

Halloween is an interesting metaphor for the healthcare industry. Some imagine the federal government as a kind of Dracula, sucking the lifeblood out of the providers through a series of small cutbacks, followed by the BIG BITE of the Balanced Budget Act. Meanwhile the Frankenstein monster of managed care has embraced and is beginning to crush the once mighty providers even as some of them attempt to transform themselves into the monster itself by developing their own managed care products. Still, it would be much too early to tell whether eternal night has fallen over the financing of the healthcare industry or if the 1990s was just a bad dream that we will all soon wake from.

Yet, between shaking off some of the real and imagined monsters of Halloween and preparing to give thanks for all the good things that have taken place at the end of the month, the RHMC finance staff and managers remain hard at work. They are not worrying about what may be in the larger context of the industry as much as concerned about performing the very real technical duties for their employer.

PREPARATION AND DELIVERY OF THE BUDGET RESULTS BACK TO THE DEPARTMENT MANAGERS

If there were one month during the year that the RHMC finance staff can sit back for a moment and take a break, that month would be November. While the routine work continues as always, the budget project, which has consumed over five months, is now relatively complete. The finance committee and the board of directors gave their approval and their blessing to the upcoming year's assumptions in October. Now the final set of assumptions, down at the department level, must be communicated. This creates an effective feedback loop allowing the managers to be cognizant of the goals and expectations placed on them.

The finance staff has certain jobs to perform before they can transmit the departmental budgets back to the managers. These jobs include the following.

- Spreading the total approved financial information across certain time periods, such as the following.
  - Twenty-six periods of time that will allow them to determine salary variances within each biweekly pay period. If the organization produced weekly paychecks, this budget spread would need to be for 52 periods.
  - Twelve periods of time to determine the monthly variances for inpatient and outpatient *volume statistics*. This will be used to determine statistical variances that often help to explain financial variances for gross revenues and expenses. The budget spread is a function of historical trends. Data is reviewed for the previous three years, by month, to develop percentages. In some cases, the financial analysts will use their experience and the prior year's trends to develop the volume spreads.

  In other cases, and depending on the culture of the organization, some of these 36 months of statistical data are put through a regression analysis program to help improve the projections. The regression analysis plots the future months volumes based on the past statistical performance. As with any projection, the results are only as good as the underlying data and the quality of the upcoming assumptions. The greater the amount of historical data that can be loaded into the system increases the possibility that the projected outcomes will have greater validity. Therefore, for a very modest cost, the results achieved from these programs can add a small amount of scientific rigor to the process.

- Producing a worksheet that lists all the appropriate budgeted line items for gross revenues, contractual adjustments, salary, fringe benefits, and all other nonsalary costs spread across the 12 monthly periods. Table 11–1 is an example of the budgeted spreadsheet produced by the finance staff for the radiology department. As you can see, the departmental line items match those in the organization-wide budget shown in Table 10–5. In fact, these lines are a summary of a number of more detailed revenue and expense categories. For example, the patient care supplies line is an aggregation of the following.
  - Bandages and dressings
  - Catheters and tubing
  - Disposable garments
  - Drugs
  - Instruments
  - IV sets and supplies
  - IV solutions
  - Needles and syringes
  - Radiology film
  - Contrast media
  - Processing chemicals
  - Other supplies

What these items all have in common is that they all vary with volumes. Because they are variable expenses, they behave similarly from a budgeting perspective. This makes it easy to determine the budget spread methodology that needs to be employed. Because the finance staff has already spread the inpatient and outpatient volumes based on historical trends, it is now simply a matter of using those budgeted monthly volume spread percentages to spread these variable expenses. Thus, all variable nonsalary expenses are spread using the already established volume spreads. Similarly, nonvariable expenses (fixed) are generally spread evenly across the 12 months, one-twelfth of the total per month. Salary and fringe benefit expenses are usually spread based on the number of days in the month because salary expenses are considered fixed and payable based on calendar days. Meanwhile, revenues are usually spread using the adjusted patient day methodology because revenue truly is a function of volume generation.

Budgeting and Spreading Contractual Adjustments by Department

The most difficult of the all the budget spreads is *the contractual adjustment by department.* This is the income statement line item that gives healthcare organizations the most trouble. The problem is based on the reimbursement methodologies that are employed by third-party payors such as Medicare, Medicaid, and the various managed care organizations. Inpatient reimbursement methodologies can include case-based (DRGs), per diems, various percentage of charges, and regular and global capitation.

Outpatient reimbursement methodologies can include percentage of charges, fee schedule, capitation carve-outs, and ambulatory payment groups.

On the inpatient side, it is literally impossible to assign the contractual adjustment on an actual basis because the third-party payors did not create diagnostic related groups (DRGs), per diems, and capitation with actual nursing and ancillary charges in mind. Instead, the net payments made by third parties to healthcare organizations, and hospitals in particular, are based on amounts that Medicare and Medicaid can impose and managed care companies can negotiate. Therefore, in assigning contractual adjustments to nursing and ancillary departments, the best method is to use reasonable statistical relationships.

As shown on Table 11–2, RHMC attempts to be as scientific as possible while working within the above constraint. The real problem with the budgeted contractual adjustment is splitting the inpatient between the various departments. In the absence of any actual information from the payors, RHMC used a percentage of charge methodology. This involves using the budgeted *inpatient charges by department,* converting them to percentages of the total and then calculating the *contractual adjustment by department* based on the total budgeted contractual adjustment.

Thus, in Table 11–2, the $87,360,000 of budgeted inpatient gross charges in column 1 are converted into percentages of the total in column 2. These percentages are then assigned to the $40,092,000 of budgeted contractual adjustments in column 3 to calculate the inpatient contractual adjustment by department. The outpatient contractual adjustment relies less on departmental allocations because until the year 2000, most outpatient contractual adjustments are based on the actual services provided. Except for capitation reimbursement, there was a direct relationship between charges and contractual adjustments. This is even true of Medicare, which has reimbursed most outpatient services on fee schedule or an interim cost to charge basis. Thus, using the organization's contract payment analyzer, it was not difficult to establish the proper contractual adjustment by department.

Starting in 2000, however, Medicare is planning to reimburse outpatients in a manner similar to the inpatient DRG. Called ambulatory payment classifications, this method will no longer equate a single charge with a single payment. Instead, one or a series of outpatient services, procedures, or treatments will be grouped and a single payment made. This will complicate the ability to accurately budget outpatient contractual adjustment by departments.

In summary, the transmission of the budget spreadsheets is very important to the proper functioning of all the healthcare organization's departments. The department managers need to know what is expected of them so that they understand the types of volumes necessary to be run for the organization to meet its revenue and bottom line objectives. Being able to communicate the results of the budget by late

TABLE 11-1

Ridgeland Heights Medical Center
Radiology Department
2000 Monthly Budget Spread
(in thousands)

	Spreading Method	2000 Budget	Jan	Feb	Mar	Apr	May	Jun	Jul	Aug	Sep	Oct	Nov	Dec
Revenues														
Inpatient revenue	Patient days	1,984.0	164.7	146.8	160.7	156.7	158.7	158.7	182.5	180.5	160.7	184.5	158.7	170.6
Outpatient revenue	Procedures	5,657.0	486.5	413.0	446.9	463.9	463.9	446.9	509.1	486.5	458.2	480.8	469.5	531.8
Total Patient Revenue		7,641.0	651.2	559.8	607.6	620.6	622.6	605.6	691.7	667.0	618.9	665.4	628.3	702.4
Less														
Contractual and other adjustments	Adjusted patient days	(3,249.0)	(276.2)	(240.4)	(259.9)	(259.9)	(263.2)	(259.9)	(295.7)	(289.2)	(263.2)	(285.9)	(263.2)	(292.4)
Charity care			—	—	—	—	—	—	—	—	—	—	—	—
Net Patient Service Revenue		4,392.0	375.0	319.4	347.7	360.7	359.4	345.7	396.0	377.9	355.8	379.4	365.1	410.0
Add														
Premium revenue	Carved-out member month													
Investment income	Not applicable	—												
Other operating Income	Not used	—												
Total Revenue		4,392.0	375.0	319.4	347.7	360.7	359.4	345.7	396.0	377.9	355.8	379.4	365.1	410.0
Expenses														
Salaries	Number of days in month	1,041.0	88.2	82.5	88.2	85.3	88.2	85.3	88.2	88.2	85.3	88.2	85.3	88.2
Contract labor	Adjusted patient days	80.0	6.8	5.9	6.4	6.4	6.5	6.4	7.3	7.1	6.5	7.0	6.5	7.2
Fringe benefits	Even	78.0	6.6	6.2	6.6	6.4	6.6	6.4	6.6	6.6	6.4	6.6	6.4	6.6
Total Salaries and Benefits		1,199.0	101.6	94.6	101.2	98.1	101.3	98.1	102.1	101.9	98.2	101.8	98.2	102.0

Bad debts	Not applicable	—	—	—	—	—	—	—	—	—	—	—	—	—
Patient care supplies	Adjusted patient days	357.0	30.3	26.4	28.6	28.6	28.9	28.6	32.5	31.8	28.9	31.4	28.9	32.1
Professional and management fees	Even	17.0	1.4	1.3	1.4	1.4	1.4	1.4	1.4	1.4	1.4	1.4	1.4	1.4
Purchased services	Even	120.0	10.2	9.5	10.2	9.8	10.2	9.8	10.2	10.2	9.8	10.2	9.8	10.2
Operation of plant (including utilities)	Number of days in month	11.0	0.9	0.9	0.9	0.9	0.9	0.9	0.9	0.9	0.9	0.9	0.9	0.9
Depreciation	Even	—	—	—	—	—	—	—	—	—	—	—	—	—
Interest and financing expenses	Even	—	—	—	—	—	—	—	—	—	—	—	—	—
Other	Even	158.0	13.4	12.5	13.4	13.0	13.4	13.0	13.4	13.4	13.0	13.4	13.0	13.4
Total Expenses		1,862.0	157.8	145.2	155.7	151.8	156.1	151.8	160.5	159.6	152.2	159.2	152.2	160.0
Operation Margin		2,530.0	217.2	174.1	192.0	208.9	203.3	193.9	235.5	218.3	203.6	220	213	249.9

Spreading Method Expressed as a Percentage of Total

Patient days		1.00	0.0830	0.0740	0.0810	0.0790	0.0800	0.0800	0.0920	0.0910	0.0810	0.0930	0.0800	0.0860
Procedures		1.00	0.0860	0.0730	0.0790	0.0820	0.0820	0.0790	0.0900	0.0860	0.0810	0.0850	0.0830	0.0940
Number of days in month		1.00	0.0847	0.0792	0.0847	0.0820	0.0847	0.0820	0.0847	0.0847	0.0820	0.0847	0.0820	0.0847
Adjusted patient days		1.00	0.0850	0.0740	0.0800	0.0800	0.0810	0.0800	0.0910	0.0890	0.0810	0.0880	0.0810	0.0900
Even		1.00	0.0833	0.0833	0.0833	0.0833	0.0833	0.0833	0.0833	0.0833	0.0833	0.0833	0.0833	0.0833

TABLE 11–2

Ridgeland Heights Medical Center
Monthly Spread of Budgeted Contractual Adjustment
For the Budget Year Ending December 31, 2000 (in thousands)

Department	Inpatient			Outpatient			Total	
	Gross Revenue	Gross Revenue as a Percentage of Total	Computed Contractual Adjustment	Gross Revenue	Gross Revenue as a Percentage of Total	Computed Contractual Adjustment	Gross Revenue	Computed Contractual Adjustment
2 East (Medical/Surgical Nursing Floor)	$ 3,400	3.89	$ 1,560	$ 800	0.89	$ 331	$ 4,200	$ 1,891
2 Southwest (Medical/Surgical Nursing Floor)	2,170	2.48	996	300	0.34	124	2,470	1,120
3 Northwest (Medical/Surgical Nursing Floor)	5,000	5.72	2,295	600	0.67	248	5,600	2,543
Labor, Delivery, and Post-Partum (LDRP)	7,350	8.41	3,373	400	0.45	166	7,750	3,539
Pediatrics	800	0.92	367	100	0.11	41	900	409
Critical Care Step-down Unit	5,220	5.98	2,396	400	0.45	166	5,620	2,561
Critical Care Unit (CCU)	3,870	4.43	1,776	200	0.22	83	4,070	1,859
Skilled Nursing Facility (SNF)	2,680	3.07	1,230	—	0.00	—	2,680	1,230
Psychiatric Unit	4,720	5.40	2,166	—	0.00	—	4,720	2,166
Surgical Suites (Operating Rooms)	7,880	9.02	3,616	13,240	14.80	5,478	21,120	9,095
Post-Anesthethesia Care Unit (PACU)	1,270	1.45	583	2,000	2.24	828	3,270	1,410
Same Day Surgery	0	0.00	—	4,000	4.47	1,655	4,000	1,655
			$40,092			$ 37,008		$ 77,100

Outpatient Procedures and Treatment Center	0	0.00	—	5,000	5.59	2,069	5,000	2,069
Anesthesia	1,470	1.68	675	3,000	3.35	1,241	4,470	1,916
Emergency Department	2,770	3.17	1,271	6,200	6.93	2,565	8,970	3,837
Renal Dialysis	320	0.37	147	3,500	3.91	1,448	3,820	1,595
Home Health Services	0	0.00	—	4,500	5.03	1,862	4,500	1,862
Eye Center	0	0.00	—	400	0.45	166	400	166
Respiratry Care	3,000	3.43	1,377	1,200	1.34	497	4,200	1,873
Fertility Center	0	0.00	—	3,500	3.91	1,448	3,500	1,448
Physical Therapy	1,550	1.77	711	3,400	3.80	1,407	4,950	2,118
Occupational Therapy	750	0.86	344	400	0.45	166	1,150	510
Cardiology	1,400	1.60	643	2,700	3.02	1,117	4,100	1,760
Cardiac Rehabilitation	0	0.00	—	500	0.56	207	500	207
Cardiac Catheterization	1,320	1.51	606	1,700	1.90	703	3,020	1,309
Radiology	2,210	2.53	1,014	5,400	6.04	2,234	7,610	3,249
CT Scan	1,610	1.84	739	5,000	5.59	2,069	6,610	2,808
Ultrasound	260	0.30	119	1,500	1.68	621	1,760	740
Magnetic Imaging Resonance (MRI)	560	0.64	257	3,500	3.91	1,448	4,060	1,705
Laboratory	8,700	9.96	3,993	7,000	7.83	2,896	15,700	6,889
Pharmacy	10,340	11.84	4,745	6,000	6.71	2,483	16,340	7,228
Nuclear Medicine	1,000	1.14	459	2,400	2.68	993	3,400	1,452
Central Supply	5,740	6.57	2,634	600	0.67	248	6,340	2,883
Total	$87,360	100.00	$40,092	$89,440	100.00	$37,008	$176,800	$77,100

November allows the department managers enough time to prepare for the upcoming year. This could mean that the manager needs to do the following.

- Recruit a new staff member because a new budgeted position has been approved to absorb significantly increased volumes
- Plan to downsize or lay off a staff member because volumes have been declining and fewer staff are needed to perform the duties
- Prepare for the acquisition of new equipment to enhance the department's ability to handle sicker patients (higher acuity) or perform more tests and therapies

Having the budget back in a timely manner is essential to the efficient and effective operation of the organization.

ISSUES INVOLVING RHMC'S COST STRUCTURE

Meanwhile, as the department managers prepare for the new year, the administration is debating a problem that has become more evident over the past year or so as the organization's bottom line has begun to shrink. There has been a lot of talk by the administration to the managers about diminishing returns. Although the *best* way to improve the organization's financial situation is to increase volumes and net revenues, many of the efforts that have been tried thus far have proven to be unsuccessful. In this light, managers have been asked to, once again, review the cost structure of their departments and reduce spending wherever possible even beyond the level of the approved 2000 budget. Over the past few years, several different methods have been used to deal with the organization's costs. Some of the efforts were highly successful while some were not.

Some of the successful efforts have included the following.

- Creation of organization-wide teams charged with reviewing specific issues leading to the reduction of definitive costs. For example, a group was organized to review the types of gloves being purchased throughout the organization. It was determined that the same types of gloves were being purchased from three different manufacturers. The group's analysis concluded that the quality of all the manufacturers were comparable and there would be no resistance by the nursing, clinical, or physician staff to making a change. Thus a three-month trial period was established to use a single glove manufacturer's product. Because the trial was successful, a change to a single manufacturer was made at total organizational savings of *$50,000 a year!* This was based on the additional volume discounts available and the ability to negotiate more aggressively. And this was just one item of potential savings.
- Creation of a formalized "suggestion box" whereby each employee was required to submit at least two cost reduction suggestions over a one-month time frame. This method is based on the assumption that the

employees working at the detailed level, such as nurses, technicians, therapists, and clerical staff, have a much better idea of the waste that is taking place and the improvements that are possible if they are addressed. RHMC's 1,000 employees yielded almost 2,000 suggestions. An organization-wide manager-led committee was established to review the ideas and bring the most promising forward for swift implementation. There were many detailed steps that were taken to move from idea to implementation but the result was a $4 million cost savings. These savings were particularly valuable because they not only positively impacted the year of their implementation, they were ongoing into all future years.

Meanwhile, unsuccessful efforts have usually all had the same elements:

- No well-defined goals
- No departmental manager involvement in establishment of the goals
- No staff involvement in the establishment of the goals
- No accountability
- No follow-up by the administration

RHMC's administration was aware of the successes and the failures. In addition to the above five reasons for the failures, some of the other distinguishing characteristics include lack of appropriate staffing, lack of political will, distractions, differing priorities, and outright resistance to change. The administrators knew they needed to enhance cost reduction efforts and were determined to achieve a lower level of unit costs while going beyond their previous successes.

The first step RHMC took to determine its current cost structure was to attempt to understand it in a macro sense. In other words, before it decided to look at the components of its cost (the micro level), it looked at its global cost structure to determine if, in fact, it was out of line with the rest of the industry. To do this, RHMC had to benchmark its costs against those of its peers. Benchmarking is "a standard of excellence, achievement, etc. against which similar things [can] be measured or judged."[1] Therefore, it needed to obtain benchmarking data on overall costs for healthcare organizations. Because RHMC was no longer only a hospital, it felt it needed to benchmark against organizations like itself, which had hospital-based programs such as psychiatric services, SNF units, and a full-scale home health agency. Furthermore, it was also interested in organizations that were managing physician practices as well.

To obtain benchmarking data on overall hospital cost, RHMC reviewed information on the available benchmarking services. Although benchmarking services are available for every industry in America, RHMC was interested only in those representing the healthcare industry. Its review turned up a number of companies that performed just these sorts of services. Many of them were dedicated solely to the healthcare industry. The review identified some healthcare benchmarking

---

[1] Random House Unabridged Dictionary, 2nd ed., 1993.

companies that specialized in only the financial aspects of the industry, others that specialized in only the clinical aspects of the industry and others that performed in both segments.

There were other distinguishing characteristics that separated the various healthcare benchmarking companies. Included among these would be the following.

1. The number of healthcare organizations that are participating in the review. (This will have a significant impact on the sample size.)

2. Whether the benchmarking company is obtaining its data from healthcare organization's themselves (which would give them access to a greater amount of data at the micro level).

3. Whether the information is being obtained from governmental sources at the federal or state level (which means that more assumptions are being made in attempting to standardize the cost information).

4. The quality and extent to which the benchmarking companies have supplied the organization's financial analyst with explanations on how to aggregate the departmental data will heavily weigh on the quality of the outcomes reported for all the peer organizations being benchmarked. It will also help or hinder the financial analyst in his or her ability to convince the department managers that the data quality is good. Good data will allow the department manager to concentrate on the results of the benchmark study rather than the on the quality of the data itself.

After selecting two different types of benchmark companies to work with, RHMC discovered some very interesting findings. The most intriguing to the administrators was that the organization had a high expense base according to both sources. This was further validated by a third benchmarking outcome. Expense in this case was measured as a function of a unit of measure. The two most frequently used units of measure for expenses are patient days or patient discharges, adjusted for outpatient volumes. These are commonly called expense per adjusted discharge (EPAD) or expense per adjusted patient day (EPAPD).[2]

Figure 11–1 represents the graph of RHMC's EPAD over the previous four years. Even more interestingly than the slope of the line, which is not decreasing but needs to be, is the position of the organization's line compared to the median EPAD of the benchmark peer group. An organization can easily delude itself into thinking that it is cost-efficient and even getting better if all it can use as a guide is the analysis of its own results. Only by looking at other organizations and finding out which are performing 'best practices' can valid comparisons be drawn.

Each healthcare organization may set the benchmark target differently. Some may aspire to be the best, thereby setting the target at the 90th percentile. Other or-

---

[2] As an aside, the words *cost* and *expense* are used interchangeably. Further, the use of discharges or admissions has almost no impact on the final calculation because in any given period (month, year), there should never be a material difference.

FIGURE 11–1

Expenses per Adjusted Discharges (EPDA) Actual versus Top 100 Benchmark Medians 100–250 beds

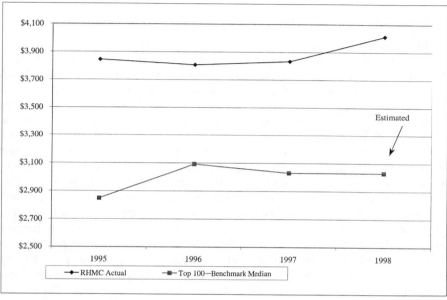

Source: HCIA, Inc., and William Mercer, Inc.

ganizations may be satisfied to be at the 50th percentile or median level for the benchmark group. This usually depends on the organization's culture and its leadership. It may also be a function of the level of competition in the area and whether or not there is a pressing need to set a high target.

RHMC is feeling the need to improve its cost structure given the negative reimbursement changes it is experiencing. The cost graph in Figure 11–1 is convincing enough for the administration to begin a series of evaluation steps that it expects will conclude in a serious improvement in its cost structure. This will come in conjunction with the new budget year and will be led by all the division heads, each of whom are responsible for departments where additional cost reductions can be made.

HOW TO IMPROVE THE ORGANIZATION'S COST STRUCTURE

There are several ways to improve the cost structure of the healthcare organization.

1. Enhance communication with physicians
2. Standardize the organization's supplies

3. Reduce utilization of services and supplies
4. Obtain best pricing for supplies and products
5. Establish and implement optimum productivity and staffing levels

Enhance Communication with Physicians

In all hospitals, the physicians control most of the cost of supplies. Physicians place orders for pharmaceutical and medical supplies to be used for patients. In many healthcare organizations, physicians often do not know the cost of these supplies because it has never been shared with them. Physicians will very often make rational and reasonable choices in the use of supplies as long as they have an understanding of the issues. Thus, it is important to create formal and informal communication channels with physicians.

There are several ways to establish communication channels. One way would be for the healthcare organization to publish its charge master, with the actual cost of each item also included in prominent places, such as the physician's lounge. This would allow physicians to review the cost of an item before writing an order, especially when there may be less expensive alternatives available. A better way could be employed if the healthcare organization requires its physician to order his or her own supply and ancillary service online. In this case, the organization could list the cost of each requested order on the computer monitor, along with the charge. When the physician places the order, an alert could pop up showing possible alternatives that are clinically appropriate. This point-of-service alert offers the greatest opportunity for changing the physician's ordering pattern. The biggest problem is that physicians in most healthcare organization do not enter their own orders either because they do not want to or the organization believes they do not want to. This is an area ripe for change. There are numerous benefits to physicians entering their own orders and using the computer for more than just looking up the location of their patients. Future issues of this sort will be explored further in Chapter 12.

Standardize the Organization's Supplies

The concept of standardizing supplies is once again wrapped around physician ordering patterns. Physicians often practice medicine the way they were taught in medical school and in their residency programs. They are often taught only one way of performing their duties. The interesting aspect of this educational feature is that medicine is taught differently at different schools. In fact, there are many different ways to practice good medicine. However some of the ways are less expensive than others, yet the clinical outcomes are very often similar.

Thus, physicians from the same hospital often want to practice medicine the way they were taught, even if it means having a wide variety of practice and ordering patterns abound at the healthcare organization where they are currently working. This is particularly true for surgeons who become very attached to the instruments of specific manufacturers that were used in the residency program they attended.

Because the look, feel, and function of each manufacturer's surgical instrument is different, the surgeon often bonds with that manufacturer's instruments for life. The problem for the healthcare organization is that this creates a group of nonstandard surgical supplies that may be quite expensive.

For example, consider that the major supply item for hip replacement surgery is the artificial hip. At RHMC, there were actually seven different artificial hips ordered by the organization's nine orthopedic surgeons who perform this procedure. Ordering from seven different manufacturers does not allow that organization to partake in discounts for volume buying and it also necessitates an inflated level of inventory because it must keep a complete set of hips for each size from each of the seven manufacturers. This nonstandardization is quite obviously inefficient and costly to RHMC. Yet none of the surgeons wants to give up the product on which he or she had trained and performed all of these surgeries throughout their careers.

What to do? It is like the irresistible object meeting the immovable force. What gives? There are a couple of potential solutions that may be considered. The first involves a *mandate* from the organization's administration that standardization must take place in the interest of cost reduction. The timing of this type of mandate is always interesting. It could come when the organization is already hemorrhaging red ink, in which case the surgeons may recognize the financial need. This may allow them to acquiesce without controversy, banding together to help the organization survive. Or the mandate could come while the organization is still financially sound and the standardization could help them stay that way.

Still, the financially sound organization faces a problem convincing the surgeons to abandon their "comfort zone." To do so successfully, the organization should facilitate a group meeting with the physicians led by the clinical chair of the surgery service. The clinical chair should explain the financial problems caused by multiple vendors and the need to economize because of the reduction in reimbursements. It is extremely important that the physicians be allowed to determine which one or two vendors should remain. Administratively imposed decisions in this regard would be suspect and challenged by the physicians.

If the first solution is politically untenable, a second potential solution involves a compromise whereby all the physicians agree to help the organization negotiate for the best artificial hip price without changing vendors. They do this by letting each of the seven salespeople know that they are seriously considering changing their hip preference unless a significant discount is offered to the healthcare organization. This discount should be equal to the price that would be available if the organization used only one type of artificial hip. Each of the vendors needs to get the same message and any vendor that does not comply needs to be dropped by the surgeon and the organization. While this solution allows the organization to obtain significant pricing concessions, the lack of standardization still means that the inventory will be too large. Still, it is better than nothing and keeps the physician's relatively happy about not having to change hip vendors.

Standardization throughout the organization holds great potential for savings. In many cases it involves very little pain to most of its users of supplies. It allows the organization to reduce its inventory of many high priced supplies and to deal with fewer vendors, thereby creating efficiencies for the material management (purchasing) department. To achieve effective standardization however, a lot of work is required by the clinical users and the purchasing agents.

- Evaluation of the opportunities for standardization
- Determination of which vendor's product they want to standardize
- Organization of a clinical trial or test of the product in those areas that will be using it
- Evaluation of the results of the trial
- Implementation of the standardization.

Reduce Utilization of Services and Supplies

This is another way achieve significant cost reductions in a hospital. The organization needs to perform analyses to help it understand the types of supplies and services that are being overutilized and who is placing the orders to do so. Rational improvements cannot be made without the data. This is especially true because the primary group that orders supplies are the physicians, and they demand data when their efforts are being reviewed. Box 11–1 summarizes the types of steps that should be taken to effectively analyze, develop, and implement improvements in supply utilization.

B O X   11–1

STEPS NEEDED TO ANALYZE, DEVELOP, AND IMPLEMENT SERVICES AND SUPPLY UTILIZATION IMPROVEMENTS

Using the organization's decision support system, or an outside agency specializing in clinical decision support:

- Segregate the inpatient discharges by DRGs
- Then, further segregate the inpatient discharges by ICD-9 diagnosis level
- Determine the levels of supplies being utilized at the ICD-9 level
- Then analyze the utilization
  - Against outside benchmarks
  - By the organization's physicians
- Identify "best practice" treatment protocols
- Utilize these best practice protocols (either internal or external) as standards of practice
- Measure individual physician variances from above
- Determine the reasons for the variances
- Develop action plans to achieve changes
- Implement practice changes

These steps are critical to a successful conclusion. There are some very interesting findings that may be uncovered using these techniques. Also, the use of benchmarks is essential to successful outcomes.

Consider the following case study from RHMC. A national clinical benchmarking firm was retained to review the utilization levels of a specific number of DRGs. The were reviewing the differences between RHMC's actual utilization and the available benchmark group utilization. The DRGs were selected based on the high number of cases seen at the organization. One of the DRGs selected was DRG 89, which is a medical DRG consisting of simple pneumonia and pleurisy, age greater than 17 with at least one comorbidity or complication (CC; if present, CCs generally mean that the patient is sicker and requires more care than a patient without CCs). The benchmarking firm first sorted all of RHMC's DRG 89 pneumonia cases into their ICD-9 components because usage at the diagnosis code level represents a much more homogenous mix than aggregated at the DRG level (Table 11–3).

The variance analysis was then sorted by price, frequency, distribution, and other factors. The positive price variance means that RHMC's unit cost of products is higher than the benchmark. The frequency variance measures how often each patient is receiving a particular type of service or supply. For example, in the case of a complete blood count lab test, this category would measure whether the test was ordered and performed more or less for RHMC's actual patients versus the benchmark group. The distribution variance represents the number of patients within the diagnosis code who are getting the service. For example, what percentage of the total patients in DRG 89 is receiving antibiotics at RHMC versus that percentage for the benchmark group.

T A B L E 11–3

Ridgeland Heights Medical Center
Utilization Analysis of DRG 89–Pneumonia
Subset: No Substantial CCs* or Moderate CCs

DRG Subset	Average Dollars				Unit Total	No. of Cases	Grand Total
	Price	Frequency	Distribution	Other			
1. No substantial CCs or moderate CCs	1,900	200	1,400	1,500	5,000	150	750,000
2. Major CCs	1,800	1,300	4,000	2,000	9,100	20	182,000
3. All other	100	(1,000)	(20)	400	(520)	10	(5,200)
Total DRG 89	1,789	256	1,610	1,494	5,149	180	926,800

*CC, comorbidities and complications. If present, CCs generally mean that the patients are sicker and require more care than patients without CCs.

When stratified, it is clear from the 'unit total' variance and the number of cases that further analysis is warranted for the subset of "no substantial CCs or moderate CCs." Next, using that subset as the new variable, they determined variances between RHMC and peer and benchmarking groups for the major ancillary services, such as laboratory, radiology, cardiology, and pharmacy. They also reported variances in the average lengths of stay.

This review immediately highlighted one interesting variance in the radiology (or imaging) service. The CT scan service appeared to be costing the organization a much greater amount of money than that reported by the peer and benchmarking group. Upon further review, it was noted that although the percentage of patients receiving services for the benchmark group was 3% and for the peer group was 6%, RHMC's utilization rate was over 18.7%, six times that of the benchmark group (Figure 11–2).

Upon learning of this, further analysis was performed at RHMC. It was discovered that a long-standing practice at the organization was for the radiologists who read the routine chest X-ray to "recommend" a CT scan for many patients, in the case of a negative finding, as a precaution for the patient. Because of this recommendation from the radiologist, the attending physician had to order the test, from a

F I G U R E   11–2

Ridgeland Heights Medical Center
Analysis of CT Scans
DRG 89–No Substantial CCs or Moderate CCs
For the 12 Months Ended December 31, 1998

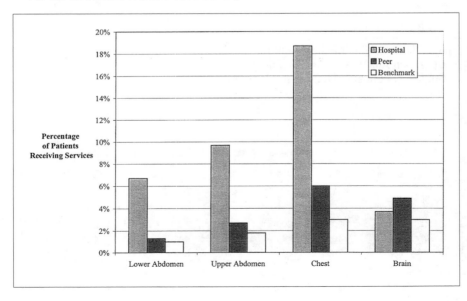

medicolegal standpoint. Now that the organization had the national data, it questioned the radiologists about this recommendation. Although surprised by the data, the radiologists did not hesitate to change their recommendation on the spot.

There was one cost saving and one revenue enhancement that accrued from just this change. First, the variable cost of the CT scan was saved. Second, because there was a waiting list for the organization's CT service, they were able to replace the unnecessary and generally unreimbursed tests with reimbursed outpatient services. The quality of the data and the depth of the analysis impressed the physicians. They became more than willing to listen to the results of subsequent review because of the outcomes in the pneumonia case.

Obtain Best Pricing for Supplies and Products

This concept is the most mundane of the cost-saving ideas. It is time-tested and the easiest to achieve. There is very little magic to obtaining best prices for the supplies and products being acquired by healthcare organizations. One of the primary methods to achieving best product pricing is to understand and practice the fine art of negotiation. But, there may be some problems with this approach if used alone.

First, the negotiator, often the purchasing agent, may not have had enough experience or training to negotiate the best available price from the salesperson. Second, the negotiator may not have any leverage to exert to command the best price. This is true in the artificial hip example presented above. If physicians tell the salesperson that they have no intention of switching to another hip regardless of what they are told by the healthcare organization, the purchasing agent will never be able to obtain a good price from the salesperson. Third, and most important, the healthcare organization may not be big enough to command the best prices from the manufacturer or distributor of the product. The best prices are usually given to those purchasers who purchase the greatest quantity of goods. Most stand-alone healthcare organizations do not look or act like a major purchaser.

Thus, it is important to look like a much bigger purchaser than they really are. In order to do this, various healthcare providers decided to band together to form purchasing alliances. Three of the biggest current alliances (also known as group purchasing organizations or GPOs) belong to the Amerinet, Voluntary Hospitals of America, and Premier, Inc.

For the price of membership, healthcare providers are permitted to participate in supply and service contracts. The GPO has already negotiated the prices for the goods. In most cases, the healthcare provider merely has to agree to purchase a minimum number in order to get pricing at a cost far less than would have been available had they negotiated as a freestanding entity. This is possible because the GPO comes to a negotiating table with tremendous purchasing clout—the ability to deliver millions of dollars of sales to the manufacturer or distributor of supplies.

In any case, the GPO member is often assured of obtaining the best or close to the best prices for much of the clinical and nonclinical goods that are required in the efficient running of their organizations. This is a primary tenet to the management of supplies in a healthcare organization. Other materials management concepts will be discussed later in this chapter.

Establish and Implement Optimum Productivity and Staffing Levels

Productivity management is a technique that was established and used for many years in nonhealthcare industries. Healthcare was late to adopt many of the techniques because until recently cost management has not been a top priority. As stated earlier in the book, prior to 1983, Medicare reimbursed the hospital segment of the industry based on their cost. The system rewarded higher costs. Labor costs represent the highest portion of costs in healthcare industry. Because there was actually a disincentive to reducing costs prior to 1983, most healthcare companies did not practice labor productivity management.

Subsequent to 1983, these incentives changed. For inpatient care, Medicare's decision to pay a specific rate according to diagnosis regardless of the patient's length of stay or resources consumed, led administrations to take some notice of the cost. Still, many organizations had a small number of Medicare patients and a reasonable percentage of charge-based payors. They were therefore insulated from most financial disasters throughout the 1980s. But, the rapid rise of managed care plans in the 1990s in most of the country has made almost no healthcare organization immune from cost pressures. They started to recognize a need for cost reductions and identified labor as the most likely area to attack.

A typical method for identifying optimum labor and productivity levels was to do the following.

- Develop a list of the tasks performed by each employee
- Determine the amount of time it took the staff to do each task
- Determine the appropriate unit of service to be used by which to multiply the task
- Do the multiplication to determine the amount of total staff time needed according to the projected volumes
- Compare the staff needed according to the calculation to the actual staffing
- When the actual staffing exceeded the calculation, reassign the staff that made up the excess; when the calculation exceeded the actual staffing, maintain the status quo

Many organizations either performed these steps on their own or engaged consulting firms to do so. When RHMC did this, the results were mixed. Some departments were able to determine that they may have been performing tasks that were nonvalue added. When this was discovered, these tasks were often eliminated, thereby freeing up staff time, where in the best case, it could be used to treat patients who were waiting for revenue-producing care. In the worst case, staff was downsized, either through attrition, relocation, or position elimination. Over a short period of time (six months) and over a small number of departments (12) and over a moderate number of staff members (400), RHMC was able to reduce its staff by 12 staff members, or 3% of staff members. While this is not an overwhelming reduction, it was achievable and it taught the organization and its administration and managers some valuable lessons.

- Understanding the actual tasks and job assignments improves the relationships between the managers and their staff. It allows a dialogue based on objective data. It enables more rational discussions. For example, if the staff feels overworked, the manager and staff can review the task list and determine whether there were any additional nonvalue-added tasks that could be eliminated without sacrificing core values.

- It is important to monitor productivity on an ongoing basis. Once the tasks are known and the units of service standards are set, the organization needs to maintain a system whereby variances are monitored on a pay period basis. This will allow them to maintain vigilance on these very important costs.

Thus, the importance of understanding, measuring, and managing labor costs is critical to maintaining a healthcare organization's cost structure. The level of labor and nonstaffing costs will play a great role in whether the organization remains financially viable or struggles to survive. Cost management is crucial in an era when volumes are stable or slightly declining and reimbursement rates are declining. RHMC has chosen to place great emphasis in these areas and has been successful using the techniques described above.

MATERIALS MANAGEMENT IN HEALTHCARE

Integral to the concept of cost management is the field of materials management or supply chain management. Materials management in healthcare is generally defined as the management of supplies and goods, both clinical and nonclinical in nature, used by the organization's staff to perform their duties. In theory, materials management is the responsibility of every employee and nonemployed physician in the healthcare facility. In practice, the materials management function is performed by the following staffs.

- Purchasing staff that negotiates and contracts with outside suppliers and distributors
- Receiving staff that accepts and logs in all the supplies offloaded at the receiving dock
- Central supply staff that maintains the organization's inventory and distributes it out to the all the users around the facility

The staffs that work in these materials management areas are aware of the magnitude of their job. At RHMC, for example, they are responsible for the acquisition of the $16,600,000 in patient care supplies budgeted for 2000. That's 16% of the

RHMC's total expenditures, which is comparable to many healthcare organizations around the country.

There are several basic tenets that good materials managers follow in order to maximize returns for their employers.

1. *Obtain best pricing for goods and supplies*—This was discussed at length in the section above. It is the primary method to contain the cost of goods. But it is not the only one.

2. *Develop close relations with distributors*—Distributors are the middlemen in the supply chain. One of their basic functions is to consolidate the medical and surgical supplies of many different manufacturers and resell them to healthcare providers for a small mark-up. This distributor/consolidator simplifies the procurement process through this "one stop shopping" approach. Distributors that do a good job of performing their tasks are often taken for granted by the materials manager. But, it is important for the materials manager to develop close relations with distributors for a number of reasons.

   Over the past couple of years, the number of major distributors has decreased as that segment of the industry experienced significant alliances and combinations. The materials manager is responsible to assure that the goods needed by the clinical and nonclinical users are available when needed. The distributors control the availability, receiving schedule, and pricing for these goods. And although the materials manager has the choice of distributors, this choice is dwindling. Good management technique would obligate the materials manager to maintain close and effective relations with the one or two distributors that supply a majority of the organization's goods.

3. *Adopt just-in-time (JIT) inventory management*—This has become extremely important over the past 10 years as healthcare providers adopted techniques pioneered in the automotive industry. Prior to adoption, this healthcare provider maintained its entire inventory within the four walls of the facility. The provider therefore bore the risk for the holding cost for all the goods being warehoused in the facility as well as an increased opportunity for obsolescence and shrinkage (theft).

   JIT allows the healthcare organization to significantly downsize its storerooms or warehouse. This produces significant savings to the organization. It can use an on-site, vacated, or downsized storeroom for more productive or revenue producing activities, or it can vacate warehouse space that it may be leasing outside its four walls, thereby saving significant rent expenses.

   JIT shifts the risk of these holding costs and shrinkage back onto the supplier or the distributor. These companies now become responsible for warehousing the products and shipping them to the organization in a timely basis. JIT increases the frequency of delivery to the organization, often from once a week to three to five times per week. It becomes imperative that the suppliers' trucks appear at the provider's receiving dock at the time that it is expected each day. Otherwise, patients' tests or surgeries may need to be postponed. Therefore, the caveats to using a JIT method are as follows.

- The supplier or distributor must be extremely reliable in its delivery schedule.
- The supplier or distributor must also have a reliable pipeline to obtain or manufacture the goods.

Because the holding costs and risk of shrinkage have been shifted back to the distributors or suppliers, they generally charge a slightly higher rate for this service and the risk it entails.

4. *Create and maintain an in-service program for the organization's entire management group*—This training program is fundamental to the efficient running of the materials management program. It allows the materials manager to communicate and educate the managers and their staff on the major internal and external issues surrounding their role in materials management issues. These issues include the following.

- Understanding the material management/central supply process
- Instructing the managers on the proper procedures for requesting a purchase order number, which when assigned, is a legal contract obligating the organization to pay for the supply or service ordered
- Whether the managers should attempt to do there own negotiating with vendors or refer these salespeople back to the organization's purchasing agents
- How to deal with salespeople who have been known to break the organization's rules about the steps they need to take before contacting specific department managers

This type of in-service will help the organization to maintain a better materials management system.

5. *Adopt consignment as a business model*—In most cases, healthcare organizations acquire goods by purchasing them from distributors or suppliers. The goods are ordered by the healthcare provider, sent by the supplier, received by the provider, billed by the supplier, paid by the provider, stored for a short time in user department, and then finally consumed. Under the consignment method, the methodology changes because while the provider acquires the goods for use, it is paid for only if used. If it is not used, it can be returned to the supplier. Consignment is most often used for relatively expensive, specialized equipment usually consumed in the surgical suites (operating rooms).

Consignment is an economical model that benefits the organization in a very positive way. It allows the organization to have access to a variety of high cost equipment without the monetary outlay usually associated with the acquisition. There is no significant downside to the provider and so it is likely to grow in popularity.

It is clear that sound materials management policies and practices within healthcare organization can have a positive impact on the facility's cost management. It is an area that needs to be highlighted whenever the concept of cost reduction is proposed.

BENEFITS OF TAX STATUS TO HEALTHCARE ORGANIZATIONS

Back in Chapter 2 the issue of not-for-profit versus for-profit healthcare was briefly touched on. Throughout the book, the not-for-profit model has been continuously highlighted because RHMC, like over 80% of hospitals or health systems, operate under this Internal Revenue Code designation. There are several very positive financial implications associated with this designation and one very large drawback. Box 11–2 summarizes the various financial benefits associated with the two designations.

If we were just counting the number of benefits in Box 11–2 it would appear that the not-for-profit entities have an advantage. After all, they get to benefit from a great amount of operating cost savings throughout the year that translate into a greatly improved bottom line. Using RHMC's 2000 budget as an example,

---

BOX 11–2

BENEFITS OF NOT-FOR-PROFIT VERSUS FOR-PROFIT DESIGNATION

Not–For–Profit	For–Profit
• Exempt from federal income taxes on profits	• Ability to issue stock in order to raise capital
• Exempt from state income tax on profits	• Ability to offer stock options to recruit and retain staff at various levels
• Exempt from property taxes (in most cases)	• More limited obligation to provide indigent/uncompensated care
• Exempt from state and local sales taxes (not exempt from excise taxes)	
• Ability to issue bond debt whose income is tax exempt to the purchaser of the debt, in order to raise capital	
• Ability to accept donations through which the donor can reduce their income tax	

Table 11-4 shows that the organization will benefit by saving $10,924,800 in taxes. That is an enormous benefit to the not-for-profit organization.

The government has granted this benefit because, historically, not-for-profit healthcare organizations have taken care of the poor, needy, and indigent who needed healthcare. These healthcare organizations did not discriminate against anyone who presented himself or herself in an emergent care situation and often they would provide care even in an urgent or elective situation. Much of this has changed over the years as the government imposed greater and greater requirements on

TABLE 11-4

Ridgeland Heights Medical Center
Operating Tax Benefits for a Representative Not-For-Profit
Healthcare Organization

		Total Potential Tax Liability Savings
2000 Projected net income	$ 3,920,000	
Federal corporate tax rate	34.00%	
Potential federal income taxes	$ 1,332,800	$ 1,332,800
State corporate tax rate	10%	
Potential state income taxes	$392,000	$ 392,000
Potentially taxable property @ estimated appraised value	$ 200,000,000	
Approximate property tax rate	2.5%	
Potential property taxes	$ 5,000,000	$ 5,000,000
Value of goods to be purchased including supplies and capital equipment	$ 30,000,000	
State and local sales tax	8%	
Potential sales taxes	$ 2,400,000	$ 2,400,000
Amount of tax-exempt bond debt issued	$ 150,000,000	
Average difference between taxable and nontaxable interest rates	1.2%	
Actual annual interest expense savings	$ 1,800,000	$ 1,800,000
Total potential and actual annual operating expense tax savings due to not-for-profit status		$ 10,924,800

healthcare providers both voluntarily (if the organization accepted 1948 Hill-Burton grants) and involuntarily (the COBRA and EMTALA regulations of 1988).

A requirement for providing services to the indigent was imposed in the late 1940s, with the passage in Congress of the Hill-Burton Act. This Act allowed the government to grant or lend monies to healthcare organizations for the express purpose of building or renovating their facilities. Aside from the fact that this legislation was the first time the federal government had really opened the spigot to a great flow of funds to the healthcare industry, this Act required the recipient organization to assure that a minimum number of dollars were spent on care for the indigent. It generally amounted to 10% of the amount borrowed each year over a 20-year period. This was the equivalent of a 200% return on the borrowed funds in aid to community residents who could not afford this healthcare.

Although the reporting requirements were onerous, the actual requirements to treat indigent patients were not a problem for most not-for-profit institutions. This, after all, was part of their mission. Keep in mind that this program was begun almost 20 years before Medicare and Medicaid in order to spur the growth of healthcare facility availability for the soldiers returning from World War II and the soldiers' families. There were also almost no for-profit healthcare facilities in the country at that time. It allowed the not-for-profit organizations to share in the largesse of the government.

The advent of Medicare and Medicaid in 1966 considerably changed the equation. There was now far greater coverage for the poor, the elderly, and the poor elderly. While these programs did not cover all the needy, it initially shrank the pool. Depending on the location of the healthcare provider, there could be a large or small number of indigent that required care. Residents whose annual income falls below the government's Federal Poverty Guidelines often populate the inner cities and rural areas. Higher earning individuals are often located in suburbs. Thus, there are varied opportunities for not-for-profit healthcare organizations to provide free or low-priced service to residents of its community.

There is an interesting counterpoint to the concept of providing community services. The late 1960s saw the first great wave of for-profit healthcare spring up. Hospital Corporation of America incorporated at this time with a mission to maximize shareholder wealth. This was in stark contrast to the not-for-profit mission to provide healthcare to all members in the community who needed it. For-profit healthcare organizations are not obligated to seek out indigents within their community. Their mission therefore differs from that of the not-for-profit healthcare organization.

In many communities where the for-profit organization's set up their operations, they sought out the best paying patients. This is known as "skimming." To maximize profits, they specifically attempted to avoid providing services to less-than-full-paying patients except where it was required by law. This occasionally led to the practice of "dumping," which is defined as discharging or transporting patients without insurance to their home or to county facilities before any treatment has been rendered.

To some extent, the desire by certain healthcare providers not to treat patients that could be a financial drain led to a new law to combat dumping. The Consolidated Omnibus Budget Reconciliation Act of 1988 set up requirements that all healthcare facilities, for-profit or nor-for-profit, must treat and stabilize any patient who presents for care in a healthcare organization's emergency department. Thus, in the case of skimming and dumping, there are no longer any advantages or disadvantages to healthcare providers based on tax status.

PREPARATION AND IMPLICATIONS OF THE ANNUAL IRS 990 REPORT

Not-for-profit, tax-exempt status confers certain responsibilities. One of these is submission of an annual corporate tax return. This IRS 990 tax form is similar in many respects to for-profit tax returns. It requests information on the organization's income and expenses just like other corporations. But unlike these other organizations, there is no tax assessment on any revenues that exceed total expenses. This is true for the operating margin as well as any total margin that includes income in investments. While the IRS 990 is initially due in March, RHMC took advantage of allowable extensions until November.

Part III–Statement of Program Service Accomplishments of the IRS 990 encourages the not-for-profit organization to highlight their community services activities over the prior year. Hospitals have developed Community Service Benefits Reports that summarize their large and small contributions made to the community. These activities include annual health screenings and immunization clinics, and community health programs such as first aid classes, school health fairs, CPR classes, stress management and nutrition programs, prenatal care programs, support groups, and sponsorship.

The Community Service Benefits Report was developed and promoted by the Catholic Health Association as a way to advocate the social value of its mission of caring and healing. During the 1980s, many of the ideas and features of the report were adopted by other not-for-profit healthcare organizations as a defined method to report their contributions to the community. Table 11–5 is a summary of the Community Service Report included in the IRS 990 of RHMC. The report is separated into several categories.

- Value of traditional charity provided to the community—the *cost* of providing free or discounted care to patients in accordance with the organization's policies
- Unpaid costs of public programs—represent the net loss (or cost) of providing care to patients insured by government programs such as Medicare or Medicaid
- Nonbilled community services—the organization's cost of providing community health education and outreach services
- Medical education—the net cost to the organization of providing teaching and education for health professionals
- Subsidized health services—the organization's cost of providing specialized or free health services to the community
- Research—self-explanatory and usually limited to academic medical centers
- Cash and in-kind donations—reportable when the organization donates cash, goods, or services of their staff for community services

TABLE 11-5

Ridgeland Heights Medical Center
1998 Community Benefits Report
Summary of Quantifiable Benefits

	Persons Served	Total Expenses	Offsetting Revenues	Net Community Benefits	Percentage of Hospital	
					Expenses	Revenues
Traditional charity care	506	$ 567,000	$ —	$ 567,000	0.58%	0.39%
Unpaid costs of public programs						
Medicare	80,000	40,000,000	30,000,000	10,000,000	10.21	6.90
Medicaid	1,500	1,400,000	800,000	600,000	0.61	0.41
Subtotal unpaid cost of public programs	81,500	41,400,000	30,800,000	10,600,000	10.83	7.31
Community services						
Nonbilled services						
Community health education and outreach	24,000	330,000	90,000	240,000	0.25	0.17
Patient education on disease prevention	2,000	40,000	10,000	30,000	0.03	0.02
Other nonbilled services	8,000	30,000	—	30,000	0.03	0.02
Subtotal community services	34,000	400,000	100,000	300,000	0.31	0.21
Medical education						
Physicians, nurses, technicians, other	—	—	—	—		
Scholarships, funding for health professionals	—	—	—	—		
Other medical education	—	—	—	—		
Subtotal medical education	—	—	—	—		
Subsidized health services						
Emergency and trauma care	—	—	—	—		
Neonatal intensive care	—	—	—	—		
Free-standing community clinics	5,200	400,000	—	400,000	0.41	0.28
Collaborative efforts in preventive medicine	—	—	—	—		
Other subsidized health services	—	—	—	—	0.00	0.00
Subtotal subsidized health services	5,200	400,000	—	400,000	0.41	0.28
Research	—	—	—	—		
Cash and in-kind donations	—	45,000	—	45,000	0.05	0.03
GRAND TOTAL	121,206	$42,812,000	$30,900,000	$11,912,000	12.17	8.22

RHMC adopted this reporting practice several years ago because of its highly structured definitions. It allows them a defendable reporting mechanism and a framework for year-to-year comparisons. The administration uses this report in an effort to understand and budget for community service benefits.

It is important for tax-exempt organizations to be clear, concise, and complete in their descriptions of their tax-exempt achievements because it is likely to be reviewed by community and noncommunity members interested in the sources and uses of the organization funds.

There are some very specific rules regarding the public's access to the IRS 990. The document is available through the IRS or through the tax-exempt organization to anyone requesting public inspection or copying. If requested through the organization, all parts of the return and all required schedules and attachments other than the schedule of contributors to the organization must be made available. It must be available during regular business hours at the organization's principal business office and at each of its regional or district offices having three or more employees.[3] Failure of the organization to properly respond to requests will result in significant fines to the organization.

The not-for-profit 990 tax return has one particular piece of information that is often scrutinized by certain segments of the public more than any other. Schedule A of the 990 requires the organization to report the names, occupations, and salaries of the five highest paid employees of the organization who are not officers of the corporation. On another page the salaries of any paid officers of the corporation are reported. Therefore salaries of the organizations top officials are likely to appear on one or the other page. Additionally, compensation of the five highest paid independent contractors for professional services are required on Schedule A. The organization's auditors, lawyers, and consultants often dominate these lines. Many local newspapers around the country have regular features reporting these wages and contract services at not-for-profit corporations.

Thus, the IRS 990 report has many uses, both for the organization and the public. As with any tax return, it is imperative to report the required information in a timely and accurate manner following the rules and regulations set down by the government. In the case of the 990, it is also important to understand the potential implications of the need to report the salaries of the highest paid employees as well as the five highest paid service providers. The RHMC finance staff and managers responsible for the preparation and submission of these tax returns are aware of the rules for reporting and filling requests for information. In fact, they use outside tax experts to review their preparations each year before the filing dates to assure that they have made no errors. This also assures that they have complied with any new rules that may have become effective in the tax year in question.

---

[3] Section M. Public Inspection of Completed Exempt Organization Returns and Approved Exemption Applications, Returns for Organizations Exempt from Income Tax Under Section 501(c)(3) of the Internal Revenue Code, Department of Treasury, Internal Revenue Service, General Instructions for Form 990 and Form 9990-EZ, page 8.

12
CHAPTER

December

Self-doubt dominated the dreams of Sam Barnes. He was worried. He was trying to move along a clearly marked road, his destination shining in the distance. But he was mired in mud, unable to make any progress. And he did not know why.

"Come on, come on, let's go," he thought to himself. "I can do this. I can get there!"

"What do I need to do to break out of this rut and get going?" rumbled through his mind.

Just then a booming voice echoed through his thoughts, "And just where is it that you think you are going?" asked the Voice.

"Whaddya mean, where am I going?" responded the incredulous Sam. "Obviously, I'm heading out there. It's my destination, my goal."

Now it was the Voice's turn to act incredulous. "Oh really Sam, and just what does that destination represent to you?"

"Huh?!?" Blinked Sam.

"Come on, Sam, don't be so obtuse. You can see the beacon out there on the horizon and you can even see what looks like a path. But if you look closer, you'll notice that there are some gaps along that paved road. In fact, you are standing in one of those gaps right now, a patch of mud so deep that it'll take you quite a bit of hard thinking to get out of it," the Voice said pretty adamantly.

"Well, I still don't know what you're talking about. Me, obtuse? I don't think so. Never was, never will be," Sam said, somewhat defensively.

"Oh really," smiled the Voice. "If you're so smart, then you tell me where you're heading, and why."

With that Sam hesitated just a moment. "Oh yeah, well of course I know where I'm heading. Out there is STABILITY for me and this crazy industry I'm in. We're going through some pretty unstable times at the moment in the financing of health-care. Not only are a lot of these reimbursement cutbacks destabilizing to the delivery of patient care, there is also a big problem for many families who stand to lose their take-home pay if they are laid off because of these cutbacks. So yeah, I'm worried. Wouldn't you be?"

"Now that you ask, yeah I guess I would be," said the Voice. "But, Sam now that you've been able to pinpoint the problem, the next question is what are you going to do to work out a solution so that you can begin the move forward again?"

Sam was mad. "Oh man, you are one big pain. Question, questions. I answer one but is it good enough for you? No! Right away you hit me with another big one. I'll tell you, no rest for the weary."

"Hey, hey, nice try, but I can see right through you. Stop avoiding the question. What are YOU going to do about the financial instability in the industry?"

"Me, why me? Why do I have to be the one to do anything about the financial instability in the industry? Who am I? I'm no politician. I can't make the managed care companies pay providers any more money. I can't make the Feds reduce their cutbacks to the industry. Not only do they think we already make too much money, they really don't have the money to fully fund the industry even if they wanted to. Their funding source is going broke. Also, those politicians always take the expedient way out. They don't lead. They react. They are afraid to alienate any constituency that votes, so they refuse to make decisions that would put the right kind of incentives in place that would begin to minimize Medicare Trust Fund disbursements."

"Oh really, tell me more," said the Voice.

"Well it doesn't seem like anybody is dealing with the conflict between patients who are demanding more services and the payors who are demanding less payments. The patients want to get better but want someone else to pay. The payors want to limit benefits so they don't have to pay. They need to raise their premiums in order to produce a bottom line margin for their own health plans or insurance companies, but they have been stymied in that regard. After all, the employers feel like they have maxed out on medical insurance premiums," came Sam's stream-of-consciousness reply.

"And your point is?" questioned the Voice.

"We need to rationalize the financing of care. We need someone to make the hard decisions. If there is too much capacity in the healthcare delivery system, contributing to too much fixed cost, someone needs the authority to close it down. If too many providers are in a certain geographical area, a facilitectomy (removal of a facility) needs to be performed. If there are not enough facilities in certain areas, like rural settings, then appropriate additions should be made."

"Come on, Sam, grow up, you know those kind of proposals are nonstarters," said the Voice, quite sarcastically. "First, no politician is going to take you up on that proposal, it's political suicide. Second, in some cases, it's been tried. Some of what you suggest is in the hands of state-run Certificate of Need Boards. Third, it sounds like another government boondoggle, letting an authority make a decision that's better left to the free market."

"Blah, blah, blah, Voice. You sound just like every one else who throws down obstacles because its easier to maintain a bad status quo than work out a better future system. What you just said is nonsense. Most Certificate of Need Boards were disbanded by their states because of ineffectiveness, and they didn't have the authority to delete facilities. They could only decide whether or not to add healthcare facilities and services, and usually only within certain provider types, making for severe unfairness. For example, they might have to approve the addition of a MRI service for hospitals, but they might not be able to stop a physician's office from adding one. Pretty dopey stuff. So it is certainly a bad model to use.

"As far as your comment about government boondoggles and letting the free market prevail, that's very problematic. This country has over 40 million underinsured or uninsured citizens, which is about 15% of the population. Who's speaking for them? Certainly not the free market thinkers. And what about the population that's aging? Right now, Medicare covers only 100 skilled nursing home days, in many cases leaving a string of poor, uninsured older people with very few options. Medicaid has already become the payor of last resort and its already government funding. If we leave government to always be the final payor of services, then maybe we need them to participate in the initial solution discussions."

"Sam, Sam, Sam," chided the Voice, "boy, sometimes you are such a bleeding heart. How can government be the solution when they are so often the problem? Don't you remember when the president tried to do this in 1993 and 1994? It failed miserably. Nobody wanted it. Health planning was set back for years because of it."

"Ah ha," thought Sam. "I've got him now." "Oh yeah," he retorted smartly. "Well that's where you're wrong buster. The 1993 initiative failed for three reasons. One, the process was handled very badly. The lesson learned was to be less arrogant and get more constituencies involved. Second, the opposition mounted a brilliant campaign. The people responsible for providing commercial health insurance had a heavy self-interest in seeing the proposals defeated. They convinced a number of legislators through scare advertising that government-run healthcare would be as inefficient as the post office. They also convinced many people that there were no problems in healthcare finance. There motto was 'If it ain't broke, don't fix it.' But you and I know it's broke, structurally and financially. Third, the proponents were ahead of their time. While it was obvious to many of us in the industry that there was a healthcare-financing problem already in the early 1990s, it was not obvious to the legislators."

"So what, Sam, that's still a lot of rehash." The Voice's voice was starting to tire. "You're living in the past. I don't see any of that mud loosening up. I still don't see you moving ahead. You seem to have analyzed a lot of the problem. You still haven't told me what feasible ideas you have to help solve the financing instability problem and if or when you propose to present them."

"Okay, already. Maybe there are a few things I can do. I'm nothing but a small cog in a small wheel. At that moment, the best I can do is continue to do the best job possible for RHMC. That means continuing to maximize the revenues staying within all the applicable laws and helping the clinical and nonclinical department managers contain their costs through assistance with reporting and benchmarking.

"But the other thing I can do is help to get out the message about healthcare financial management and healthcare financing. They are the two sides of the same coin. It's a fact that you can't be the best healthcare financial manager without having a solid understanding of healthcare financing issues. And if you have a truly good understanding of the financing issues, it is hard to ignore them and try to improve it because of the significant impact they have on each facility's bottom line."

"So, what are you going to do?" an inquisitive Voice asked.

"I suppose I could write a book that blends theory with practice, anecdote with history and narrative with exposition. It should be something that would help in understanding the day-to-day functioning of healthcare managers and their staffs. The real efforts it takes to keep a healthcare organization running as smoothly as possible in this difficult day and age. My hope would be that it allows readers to gain this understanding and as a result, one or many of them can take the next steps to improve the financing of the healthcare delivery system in the future. None of us is going to solve this alone. It will take a concerted effort by a strong group committed to an overall solution, not just Medicare and Medicaid. Everything and everyone."

And with that, Sam was startled out of his dream. As he regained consciousness, he felt his sore feet loosen up as he jumped out of bed to get to his word processor.

December. Thanksgiving gone. Christmas and New Year's Day to come once again, and quickly. The air is brisk as it skims across the Great Plains and Canadian frontier, heading east to a rendezvous with the denizens of northern Illinois. The winter coats are out and the first dusting of snow has already been felt in the region. The winter doldrums are beginning to set in.

MORE Y2K AT THE YEAR END

But at RHMC, there is no time for those emotions. There is just too much work to do. In particular, the finance managers and staff are preparing for a special New Year, January 1, 2000, and hoping that all the work that they have performed over the past

18 months allows them to avoid any Y2K disasters. They are not only concerned about whether they have found and fixed any and all internal bugs, they are also concerned about some things that seem completely out of their control, such as the following issues.

External and Internal Utilities and Services

- Supplies of electricity, water, telecommunication, and transportation from outside providers
- Supplies of security, fire protection, and other emergency/disaster coordination provided by community resources
- Communication with suppliers and payors, including banking for cash flows and payroll
- Staffing affected by Y2K emergency/disaster (including issues such as scheduling. communications, payroll, fear of family situation)
- Staffing/consultation (i.e., additional hires/contracts to facilitate resolving Y2K problems or facilitating contingency planning)

Other Concerns

- Coordinated testing with outside suppliers and vendors to ensure that the tests themselves have not been ameliorated by unknown or unauthorized system changes or modifications
- Obtaining certification or y2k status/reengineering information and materials from outside vendors and the government
- Meeting medical services obligations
- Meeting legal, fiduciary, community, and employer responsibilities
- Meeting external financial requirements such as FASB, AICPA, and SEC
- Meeting other data and certification requirements, such as quality reviews, JCAHO review, and external auditing[1]

Y2K Contingency Planning

As we know from Chapter 10, RHMC had set up a Y2K contingency planning subcommittee earlier in the year charged with determining a course of action that would keep the organization up and running even if some of the worst case scenarios came to reality.

The subcommittee did its work and determined that if power went out for a period not to exceed 48 hours, there would be very little disruption in the operations. The organization's generators would be able to handle a minimal power load, maintaining essential patient care operations. Downtime procedures, which have always been available, would become operational. This would allow the nursing and ancillary staffs to perform physician ordered tests and treatments while retaining the

---

[1] Discussion paper on Y2K, HFMA Knowledge Network, February, 1999.

charge information on paper until the computers became available after the power was restored.

If, on the other hand, the power was not restored within 48 hours, there was a fear that a *teotwawki* (the end of the world as we know it) scenario would take over. There was great concern about how Ridgeland Heights Medical Center would be able to cope in the event of a disaster of that magnitude. Assurances that *teotwawki* would not happen needed to be relied on because RHMC could not control the utilities issue. They felt comfortable that as long as the power stayed on, they could cope with any other contingency.

The administration planned a nonalcoholic New Year's Eve party at the facility for the evening of December 31, 1999, because they had decided to have a full shift of personnel working at midnight, monitoring and fixing any internal glitch caused by Y2K. At this point, the planning was done and fate would decide the final consequences.

GETTING READY FOR YEAR-END REPORTING . . . AGAIN!

While the finance managers were attempting to deal with this once-in-a-century problem, the finance staff was performing its routine business of preparing the November financial statement and taking the first steps in getting ready for year-end reporting. During the November closing of the books, the staff takes extra time to analyze and evaluate the balances in the balance sheet and income statement accounts. They are searching for unexplainable variances.

Any variances will need to be understood and appropriately adjusted before the close of the year and it is always better to make these adjustments in November rather than December. December adjustments are more obvious to the primary readers of the financial statements, the CEO, and the board because they have become conditioned to inquire about significant December line item changes. While it is best to have no adjustments made by the auditors, it is also preferable to have no major internal adjustments in December, if it can be avoided. It's much better to make the adjustment in November.

OPEN HEART SURGERY PRO FORMA

Meanwhile, RHMC's administration has continued to analyze the future of the organization and has determined that the time had come to fill a major hole in its product offering. As a medium-sized community hospital, RHMC did not perform cardiovascular (CV) surgery (commonly known as open heart surgery). When this procedure was first developed in the 1960s, it was performed only by surgeons at major academic (teaching) medical centers that had been involved in the initial trials or who had subsequently trained and/or assisted with the original surgeons.

Over the years, many surgeons have been trained on this procedure. In addition, the steps required to perform these procedures have become well known, and in the 1980s some community hospitals began offering CV surgery. The mortality rates at many of these hospitals were equivalent to those at the teaching hospitals. This encouraged some other community hospitals to offer this service. In the late 1990s, it was important, in a competitive service area, for some community hospitals to provide this service to its patients. It indicated to patients and their physicians that the organization practiced serious medicine, surpassing other community hospitals that did not offer the service and on par with some academic programs.

RHMC administration decided it was time for them to attempt to implement one of the main tactics in its strategic plan. They knew that in order to continue to compete for patients in its core and secondary service areas, they must develop a cardiac surgery program. Heart disease is and has been the number one killer of Americans for many years. Heart disease, which leads to death, also may occasion the need for significant inpatient and outpatient services. In order for RHMC to access more of these patients for treatment, an open heart surgery program was required.

To determine the financial implications of such a program, the finance division was asked to develop a financial pro forma. Unlike the pro forma developed for the MRI, as shown in Chapter 1, which was relative easy because it involved only one department—radiology—and involved only one set of volume assumptions, the open heart surgery program involves many more departments and personnel. This creates a number of additional variables, thus increasing the complexity of the analysis, which increases to some extent the risk of uncertainty that the assumptions are sound.

Development of Volumes and Revenues

The first step to developing an open heart surgery pro forma, as with almost every other pro forma, is to determine the volumes of services that can be provided. In this case there are two prevalent procedure types. Coronary artery bypass grafts (CABGs) are often pronounce cabbages and are generally the procedures referred to when people talk about open heart surgery. Percutaneous transluminal coronary angioplasty (PTCA) is a procedure that cleans out plaque that has formed on the vessels that lead to the heart, also through invasive surgery.

Tables 12–1 and 12–2 show the detailed and summary volumes projections, which are based on usage rate within the organization's service area as well as the actual volume of cardiac catherization procedures currently performed at RHMC. The best way to initially determine if they will be able to achieve a CABG volume of 200 per year (a number generally agreed to be a minimum for competency in the industry) is to review the current volumes that it is generating. After that review, the medical center should look at the surrounding community volumes. Thus, the medical center's plan is to convert 100% of its current catherization patients that have been transferred to other facilities into its own CABG patients. That, however, will give them only 120 potential patients a year. So, it then reviewed that patient origin data of all CABG patients within its surrounding community, which is available from a state database, to determine which other hospital's volume it could divert. This is called a market-based solution.

After determining the volumes, the financial analyst estimates the gross revenues it can charge for the service *based on* current market rates. In addition to gross revenues, RHMC needs to estimate the mix of payors that will represent the CABG and PTCA patients. It does this based on surveys of area hospitals that are willing to share such data. It can also validate this data by reviewing the payor mix of its catherization patients. RHMC needs to perform this estimate in order to project its net revenues, which will be based on the contractual rates that can be negotiated with third-party managed care payors as well as acceptance of the rates paid by Medicare and Medicaid for these services. Finally, in order to complete its net revenue projections, the medical center will need to estimate these contractual rates. This is also based on information from other area hospitals and, in some cases, best guesses from the medical center's managed care negotiator.

Financial Analysts Should not Be Proposal Champions

To reiterate a comment from the pro forma development in Chapter 1, the absolute toughest assumption in any pro forma is the volume projection. However, the second toughest is often the net revenue rates assumptions because of the significant possibility of being too optimistic.

It is important to be conservative when estimating both the volumes and the net revenues. In this industry, as well as most others, optimistic pro forma projections have often given way to *greenlighting* a project that subsequently fails because of problems within these two areas. Nobody, particularly the financial analyst, wants a finger pointed because of overly optimistic projections. The finance pro forma developer needs to use their best judgment in critically evaluating the numbers that are presented to them from the operations representative. Keep in mind that the operations representative has a bias towards getting a project approved. It allows them to grow their area of responsibility.

The finance representative should never have such a bias. They need to remain independent and objective at all times. If the pro forma shows a very good internal rate of return, then it will be obvious to all reviewers and the project will be approved on its merits. Do not help the result by improving these critical pro forma elements just because it seems like a good project to do or because the operations representative is pushing to do so. Also, the pro forma finance representative developer should not become a "champion" of the project. That is the role of the operations or business development representative. Always stay objective!

Development of Expenses

After completing the volume assumptions, the projection of expenses can begin. Like revenues, expenses are both fixed and dependent on the volume projections. Because most project expenses are variable (i.e., they vary with volume), it is important to have the volume assumptions completed before an estimate of staffing and supplies can begin. Table 12–3 is the CV surgery projected income statement (pro forma). In addition to its summarization of gross and net revenues, it shows summarized expenses by specific categories.

T A B L E 12-1

Ridgeland Heights Medical Center
Cardiac Surgery Program
Projected Cardiac Procedures, Gross Revenues & Net Reimbursement
Years 1–5

DRG Number	Year 1	Year 2	Year 3	Year 4	Year 5
103 Heart transplant	0	0	0	0	0
104 Cardiac valve proc with cardiac cath	7	7	20	20	20
105 Cardiac valve proc without cardiac cath	8	8	20	20	20
106 Coronary bypass with cardiac cath	30	55	80	80	80
107 Coronary bypass without cardiac cath	30	55	80	80	80
108 Other cardiothoracic procedures	0	4	4	4	4
110 Major cardiovascular procs with cardiac cath	0	14	14	14	14
111 Major cardiovascular procs without cardiac cath	0	4	4	4	4
112 Percutaneous cardiovascular procedures	85	100	100	100	100
116 Other perm cardiac pacemakers implant or PTCA with stent	0	0	0	0	0
Total cardiac procedures	160	247	322	322	322
Total CABG and valve procedures	75	125	200	200	200
Total PTCAs	85	100	100	100	100
Total other procedures	0	22	22	22	22
Total cardiac procedures	160	247	322	322	322

DRG Number	Year 1	Year 2	Year 3	Year 4	Year 5	Medicare Reimburse	Contractual Percentage
103 Heart transplant	0	0	0	0	0	0	
104 Cardiac valve proc with cardiac cath	80,000	80,000	80,000	80,000	80,000	31,823	60.22
105 Cardiac valve proc without cardiac cath	74,000	74,000	74,000	74,000	74,000	24,345	67.10
106 Coronary bypass with cardiac cath	74,000	74,000	74,000	74,000	74,000	24,156	67.36
107 Coronary bypass without cardiac cath	65,000	65,000	65,000	65,000	65,000	17,687	72.79
108 Other cardiothoracic procedures	65,000	65,000	65,000	65,000	65,000	17,687	72.79
110 Major cardiovascular procs with cardiac cath	67,000	67,000	67,000	67,000	67,000	18,080	73.01
111 Major cardiovascular procs without cardiac cath	67,000	67,000	67,000	67,000	67,000	18,080	73.01
112 Percutaneous cardiovascular procedures	33,000	33,000	33,000	33,000	33,000	9,106	72.41
116 Other perm cardiac pacemakers implant or PTCA with stent	33,000	33,000	33,000	33,000	33,000	10,498	68.19

DRG Number	Year 1	Year 2	Year 3	Year 4	Year 5	Medicare Reimburse	Contractual Percentage
103 Heart transplant	0	0	0	0	0	0	
104 Cardiac valve proc with cardiac cath	560,000	560,000	1,600,000	1,600,000	1,600,000	21,824	72.72
105 Cardiac valve proc without cardiac cath	592,000	592,000	1,480,000	1,480,000	1,480,000	17,526	76.32
106 Coronary bypass with cardiac cath	2,220,000	4,070,000	5,920,000	5,920,000	5,920,000	20,782	71.92
107 Coronary bypass without cardiac cath	1,950,000	3,575,000	5,200,000	5,200,000	5,200,000	17,795	72.62
108 Other cardiothoracic procedures	0	260,000	260,000	260,000	260,000		
110 Major cardiovascular procs with cardiac cath	0	938,000	938,000	938,000	938,000		
111 Major cardiovascular procs without cardiac cath	0	268,000	268,000	268,000	268,000		
112 Percutaneous cardiovascular procedures	2,805,000	3,300,000	3,300,000	3,300,000	3,300,000	7,660	76.79
116 Other perm cardiac pacemakers implant or PTCA with stent	0	0	0	0	0		
Total cardiac procedures	8,127,000	1,356,3000	18,966,000	18,966,000	18,966,000		
Total CABG and valve procedures	5,322,000	8,797,000	14,200,000	14,200,000	14,200,000		
Total PTCAs	2,805,000	3,300,000	3,300,000	3,300,000	3,300,000		
Total other procedures	0	1,466,000	1,466,000	1,466,000	1,466,000		
Total cardiac procedures	8,127,000	13,563,000	18,966,000	18,966,000	18,966,000		

Payor Mix

	DRG Number #106	DRG Number #107
Blue Cross	2	1.57	2	2.56
HMO	23	18.11	50	64.10
HMO Sen	28	22.05	14	17.95
Medicare	55	43.31	4	5.13
Medicaid	2	1.57	2	2.56
PPO	17	13.39	6	7.69
Total	127	100.00	78	100.00

T A B L E 12–2

Ridgeland Heights Medical Center
Cardiac Surgery Program
Summary of Assumptions
December, 1998

Capital costs	CV Program					
Equipment	$1,092,553					
Renovations	$ 5,000					
Total capital costs	$1,097,553					
		Year 1	Year 2	Year 3	Year 4	Year 5	Total
Volumes						
CABG and valve procedures		75	125	200	200	200	800
PTCA/other valve procedures		85	122	122	122	122	573
Total volumes		160	247	322	322	322	1,373
Total volumes per day @ 260		0.62	0.95	1.24	1.24	1.24	1.06
Charge per test						
CABG and valve procedures		70,960	70,376	71,000	71,000	71,000	
PTCA/other valve procedures		33,000	39,066	39,066	39,066	39,066	
Gross revenues						
CABG and valve procedures		5,322,000	8,797,000	14,200,000	14,200,000	14,200,000	56,719,000
PTCA/other valve procedures		2,805,000	4,766,000	4,766,000	4,766,000	4,766,000	21,869,000
Total revenues		$8,127,000	$13,563,000	$18,966,000	$18,966,000	$18,966,000	$78,588,000

Payor Mix

Medicare	40.00%	40.00%	40.00%	40.00%	40.00%
Managed care	55.00%	55.00%	55.00%	55.00%	55.00%
All other	5.00%	5.00%	5.00%	5.00%	5.00%
Total payor mix	100.00%	100.00%	100.00%	100.00%	100.00%

Contractual allowances

CABG and valve procedures

Medicare	72.80%	72.80%	72.80%	72.80%	72.80%
Managed care	72.60%	72.60%	72.60%	72.60%	72.60%
All other	20.00%	20.00%	20.00%	20.00%	20.00%

PTCA/other valve procedures

Medicare	72.00%	72.00%	72.00%	72.00%	72.00%
Managed care	77.00%	77.00%	77.00%	77.00%	77.00%
All other	20.00%	20.00%	20.00%	20.00%	20.00%

NOTES:

-Volumes and service mix are based on research from current RHMC cath lab volumes and external sources.

-Payor mix is based on Smith Memorial Hospital actual data for DRG numbers 106 and 107.

-Gross revenue is based on full year operations for DRGs 106 and 107. All other DRGs are estimated based on 106 and 107.

-Contractual allowances are based on Medicare and Managed Care approximate rates from other regional hospitals.

-Gross charges are projected to increase at 0% per year.

-Variable expenses are projected to increase by an inflationary rate of 5% per year.

-Equipment is depreciated over 8 years.

-Spin-off revenues and expenses are provided at a 5% increase over the 1997 actual cardiovascular service line.

TABLE 12-3

Ridgeland Heights Medical Center
Cardiac Surgery Program
Income Statement Proforma
December, 1998

	Year 1	Year 2	Year 3	Year 4	Year 5	Total
Revenues						
Gross revenues	$8,127,000	$13,563,000	$18,966,000	$18,966,000	$18,966,000	$78,588,000
Less: contractual allowances	5,751,656	9,600,616	13,385,201	13,385,201	13,385,201	55,507,874
Net revenue before spin-off	2,375,344	3,962,384	5,580,799	5,580,799	5,580,799	23,080,126
Marginal spin-off revenue	207,500	311,250	415,000	415,000	415,000	1,763,750
Total net revenues	2,582,844	4,273,634	5,995,799	5,995,799	5,995,799	24,843,876
Expenses						
Staffing	1,008,296	1,156,089	1,285,934	1,336,223	1,388,524	$ 6,175,066
Fringes @ 30%	302,489	346,827	385,780	400,867	416,557	$ 1,852,520
Total staffing and benefits	1,310,785	1,502,916	1,671,714	1,737,090	1,805,081	$ 8,027,586
Variable start-up staffing costs	131,532					
Variable expenses:						
Laboratory	75,337	120,587	174,419	174,419	174,419	$ 719,182
Radiology	31,912	52,027	78,924	78,924	78,924	$ 320,711
Pharmacy and IVs	51,293	82,539	121,082	121,082	121,082	$ 497,078
Other ancillaries	19,814	31,725	45,928	45,928	45,928	$ 189,322
Supplies—RHMC direct variable	683,519	1,004,343	1,627,793	1,627,793	1,627,793	$ 6,571,240
Marginal spinoff cost	112,500	168,750	225,000	225,000	225,000	$ 956,250
Total variable expenses	974,375	1,459,970	2,273,146	2,273,146	2,273,146	$ 9,253,783

Fixed expenses						
Franchise fee—teaching hospital	250,000	175,000	100,000	100,000	100,000	$ 725,000
Contract labor—perfusionists	18,750	31,250	50,000	50,000	50,000	$ 200,000
M.D. house coverage	327,840	340,954	354,592	368,775	383,526	$ 1,775,687
Medical director fee	25,000	25,000	25,000	25,000	25,000	$ 125,000
Education	44,480	13,480	13,480	13,480	13,480	$ 98,400
Maintenance costs	64,154	64,154	64,154	64,154	64,154	$ 320,770
Marketing	250,000	200,000	100,000	100,000	100,000	$ 750,000
Equipment depreciation	140,319	140,319	140,319	140,319	140,319	$ 701,596
Building renovation depreciation	0	625	625	625	625	$ 2,500
Total nonstaffing expenses	1,120,543	990,782	848,170	862,354	877,105	$ 4,698,953
Total expenses	3,537,235	3,953,668	4,793,030	4,872,590	4,955,332	21,980,322
Contribution to overhead	($ 954,391)	$ 319,967	$ 1,202,769	$ 1,123,209	$ 1,040,467	$ 2,732,022
Internal rate of return						28.08%
FTEs	16.7	18.8	20.5	22	23.5	23.5
Cash flow	−1,097,553	460,911	1,343,713	1,264,154	1,181,412	3,436,117

Staffing Expenses

A key expense assumption is estimating the number and type of staff required to perform the services. In the case of the open heart surgery program, there are several different types of employees required, such as specialized operating room nurses and technicians; intensive care unit nurses; additional cardiac catherization nurses and technicians; as well as cardiology, respiratory therapy, and cardiac rehabilitation technicians. In this case, RHMC estimates it will need an total of 16.7 additional full time equivalent (FTE) employees in the first year of the program rising to 23.5 FTEs in the fifth year.

Fringe Benefits

RHMC is consistent in its use of a 30% fringe benefit rate on all of its pro formas. The derivation of this rate was explained in detail in Chapter 1, and in this pro forma they continue to do so.

Variable Start-up Staffing Expense

As with most new programs, there will be expenses incurred to start-up a program before any revenues are generated. These start-up costs are usually related to the training of the new program staff, whether new employees from the outside or re-training of existing staff from other departments. This training is obviously important because the staff must be ready to perform in a competent manner on the day that the service opens to the public.

In the case of the open heart surgery program, training is extensive for all levels of staff involved. Most new staff will receive eight weeks of intensive training, both in the classroom and on the job, at other hospitals that already are performing the service. In addition, currently employed staff will receive the necessary training to treat and service the new patients. The cost of their training, as well as the cost of the replacement staff paid while they are training outside the unit will be included in this start-up cost.

Variable Expenses

To determine variable expenses of the new service, which involves several different hospital departments, it is essential to be able to estimate two items to the greatest precision possible. These two items are the *volumes* (units of service) of the new services to be rendered (which we know is already available because of the work performed to determine revenues) and the *cost per unit of service.*

Determining the cost per unit of service does not have to be an onerous task. If the organization has developed a cost accounting system, then it should not be difficult to use the cost that has already been established for each individual service code (procedure code). These procedure code costs should then be applied against the projected volumes to determine the variable expenses of the new service. If the organization has not developed a cost accounting system, it can still use the simple, though less sophisticated, method called the ratio of cost to charges, available to all healthcare organizations that file a Medicare Cost Report. The ratio of costs to charges was reviewed in detail, in Chapter 4.

Fixed Expenses

The fixed expenses are generally very specific to the program and, of course by definition, they do not vary with volume. In this case, there are three key fixed expenses.

1. A franchise fee
2. A cost for 24-hour physician coverage of the cardiology patients in the hospital
3. Marketing costs

Franchise Fee—Because RHMC is a community hospital and does not have prior experience or expertise in open heart surgery, it has decided to affiliate with a respected academic medical center just on the fringes of the RHMC service area, to provide the experience and expertise. The academic medical center decided to charge RHMC a franchise fee for its services that include on-site and off-site training of RHMC staff, any and all required technical assistance, and the use of their CV surgeons.

24-Hour Physician Coverage—Again, because RHMC is itself not a teaching hospital, it does not have interns and residents to cover its inpatients throughout the day and night. The RHMC administration decided that in order to promote and market its new service to primary care and specialist physicians (especially cardiologists) in its service area and beyond, it needs to offer this 24-hour on-site coverage by hiring its own set of physicians to cover the inpatients. This coverage allows the referring cardiologists to increase their comfort level that their patients have adequate care available, especially at night.

Marketing Costs—As can be seen in the projected income statement, this program is projected to earn net revenues of almost $25,000,000 over the first five-year period. The administration has determined that it is worth $750,000 over that same time period to bring this new program to the attention of its prospective customers, primarily the referring physicians such as primary care physicians and area cardiologists. While there will be a small amount of marketing directed to the consumer, this is considered only a secondary consideration because most patients in the late 1990s are unable to self-refer for nonprimary services.

Financial Conclusion—Open Heart Surgery Program

The contribution margin or contribution to overhead over the five year period is a positive $2,732,022 including depreciation charges. On its face, this would appear to be a good return. But, this does not tell the whole story. As was explained in Chapter 1, many healthcare organizations use either the net present value calculation or the internal rate of return. RHMC prefers the percentage methodology inherent in the internal rate of return. The 28.08% internal rate of return on the initial investment for the open heart surgery program justifies the administration to take this program and its $1,092,553 initial investment to the December finance committee and the board of directors.

It is important to note that the finance division did more than just present the models in Tables 12–1, 12–2, and 12–3. They also built sensitivity models that assign more optimistic and pessimistic volumes in order to assess the impact of other possible scenarios. The finance committee requires these sensitivities because they are aware that pro formas are only as good as the volume assumptions made.

DECEMBER FINANCE COMMITTEE AGENDA ROUTINE ITEMS

In addition to the CV surgery program that the administration will present at the December finance committee and the regularly scheduled monthly financial statements and accounts receivable report, there are two more routine reports that will be presented. There will be a review of the organization's insurance coverages and a request for approval of the external auditors and their fees for the following year.

Review Malpractice Insurance Coverages

An important feature and function of RHMC's cost structure and risk management program, professional liability insurance (or malpractice insurance, as it is commonly known), is reviewed with the finance committee once a year. They are concerned about the level of coverages as well as the premium costs. Table 12–4 shows the report that is presented to the committee. As with most insurances, the cost of coverage decreases on each layer above the primary or first layer because there is less chance for claims being made against these additional layers. RHMC was fortunate to have experienced a reduction of premiums in 1996 and 1997 as a result of a small number of claims being filed. In addition, there were even fewer payments, or losses, against claims made. Still, it is incumbent on the organization to guard itself against potential claims of poor treatment or poor outcomes. It is within the fiduciary responsibility of the finance committee members to be apprised of and understand the significance of the level of malpractice coverages. They are comfortable with the current levels and understand the need to pay these self-insurance premiums.

Review and Approve Auditors and Their Fees for the Current Year

The final action that will be made by the finance committee this year is approval of the auditors along with their proposed fees. The audit partner and manager of the CPA firm that RHMC has been using for a number of years have been invited to present their proposal indicating the scope of the audit, a high-level discussion of how they plan to conduct the audit, and the various responsibilities of the client. They present the *arrangement letter* that spells out, in detail, the responsibility of the

T A B L E 12–4

Ridgeland Heights Medical Center
Professional Liability Self-Insurance Status
Premium Update
December, 1999

RHMC's self-insurance administrator has estimated the premiums required to maintain our coverage for professional liability over the period through December, 2000. The coverage will be identical in amount and structure to that which was in effect in 1999. An optional third layer of excess coverage was added effective January 1, 1997.

	Per Occurrence Limit	Aggregate Limit	Funding
First Layer	$1,000,000	None	Primary Trust
Second Layer	$10,00,0000	$20,000,000	Excess Trust
Third Layer	$10,00,0000	$10,000,000	Excess Coverage

The schedule below indicates the premiums that have been paid for the policy years beginning in 1995:

	1996	1997	1998	1999	2000
First Layer	$450,000	$400,000	$600,000	$650,000	$680,000
Second Layer	250,000	250,000	280,000	300,000	310,000
Third Layer	—	100,000	95,000	90,000	90,000
Total	$700,000	$750,000	$975,000	$1,040,000	$1,080,000
Budget	$900,000	$800,000	$900,000	$10,00,000	$1,100,000

audit firm and RHMC. It also spells out any additional services that the organization has commissioned the auditors to perform and the fees for these services. These arrangement letters are standard and have evolved over time as the auditors have had to defend themselves and their firms in court, particularly when the auditor's client went bankrupt, leaving a line of creditors looking for some recourse.

The audit partner will spend some time pointing out current items of interest in the industry (hot topics!) and comment on any topics that the finance committee members might want to know more about. The finance committee at RHMC is charged with selecting an audit firm each year. It is important for the members to feel comfortable with their choice because the auditors will be passing judgments on the quality of the work of the finance managers. They want a professional and unbiased opinion of the financial statements and of the financial managers and staff. It is an important decision that is made easier if an ongoing relationship has been established over the years.

The audit fees are reviewed for consistency by the committee. They are interested in any rates of increase over the prior year. In addition, the committee will periodically request that management perform a comparison of pricing with other audit firms in the region to determine if they are being charged more than their peers. While the committee values a long-standing relationship, they do not want to overpay for it. Thus it is in the best interest of the current audit firm to stay competitive because they know it will be checked.

Finance Committee Annual Achievements

The December finance committee meeting concludes the work of the committee members for the year. They have had a productive year, reviewing the work of the organization's management across most aspects of healthcare financial management. They touched on the following topics.

- Monthly financial statements reporting and analysis, particularly the variances between the actual results and the approved budget
- Special reviews regarding the ongoing payment reductions by the Medicare and Medicaid programs through the Balanced Budget and the Managed Care plans
- Accounts receivable issues and analysis
- Bond debt status
- Health and malpractice insurance analysis
- Approval of the auditors, their fees, and the annual audit and auditors management letter
- Pension status and the actuary's report
- Materials management analysis
- Information systems plans, particularly concerning the y2k issues and the new systems needed by the organization
- Approval of the five year strategic financial plan linked to the organization's strategic plan early in the year
- Approval of the annual budget for the upcoming year

Throughout the year, as part of their monthly review of the financial statements, they also were apprised of the income earned on their investments. Because of the positive market result of the past seven years, this has become the most pleasant issue for the committee members. However, their review was cursory because a separate investment committee was primarily involved with investment opportunities and results. Although the investment policies and practices are beyond the scope of this book, it has become extremely important in producing overall positive results for healthcare organizations, especially with the significant reductions in reimbursement rates by all the major payors.

Although the committee is somewhat disappointed in the overall operating margin results, management's ongoing education of the members regarding payment reductions and ongoing concerns regarding cost management have given the members a better appreciation of the challenges confronting healthcare organizations. They are in a better position to assess the year just past and the years that will follow. They are concerned about the financial integrity of the organization and worried about how to maintain and even improve the high level of patient care that currently exists. There have been discussions regarding the future of RHMC's financial position as well as that of the industry in general. While it takes on a crystal ball feel, it is a necessary step and required management technique for future planning.

LOOKING INTO THE FUTURE OF HEALTHCARE FINANCE

The future of healthcare financial management and healthcare financing is anyone's guess. It could take any one of a hundred paths, twisting and winding, approaching forks in the road not currently evident to current planners. Decisions could be made by government employees and/or politicians seeking to save the Medicare Trust Fund for future beneficiaries who may or may not achieve intended consequences. Decisions could also be made by the executives at managed care plans seeking to increase their profits at the expense of patients or providers by limiting their exposures on medical loss ratios. Decisions could also be made by the employers around the country, some of whom have grown tired of subsidizing medical insurance for their employees.

Each of these paths could continue to be taken simultaneously as they seem to be doing now, at the end of the 20th century, or they could diverge. Clues abound everywhere about the possible futures of healthcare finance. There are comprehensive industry models as well as segment models. RHMC and its administration are concerned about the financial implications of future trends. They would be delighted to recognize any particular emerging trend and be one of the first to implement services that would improve their revenues. They would also be amenable to applying any new ideas that produce efficiencies without compromising patient care or patient satisfaction.

For this discussion, it is best to look at the trends for the industry as a whole, the payors and the providers. Over the course of this book we have seen many concepts used in financial and general operations of the industry. We have seen many theories turned into practice and used to maximize the clinical, operational, and financial outcomes for RHMC. It is time to do some crystal ball gazing and see how some of the current trends might reach into the future.

General Macro Healthcare Trends

Two trends appear to be emerging faster and with more power.

1. The cutting edge research and development in gene therapy that has already produced some startlingly positive results in a few diseases in the late 1990s with the promise of landmark breakthroughs in other diseases in the very near future

2. The growing value of drug therapy in curing and/or containing illnesses that are already helping to produce some dramatic quality of life improvements in the lives of patients with certain diseases

There are some fascinating details regarding these two trends.

- *Gene Therapy*—Most likely gene therapy will be the primary medical treatment of the 21st century and have a profound affect on the delivery of medical care. Gene therapies will be the outgrowth of the 15 year $3 billion Human Genome Project funded by the federal government to find all human genes by 2005. By 1999, scientists had located about half of the 60,000 to 80,000 genes in the human genome, which is the set of genetic instructions carried within a single cell of an organism.

  According to an article in the *Chicago Tribune,* the most sweeping, near-term benefit of knowing our genes is likely to be a major improvement in health that could supersede the tremendous advances made by vaccines and antibiotics. The article quotes a physician as saying "even thought we like to think we're fairly sophisticated in medicine, we don't cure disease. We make it more bearable, or we prolong people's lives. Genomic medicine is different. It is the fact that you're getting at the root cause of the disease and you have rational new ways of treating it." In fact, another physician who is working on gene repair and gene therapy is quoted as saying "We can envision a hospital some day that is strictly a gene-therapy hospital."[2]

  Time magazine devoted 45 pages of its special January 11, 1999 edition to the genetics issue. Titled "The Future of Medicine—How Genetic Engineering will Change Us in the Next Century," it provides in-depth coverage to the history of modern genetic research, the current climate, and some of the medical advances that should be available in the near future. Possible develops on the horizon include the following.

  - Replacing defective cells to generate healthy tissue in combating Alzheimer's disease, heart disease, and diabetes

  - Developing fruits and vegetables to deliver drugs to stave off infectious diseases or treat various chronic conditions rather than rely on injections to do the same

  - Developing better vaccines to coax the body to churn out killer T-cells, which strike at offending microbes with great specificity

---

[2] Kotulak, R. (1999). Genetics Reshaping Medicine—The Future Is Now for Powerful New Tool. *Chicago Tribune,* February 21, p. 1.

- Lengthening the tips of certain chromosomes that might control the aging process (If this is determined to be correct, it could be theoretically possible to rejuvenate parts of any organ with a simple injection)

  There are great social and ethical issues at work here, and much bioethical debate is currently underway. The private sector is heavily involved in its own human genome research and some companies have already developed practical solutions to some diseases. In any event, the genie is out of bottle and the rampant development of these therapies is likely to be the number one healthcare story in the next century.

- *Drug Therapy*—This is an extension of much of the gene therapy that has already been done throughout the 1990s. Wonder drugs that significantly improve the health of patients with specific conditions are beginning to come to market, with enormous price tags attached. Many of these new drugs will reduce a patient's pain or provide cures to long-standing illnesses. Examples of these drugs were cited in an article appearing in *Modern Healthcare* in 1998. Two new drugs that lower the risk of heart attacks and death in patients with serious angina were introduced in mid-1998. These drugs are legitimate clinical breakthroughs but cost between $700 and $1,400 per episode of care.[3] The hospital and physician side of the industry and the insurance companies will be tested in their resolve for use and reimbursement of these new therapies.

  For example, Table 7–6 in Chapter 7 is a summary of projected price increases into the year 2000. This schedule clearly shows the pharmaceutical's line with the single highest percentage increase of any of the expense categories for both 1999 and 2000. And it is not expected to get better as more truly efficacious miracle drugs make their way through the FDA's testing process and become available for prescription use. So, the providers and insurers are already gearing up for the seemingly inevitable cost increases related to these new drug therapies. It remains to be seen if these high cost drugs eventually lower the overall cost of healthcare throughout the nation.

- *National Health Care Expenditure Projections*—In the first chapter of this book, it was shown that the United States spent almost $1.1 trillion on healthcare in 1997, the last year for which data are available. This accounted for 13.5% of the country's gross domestic product (GDP). Yet in an article published in the September/October issue of *Health Affairs,* it is estimated that healthcare spending will increase to $2.1 trillion, or 16.6% of the GDP, by the year 2007, an increase of almost 100% over this 10-year period.[4] These are huge dollar increases backed up by an

---

[3] Hensley, S. (1998). New Drugs Blast Budgets—Patients Benefit; Hospital Pharmacies Weigh Options. *Modern Healthcare,* June 8, p. 36.

[4] Health Care Financing Administration's Office of the Actuary. (1998). The Next Ten Years of Health Spending: What Does the Future Hold? *Health Affairs,* September/October, p. 128.

enormous movement of additional funds being spent on the nation's sick care and well care.

According to the summary of the study shown in Table 12–5, the areas with the greatest expenditure increases between 1996 and 2007 are drugs (144.6%), other personal healthcare (231.2%), and program administration (148.4%). As was recounted above, the reasons for the drug increases should be no surprise. A major part of the increase in other personal healthcare expenditures is related to alternative medicine, which has also been discussed previously. The increases in program administration can be inferred to be due in large part to the proliferation of small- to medium-sized managed care plans that charged significant administrative fees to act as middleman between the purchaser and providers of healthcare.[5]

Meanwhile hospitals (81.1%) and nursing homes (88.9%) expect much smaller increases caused in large part by the significant payment reductions by Medicare's Balanced Budget Act and managed care negotiations. Perhaps the biggest surprise is that home healthcare (118.9%) is not hit harder. This is because the need for these services are projected to continue to increase greatly even while the unit payments are being severely reduced.

No matter how this pie is sliced, $2.1 trillion is a gigantic pile of money that is going to be paid to healthcare industry providers. In no way is this an industry in decline. Not only does the gross number increase, the GDP percentage does also. In the near future, this industry will continue to play a large part in the financial wealth of this nation as it has always played the key role in its health.

Industry Payor Trends

- *Medicare*—The major player in the payor community. In its current form, it is the largest payor of healthcare services. As a government agency, it is subject to politics in a significant way. In 1999, the future of the Medicare program is being debated at the highest levels of government. The National Bipartisan Commission on the Future of Medicare debated for one year, from early 1998 to March 1999, on how to keep the Medicare Trust Fund from going bankrupt in 2008.

    Of major interest is what happens to healthcare expenditures after the 2007 projections cited above. Medicare will have to share in the brunt of the expenses. The Bipartisan Commission was charged with recommending

---

[5] Relman, A. (1998). The Decline and Fall of Managed Care. *Hospitals and Health Networks,* July 5, p. 70. "[M]anagement costs, corporate overhead, and profits are taking too large a bite out of the healthcare premium."

T A B L E 12–5

National Health Expenditure Amounts
1996 Actual–2007 Projected
Selected Years
(in millions)

	1996A	2000P	2004P	2007P	% change 2007P vs 1996A
Payors					
Private pay and insurance	552.0	696.4	923.5	1145.8	107.6
Medicare	203.1	252.9	330.2	415.6	104.6
Medicaid	147.7	188.0	260.0	337.0	128.2
Other government	132.3	157.9	197.1	234.9	77.6
Total	1,035.1	1,295.2	1,710.8	2,133.3	106.1
Providers					
Hospital care	358.5	418.4	533.1	649.4	81.1
Physician services	202.1	253.1	339.6	427.3	111.4
Dental services	47.6	60.7	78.1	95.2	100.0
Other Professional services	58.0	77.7	106.8	134.5	131.9
Home health care	30.2	38.2	52.4	66.1	118.9
Drugs and other medical Non-durables	91.4	124.5	173.5	223.6	144.6
Vision products and other medical durables	13.3	15.8	19.6	23.3	75.2
Nursing home care	78.5	96.4	122.8	148.3	88.9
Other personal health care	27.6	39.4	63.5	91.4	231.2
Program administration— Public and private	60.9	88.1	118.0	151.3	148.4
Government public Health activities	35.5	46.9	61.3	74.9	111.0
Research and construction	31.5	36.0	42.1	48.0	52.4
Total	1,035.1	1,295.2	1,710.8	2,133.3	106.1
U.S. Population	275.3	284.9	293.9	300.5	9.2
Per capita spending	3,759	4,547	5,821	7,100	88.9
Percentage change from 1992		21.0%	54.9%	88.9%	

Source: National Health Expenditures Projections, http://www.hcfa.gov/stats/NHE-Proj/tables/t01.htm
Source: National Health Expenditures Projections, http://www.hcfa.gov/stats/NHE-Proj/tables/t02.htm

changes to the current program. They were concerned that between the years 2011 and 2030, 77 million baby boomers will turn 65 and there will be fewer workers per retiree to fund the Medicare program. So their goals for 21st century Medicare was for the program to be the following things.

1. Responsive to the needs of the beneficiaries
2. Cost-effective, for both the beneficiary and the tax payor
3. Available to younger workers who expect a financially viable program when they retire
4. Fair to providers[6]

Box 12–1 is a summary of the proposed changes. Its chairman and cochairman Senator John Breaux (Democrat from Louisiana) and Representative William Thomas (Republican from California) issued the proposal as a final draft on March 15, 1999. It recommends major changes in the method by which Medicare pays for services. Although there were some very new features proposed by the chairmen and it was supported by a vote of 10 to 7, it lacked the crucial 11-vote super majority needed to formally adopt the proposal and move it on to the Congress. In fact, President Clinton came out against the proposal just before the vote, praising the commission for its work but saying that "it falls short in several respects" and that he would develop his own plan.[7]

As we know from Chapter 4, as currently formulated, Medicare pays providers, such as hospitals, physicians, nursing homes, and home health agencies, for services rendered under specific payment guidelines. Under the proposed Bipartisan Commission guidelines, Medicare would subsidize patients' purchase of healthcare coverage from managed care plans that bid to participate in the program. Called "premium support," this proposal is similar to the plan currently offered to federal employees under the Federal Employees Health Benefits Program (FEHBP). Medicare beneficiaries would have been given a voucher worth a specific amount of money from which they could purchase a basic package of benefits. Any voucher dollars left over could be used to increase benefits beyond the basic package, or the Medicare beneficiaries could pay extra out-of-pocket premiums for additional coverages.

The Commission's other major proposal was the inclusion of pharmacy benefits for some specific sets of individuals or plans as outlined in Box 12–1. This proposal was extremely delicate and yet, because it does not endorse comprehensive pharmacy benefits, President Clinton rejected it. Half the commission was adamant that the drug benefit be included out of fairness because Medicare HMO beneficiaries currently receive drug benefits. But, heavy lobbying by the

---

[6] Press Release, 1/5/99—Medicare Commission Continues Analyses; Details Criteria for Medicare for Next Millennium, http://medicare.commission.gov/medicare/med1599-2.html.

[7] McGinley, L. (1999). Medicare Overhaul Shifts to Capitol Hill—National Commission Fails to Endorse a Proposal; Clinton Criticizes It Too. *Wall Street Journal,* March 17.

B O X 12–1

NATIONAL BIPARTISAN COMMISSION ON THE FUTURE OF MEDICARE

SUMMARY OF BREAUX/THOMAS PROPOSAL

MARCH 15, 1999

MEDICARE BOARD

The board would provide information to beneficiaries, negotiate with plans, compute payments to plans (including risk, geographic, and other adjustments), and compute beneficiaries' premiums (collected via Social Security system as with Part B premiums now). Board approval would be required for plan service areas and benefit package designs.

BENEFITS

The standard benefits package specified in law would consist of all services covered under the existing Medicare statute (Medicare-covered services). Plans could establish their own rules as to how the benefits would be provided. Board approval would be required for all benefit design offerings and the board would allow variation only within a limited range as the risk adjusters were proven over time.

PRESCRIPTION DRUGS

Private Plans

All private plans would be required to offer a high option that included at least the standard benefits package plus coverage for prescription drugs. The minimum drug benefit for high option plans would be based on an actuarial valuation, with standards and examples set by the board.

Low Income

The proposal would immediately extend coverage of prescription drugs to qualifying beneficiaries under 135% of poverty under Medicaid with full federal funding of the additional cost. That coverage could be provided through high option plans when the premium support system was implemented. (A special premium support schedule could be used to combine premium and drug subsidies for low-income beneficiaries.)

Fee-for-Service

The Health Care Financing Administration (HCFA) would be allowed to contract with or enter joint marketing arrangements with private insurers offering prescription drug benefits. That would allow a public/private high option plan or plans, with HCFA providing coverage for Medicare-covered services and its private partner(s) providing

Source: Summary of Breaux/Thomas Proposal, National Bipartisan Commission on the Future of Medicare, www.medicare.commission,gov/medicare/btp31599.html.

Continued.

Continued

coverage for drugs. HCFA's share of the premium in a public/private high option plan would simply be the premium for its standard option plan. In the longer run, HCFA would be allowed to transition the government-run fee-for-service plan to a more private-managed basis overall, possibly with different alternatives available regionally.

Medigap

The National Association of Insurance Commissioners would develop new model plans immediately under a federal directive. All plans would include basic coverage for prescription drugs. One plan would be drug-only. Plans would vary regarding the degree Medicare coinsurance was covered.

PREMIUM FORMULA BASICS

Beneficiaries would pay 12% of the premium for the standard benefits package on average, pay no premium for plans less than about 85% of national weighted average, and pay all of the additional premium for plan premiums above national weighted average. (An example of this type of premium schedule was included in the estimate from February 17.)

Although all plans would be available on the national premium schedule, only the cost of standard benefits (Medicare-covered services) would count toward the computation of the national weighted average premium. Plans with only a high option would be required to separate out the cost of extra benefits in their submission to the board for that purpose.

If early versions of the risk adjuster would otherwise fail to prevent excessive premium differences between high and standard option plans, the board's actuaries could require that differences in premiums reflect the difference in value of benefits offered for private plans with multiple benefit options.

In areas where only the government-run fee-for-service plan operated, the beneficiary obligation would be limited to the lower of 12% of the fee-for-service premium or 12% of the national weighted average premium.

FEE-FOR-SERVICE BENEFITS

The government-run fee-for-service plan would have a $400 combined deductible, indexed to the growth in Medicare costs. Coinsurance of 10% would be charged for home health, laboratory services, and certain other services not currently subject to coinsurance. No coinsurance would be charged for inpatient hospital stays and preventive care.

MANAGEMENT OF THE GOVERNMENT-RUN FEE-FOR-SERVICE PLAN

All plans, private plans and the government-run fee-for-service plan, would compete in the premium support system; all plans would have premiums and would be available on the national schedule. The fee-for-service plan would have a premium like any other plan—it would adjust its premium in subsequent years based on its cost experience.

Concluded

The proposal recommends that efforts to contain costs in the fee-for-service plan continue. Toward that end, HCFA would be allowed to pursue competitive purchasing strategies in areas where its payments were not appropriate. The estimate assumes that the growth of fee-for-service spending would be moderated somewhat by a combination of HCFA and Congressional efforts. Without such ongoing savings, the fee-for-service plan could gradually lose its competitive position with private plans.

SPECIAL PAYMENTS (EDUCATION, DISPROPORTIONATE SHARE, RURAL SUBSIDIES)

Under the proposal, federal support for direct medical education (DME) would be carved out of Medicare. DME funding would continue through either a mandatory entitlement or multiyear discretionary appropriation program separate from Medicare. Depending on the nature of the replacement program for DME, the federal budget as a whole might not be affected by the carve-out. The proposal would also recommend exploring funding disproportionate share hospitals (DSH) and indirect medical education (IME) outside of the Medicare program and financing those items through a mandatory or multiyear discretionary appropriation program.

Any special payments remaining in Medicare would not be included in premiums for the government-run fee-for-service plan or private plans.

RETIREMENT AGE

The normal age of eligibility would be gradually raised from 65 to 67 to conform with that of Social Security. Congress would develop an exemption process for affected beneficiaries with special needs, such as those unable to work and otherwise get health coverage. Eligibility requirements under that exemption process would not necessarily be the same as the requirements for eligibility based on disability for those under 65, although the waiting period for eligibility based on disability could also be waived or shortened for those affected by the change.

LONG-TERM CARE

The proposal indicates that long-term care issues should be separated from Medicare (an acute care program). The proposal would require a study of various long-term care issues. The cost estimate does not include any impact on the budget from long-term care items.

FINANCING

The proposal would implement a combined trust fund, with guaranteed general revenue funding to grow at the same rate as overall program costs if it otherwise would exceed 40% of the program's cost (without further Congressional approval). The initial balance in the combined fund would equal the balance in the Part A and Part B funds at the time of enactment.

pharmaceutical industry since the inception of Medicare has kept this benefit out of the hands of most Medicare beneficiaries.[8] Still, legislative threats to impose the equivalent of price controls on the pharmaceutical industry allowed the Commission to agree to this partial yet rejected concession.

The Bipartisan Commission's recommendations, had they been adopted, would have changed the Medicare program dramatically. While the federal employees currently use this premium support system, it is unclear how it would fair with Medicare recipients. In any event, this type of radical change was sure to create upheaval in the delivery of medical care to the elderly. There was no assurance that this change would have been positive or negative. HCFA actuaries released a report during the last week of February 1999 indicating that the premium support proposal should save at least $75 billion over a 10-year period. Still it is not clear that the proposal will save enough money to keep the Medicare program solvent through the year 2030.

President Clinton criticized the Commission proposal primarily for three reasons.

1. It would have raised the age of eligibility for benefits from 65 to 67, a move that would increase the number of Americans without health insurance.

2. It would not include comprehensive prescription drug benefits, only some partial benefits to specifically targeted economic groups.

3. It would not require that 15% of the budget surplus over the next 15 years be used to help shore up Medicare.

This last item was important to the President because, in his Year 2000 budget proposal, he pledged to use $700 billion of the federal budget surpluses to ensure Medicare's solvency through the year 2020. In doing so, he did not detail whether he would expect this money to be spent using the current Medicare reimbursement methodology or a different one. As the details become known, and the fallout from the Commission's inability to vote out an acceptable proposal, healthcare financing could embrace a very interesting and different alternative future. These various proposals will continue to make the future of healthcare financial management quite entertaining.

- *Managed Care*—As we already saw in Figure 4–6, almost 67 million Americans, or 25.2% of the population, are enrolled in managed care programs. Most of these members are enrolled through their employers. Still, according the latest government statistics for 1997, 8.2% of Medicare patients, or 5.5 million, and 7.2% of Medicaid patients, or 4.8 million, are enrolled in managed care programs where the programs contract directly with the HMO to pay the appropriate annual premium.[9]

---

[8] Lagnado, L., Mcginley, L., Tanouye, E. (1999). Dose of Reality, Idea of Having Medicare Pay for Elderly's Drugs Is Roiling the Industry. *Wall Street Journal,* February 19, p. 1.

[9] Health, United States, 1998, Table 135.

Managed care emerged quickly in the 1990s to supersede the old indemnity health insurance polices that paid providers the charges that were billed to these insurance companies. When the ultimate payors, the employers, tired of premium rates rising at ever increasing levels, they moved most of their plans to managed care. Throughout the 1990s the managed care plans controlled the employers premium increases through utilization controls and a heavy emphasis on payment limitations to providers.

By the end of the century, the managed care plans' control on both these areas is under severe attack. The government has been attempting to pass patient protection legislation since 1997 and although it has not yet been achieved, there is a very good possibility that it will succeed very soon. This legislation will remove some of the utilization controls that the health plans have been using primarily to limit specialist referrals, often for highly expensive tests. In addition, employers have been hearing a loud and clear call from their employees that they want more choice in their provider selection than has been available through the basic managed care health plan. This has lead to the new point-of-service (POS) offerings in many plans' that allow the plan member to receive service from providers outside the plan's panel with very little financial disincentive. This freedom of choice, however, carries a price with it.

Inevitably, the industry is starting to see the return of healthcare inflation that outstrips the inflation inherent in the rest of the economy. In 1999 employers are already starting to feel the pinch as managed care plans have proposed 6% to 12% premium increases.[10] At the same time, it has been reported that the percentage of U.S. workers enrolled in the more restrictive types of managed healthcare plans fell for the first time in 1998 according to a survey suggesting that the managed care strategy has run its course. The report found that 47% of employees covered by U.S. companies were members of either HMOs or POS plans, down from 50% in 1997. Meanwhile enrollment in the less-restrictive PPOs climbed from 35% to 40%.[11] This is an indication that the restrictive managed care plans premise of "less access, less cost" was no longer acceptable.

These upward cost trends are a function of several items.

1. Less restrictive, more choice plans
2. The upward surge of pharmaceutical costs, which are borne in large part by the health plans
3. The increase in the health plans medical-loss ratio, which itself has been driven by lower than required premium increases over the past several years

While the short-term future of managed care is probably secure, its long-term future is questionable. Medicare's plan to provide premium support payments to

---

[10] Walker, T. (1999). Experts Predict 6% to 12% Premium Increases in 1999—Employers and Employees to Pick Up the Monetary Slack after Healthcare Cost Hikes in Recent Years. *Managed Healthcare,* January, p. 17.

[11] Winslow, R. (1999). Measure of HMO Membership Fall for First Time. *Wall Street Journal,* January 16, p. A2.

patients as well as Medicaid's drive to enroll as many of their eligible members as possible may well reinvigorate the plans. To be successful, though, the plans will need to convince a skeptical public that they care as much or more about quality as they do about cost. Otherwise, these profit-driven plans may be replaced by not-for-profit, community-based plans controlled by hospital and physician providers that can demonstrate quality above cost.[12] Or employers may well decide they do not need an intermediary adding a 20% to 25% cost factor to the premium. They may choose to contract directly with providers.[13] Any one of these propositions is possible.

Industry Segment Trends

Hospitals

In 1975 there were approximately 1.5 million hospital beds in America. By 1996, this number had shrunk to just over 1.0 million, a reduction of about 33% in just 21 years.[14] In addition, the total number of hospitals had decreased from 7,156 to 6,201 in the same time period. If the bed count is extrapolated out, there should be no need for any hospital beds by the year 2038. But the demise of the American hospital is not likely to come that soon and possibly not forever.

Here's a riddle concerning the future of hospitals and hospital care. If the healthcare community is going to practice Star Trek medicine in the future, with medical tri-corders and magic pills developed through the use of gene therapy that do away with the need for surgery, why does the Starship Enterprise have a sick bay? It may have to do not only with the technical competency and proficiency of the nurses, doctors and technicians that treat the patient, but it may also involves the compassionate care given by these same individuals. Patients have come to prize the high tech and *high touch* environment of hospital care.

There is good reason to believe that hospitals will have to reinvent themselves in the next century to provide improvements in many areas in order to remain a viable delivery system. There is also ample evidence to believe that they can do so. Improvements might include the following.

- *Patient-friendlier processes from the registration function to the clinical climate followed by the discharge planning and billing requirement.* Many hospitals have already begun to adopt systems to deal with these issues. Heavy reliance on preregistration processes and point-of-service registration has been adopted at many facilities. Most new hospitals are built with private rooms only; semi-private rooms and wards are a thing of the past in many communities. Similarly, most renovation projects of

---

[12] Relman, A. (1998). The Decline and Fall of Managed Care. *Hospitals and Health Networks,* July 5, p. 70.

[13] Ibid.

[14] Health, United States, 1998, Table 109.

patient floors adopt the private room concept. Many hospitals have also adopted more highly structured discharge planning techniques that emphasize patient and family education and a wide variety of post-hospital options. This is often called continuum of care and it improves the awareness of the patients and their caregivers.

- *Development of additional revenue sources.* For hospitals to prosper and thrive in the future, they will need to tap into new healthcare services that may not exist today. One obvious developing area would be gene therapy clinics, but it is still too early. However, there are a number of areas where hospitals could increase their inpatient and outpatient revenues. The Advisory Board has developed a list of products and services that have the potential to generate additional top line revenues for hospitals. Some of these outpatient care areas include alternative medicine centers, mid-life women's centers, and digestive disorder clinics. Additionally the list includes hospital condominium products such as stroke centers, frail elderly units, and cardiac crisis centers. Finally The Advisory Board suggests medical management products such as remote chronic monitoring and catastrophic care planning.[15]

  To survive in the future, hospitals will need to develop these new revenue sources or steal market share from competitor organizations that are also trying to do the same.

- *Cost reductions based on improved clinical decision support systems.* There is an enormous opportunity in most hospitals to improve their cost structure through the use of utilization and consumption controls along with standardization of protocols and supplies. This was covered in some detail in Chapter 11. Hospitals of the future will have to stop talking and start doing.

  The best chance these providers have to accomplish this task is through the use of clinical decision support systems that include the hospital's unit costs and volumes segregated by physicians and clinical coding (such as ICD-9 and CPT-4 codes). This could and should be incorporated into clinical (critical) pathways development and monitoring. These systems exist now. The successful providers will take a leadership position and enlist their physicians to change ordering patterns that reduce costs while maintaining or improving quality.

  According to an article in the February 1999 issue of *Healthcare Financial Management,* "Information systems can help build critical pathways, measure variations in patterns of care, perform comparative performance assessments, and provide analytical services, such as quality and utilization outcome comparative data for special units or services.

---

[15] Product Innovations: 1998 Guide to Promising Health System Products and Services—The Advisory Board Company.

Other capabilities include order entry, laboratory test results posting, alerts and reminders, and providing clinicians with access to diagnostic algorithms, treatment standards, and educational services. The computerized electronic medical record enables providers to improve data accessibility and accuracy, provide on-line reporting capabilities, reduce duplication, and improve productivity, while reducing errors and cutting labor and office supply costs."[16]

Using the clinical decision support tools provides one of the best opportunities for healthcare systems of the future to position themselves as lower cost, more efficient, more patient-friendly providers.

- *Develop the concept of a virtual hospital or a hospital without walls.* This entity may include only a small physical structure for major surgeries and critical care beds. All other activities would take place at clusters of widely (or closely) separated facilities (e.g., imaging centers, same day surgery centers, and/or ambulatory centers for activities that cannot be accomplished over the phone or through telemedicine). There would also include a communications center that would facilitate electronic monitoring of chronic patients and telemedicine capabilities.

Physician Practice Management

Physicians, of course, will continue to practice medicine and their practices will evolve with the coming wave of pharmaceutical and gene therapies. How they run their office is another matter entirely. There has been a major revolution in the way physicians have run their offices over the past five to seven years. Physician practice management companies (PPMCs), the highfliers of the middle to late 1990s, have fallen out of favor. MedPartners, previously the nation's leading PPMC, sold its PPM operations to focus on pharmacy benefits management. The second largest PPMC, PhyCor, is in bankruptcy. There is a dramatic rethinking of what it takes to success-fully operate a physician practice in the near and far future.

A clue is offered in a report published by the Medical Group Management Association (MGMA), Performances and Practices of Successful Medical Groups. This is a benchmarking study that profiles groups that show superior performance in profitability and operating costs; production, capacity and staffing; and accounts re-ceivable and collections. As summarized in a *Modern Healthcare* article, highly suc-cessful physician groups manage their practices with seven common techniques.

1. Utilizing detailed cost accounting
2. Knowing the true cost of delivering care
3. Employing zero-based budgeting
4. Applying physician incentive compensation
5. Utilizing effective managed care contracting

---

[16] Rosenstein, A. (1999). Inpatient Clinical Decision-Support Systems: Determining the ROI. *HFM Magazine,* February, p. 52.

6. Employing effective coding techniques
7. Improving service delivery[17]

Physician practice is one of many areas where good past practices will work well in the future. All the items on this list are nothing more than good management practices. Any physicians who want to be managed using good practices can do so, easily. The challenge on the physician side of the industry is to effect a major change in the thinking of many physicians who simply do not believe they need to change. In the future, because of the major reimbursement changes for physicians over the past 10 years, behavior that follows the payment rules will lead to good financial results. If followed, the industry could experience dramatic cost savings as physicians strive to maintain or enhance their bottom lines through cost-effective management.

Skilled Nursing Facilities

SNFs will either be financially profitable or be a major cost drain in the future. It depends on whether it is a freestanding facility or a hospital-based facility. Under the new prospective payment system (PPS) of reimbursement for SNFs, a single national rate will be in effect for Medicare patients by the year 2002. This payment rate, which is variable based on patient severity, should increase the revenues of many low cost freestanding SNFs while drastically cutting the revenues of higher cost hospital-based units.

The reason for this is simple. Until 1998, skilled nursing facilities were reimbursed on their cost (with a reasonable cost limit). Thus, the hospitals received higher reimbursements because of their higher cost basis, usually associated some personnel-related and overhead costs. Conversely the freestanding facilities were paid lower rates as a result of their lower costs. When the government decided to level the playing field and pay one rate regardless of ownership, they not surprisingly chose the lower rates. This will probably cause many hospital-based units to close over the next three years as the full impact of the PPS becomes onerous in 2002.

The remaining SNFs stand to be highly successful. The aging of the population will require eldercare on a much more intense scale. Not only is the baby boomer generation approaching older age, many elderly are themselves getting older. The frail elderly, usually defined as individuals 85 years and older, are increasing. Their needs are greater and the SNF operators that figure out the proper formula of care should profit, probably through facility consolidations. They should be able to be financially successful without sacrificing high quality care.

Home Health Agency Services

Home health agencies (HHAs), on the other hand, will probably continue to suffer greatly at the hands of the government rate-makers. While it is still not clear how they will design a prospective payment system for HHAs, it is clear that the

---

[17] Jaklevic, M.C. (1999). Practices with the Best Practices. *Modern Healthcare,* February 8, p. 64.

reimbursement will continue to be held down at the sub-par levels effected in 1998 under the interim payment system.

The dramatically low rates, typically less than the cost of care being rendered, will probably have negative effects on access to the care that is so greatly needed by many Medicare aged patients. In fact, the head of the American Federation of Home Health Agencies predicts that "half the nation's 9,700 agencies will close in 1999 unless the reimbursement system is changed substantially."[18]

Home healthcare is an important cog in the continuum of care in the industry. A dramatic reduction of providers, along with the reduction of SNFs, will leave a gaping hole that will be very difficult to fill. It is likely that when the lack of service providers becomes obvious, the government will step in and restore the home health rates back to a rational level. The providers and patients already left in the dust will be nothing more than a memory.

Healthcare Information Technology Trends

Information system advances hold some of the greatest opportunities for the improvements of quality and efficiency at healthcare organizations. The ability for clinicians to know more about the patient and his or her medical, social, and economic history, as captured in an electronic medical record that can store, retrieve, and display this information in a user-friendly and timely manner, is coming soon. These types of information will allow the clinicians to develop treatment plans sooner because they will be able to make correct diagnoses quicker. In fact, in the future, the computers will be assisting the clinicians in making patient diagnoses. Medical databases are being developed that can assess the probability of a diagnosis based on the input of symptoms and complaints presented by the patient. The databases will be updated continually in real time with the latest clinical findings as published in clinical journals from around the world. Once the diagnosis is made, these databases will also provide the most efficacious treatment pattern. Clearly, a targeted approach to treating a properly diagnosed illness has a better chance of clinical success with a lower cost for achieving it.

That is just one of many improvements that information technology holds. Several articles in the February 1999 issue of Healthcare Informatics discuss nine hot healthcare information technology trends and what they may mean in the future. Each of the trends was chosen on the basis that it provides at least one of three critical components to healthcare delivery—lowering overall costs, offering a competitive advantage, and/or improving patient care.[19] Some of these trends are as follows.

1. *The Internet*—It will allow broader access to healthcare information. No longer will a clinician need to be hard-wired to a system or server outside his or her office. Now, any information that is put out on the Internet will be available at no additional hardware cost. The three major groups that

---

[18] Saphir, A. (1999). SNFs Face Prospect of Major Upheaval. *Modern Healthcare,* January 4, p. 32.

[19] Elliot, J. (Ed.). (1999). Nine Hot Technology Trends. *Healthcare Informatics,* February, p. 81.

might take advantage of this information, enterprise administrators, physicians and other medical personnel, and consumers or potential consumers, all have different needs. Anticipating the desires of the potential audience and matching them with existing or proposed applications will help the healthcare organization of the future to find a balance for enabling the Internet applications.

2. *Continuous Speech Recognition (CSR)*—Major breakthroughs in 1996 and 1997 improved the quality of CSR dramatically. The addition in 1999 of 25,000 medical word dictionaries is just starting to bring voice recognition into the healthcare mainstream. CSR lends itself to anything where people's hands aren't available and in communities where dictation help is in short supply. Currently this would include physical areas such as autopsy and operating rooms. It would also include the production of operative and radiology reports. But this rapidly evolving technology could allow many more hands-free applications enabling clinicians to spend more time with patients and less on administrative functions.

3. *Wireless Computing*—This is high tech at its finest, combining gee-whiz appeal with practicality. Wireless devices can be used by clinicians to review test results, take notes during patient visits, and consult drug formularies. They can also be used to collect better clinical data thereby improving outcomes and cost-effective care. Acceptance is higher with nonphysician clinicians than the physician themselves. But as voice recognition software improves and palmtop computers become even more cost-effective, it is probable that wireless computing will hold a significant role in the future.

4. *Telemedicine*—This is the concept of using computers and telecommunications to transmit medical information to remote locations. This is a program still in its infancy and yet was on a pace to exceed 55,000 consults in 1998.[20] Although state politics and cost considerations have slowed down the spread of telemedicine, the underlying concept of matching skilled clinical specialists with the needs of areas underserved by such professionals is still paramount. The technology continues to improve, the cost continues to decrease, and the need continues to increase.

5. *Data Warehousing*—This is more than the storage of mountains of data. At its best, data warehousing allows healthcare organizations to understand more about their costs, revenue streams, and consumers. It also allows organizations to mine the endless pile of data that has been accumulated within the various computer fields and turn it into something valuable. It is all about turning data into useful information thereby using the acquired knowledge to move the organization along in a positive direction.

---

[20] Essex, D. (1999). Telemedicine. *Healthcare Informatics,* February, p. 100.

Computers have become extremely powerful in terms of their data storage and retrieval capabilities. The information stored in them will enable organizations to more effectively market to managed care companies and/or directly to consumers. The organization that successfully achieves a breakthrough with their data warehousing will have a competitive advantage. It will be worth the effort to succeed.

Thus, information technology in the future of healthcare will play a key role in helping organizations to achieve mundane or lofty goals. When it comes to technology, there will be very few limits on the improvements that can be made to the care of the patient at a reasonable cost.

Other Healthcare Trends

Integrated Delivery Systems

One of the biggest trends that has not yet been covered in this book involves the formation of integrated delivery systems in healthcare. There are many books that have been written about the who, why, where, when and how of integrated systems. Mergers and acquisitions of providers were very hot for the 10 years between 1987 and 1997. Yet in 1998, these activities among providers fell by 27% according to Irving Levin Associates. Overall, publicly announced healthcare transactions, including hospitals, physician groups, HMOs, and post-acute companies, decreased 11% to 1,131.[21]

Could reductions in these merger and acquisition activities be the start of a trend? Have providers discovered that there is no synergy in vertical and/or horizontal integration? Is there a loss of focus on core services when administrators' time is fragmented? A 1998 Environmental Assessment produced by VHA, Inc., and Deloitte and Touche LLP concludes that consolidations will continue as the numbers of mergers remain at peak levels. Thus, notwithstanding the slowdown in merger activities in 1998, horizontal integration remains strong with big provider systems getting bigger and bigger. Still, because integrated systems have high fixed costs that often put them at an economic disadvantage to nonintegrated providers, there has been a heavy movement towards cost efficiencies. This will need to continue in the future for these integrated delivery systems to be successful. It may not happen.

Fraud and Abuse

It seems clear that efforts by government agencies to weed out fraud and abuse by healthcare providers will continue at high levels for the foreseeable future. There is a good reason for this. The government is simply going where the money is. As Medicare and Medicaid expenditures approach $400 billion a year, the opportunity to achieve savings is huge. Yet as reported during February 1999, the Medicare overpayment error rate for fiscal year 1998 declined from 11%, or $20.3 billion, to

---

[21] Bellandi, D. (1999). Levin: Mergers Fell Sharply in '98. *Modern Healthcare,* January 25, p. 8.

an estimated 7.1%, or $12.6 billion, the lowest error rate since the Office of Inspector General and HCFA began comprehensive audits in 1995. About $9.3 billion of the overpayments are attributable to billing for services that were not medically necessary or upcoding services for higher reimbursement.[22]

The reduction in billing errors since the start of the audit program indicates that when processes are monitored, significant improvements are possible. The good news for the industry seems to be that the government is beginning to back off its position that all billing errors constitute fraud. This will aid the dialogue between the industry and the government in the years to come. The ability of the government to refine and simplify billing rules, and the improvement in electronic billing systems and edit programs built into these systems will greatly contribute to reduced billings errors and help to achieve the savings needed by the government to keep its healthcare trust accounts solvent.

All this prognosticating about the future holds big promises and big threats. As the healthcare industry continues to prepare for its unknown future, it faces a daunting financing challenge. It needs to decide if it truly believes that the current projected expenditure levels can be sustained. Also will the country continue to allow a disproportionate amount of its wealth to be used for healthcare in the manner it has in the past? The industry is going to have to face public schizophrenia and political posturing as it winds its way down the path leading to an unknown tomorrow. The one constant we are assured of is that there will always be change.

A study commissioned by the League of Women Voters with the Henry J. Kaiser Family Foundation shows just how great a task this will be. The study found the following results.

- Americans love Medicare, and they say they're willing to do whatever's necessary to keep it, but they are loath to raise payroll taxes or personal contributions.
- Americans say people should be responsible for themselves as much as possible, but they think the government should cover long-term nursing home care so they won't have to use personal savings.
- Americans know that Medicare is in serious trouble, but their major proposal for fixing it is to eliminate waste and fraud.
- Americans don't want to cut payments to doctors and hospitals because they are afraid that if payments are reduced, fewer providers would take Medicare patients.
- Americans think that raising the Medicare eligibility age from 65 to 67 is a bad idea that would push large numbers of people into the ranks of the uninsured.[23]

---

[22] U.S. Department of Health and Human Services. (1999). Audit Shows Dramatic Decline in Medicare Overpayment. *HHS News,* February 9. http://www.hhs.gov/news/press/1999pres/990209a.html.

[23] Quinn, J.B. (1999). Public Is in Medicare Dream World. Washington Post Writers Group, *Chicago Tribune,* February 28, Section 5, p. 3.

In the end, healthcare finance professionals will need to understand all the factors that affect the finances of the industry. Whether they are managers, accountants, financial analysts, payroll or accounts payable specialists, materials management buyers, receivers or distributors, registrars, billers, collectors, or ombudsmen, they all have a common goal. The goal is to support the patient caregivers in every way possible. This usually means using their expertise to maximize revenues or minimize costs to produce the highest possible operating and net margins so that the healthcare organization they represent can continue to buy the latest medical equipment and hire the best qualified personnel to provide the best patient care. This may be why *CFO Magazine* published an article titled "Critical Condition—Why Healthcare CFOs Have the Toughest Finance Jobs in America." In the article they quote an amalgam of healthcare CFOs. One says, "The whole industry is in turmoil, and I don't think any of us know where this is going. We have a lot of options and I'm not sure any one is the right one but decisions have to get made. It's not just a business; there are enormous social considerations. Every day we have to consider that the consequences of not doing a good job are just terrible. We take it very, very seriously."[24]

And they take it seriously at Ridgeland Heights Medical Center, with an occasional cup of humor thrown in on the side. Finally they were happy to conclude another successful year. Then the clock struck midnight, December 31, 1999. As the second hand rolled over into a new century, a new era may have dawned for healthcare finance . . . or is it just a dream?

———————

"Dad, are you finally done?" asked an overly tired Susie.

"Well honey, I guess I'm done with this book," said a greatly relieved Sam. "But I don't think I'm done getting out the message of how important the things that we do in healthcare finance are. I suppose I'll keep doing something of this sort for a while. You know I enjoy doing it, so I'll just stay with it."

"Yeah dad, that's great. But remember I just heard you tell this whole story over the last year. I'd really rather go out and kick the soccer ball around with you," said Susie with just the slightest whimper in her voice.

"Yeah, you're right," beamed her proud dad at the active little girl. "Let's go."

---

[24] McCafferty, J. (1999). Critical Condition—Why HealthCare CFOs Have the Toughest Finance Jobs in America. *CFO Magazine,* January, p. 71.

ABOUT THE AUTHOR

Steven Berger is currently the Vice President of Finance at Highland Park Hospital, Highland Park, Illinois, a suburb just north of Chicago. He has over 20 years experience in healthcare financial management, having been a finance officer at five hospital-based healthcare systems. These many diverse organizations included urban and suburban facilities, both academic and nonteaching, ranging in size from 100 to 400 beds. He began his career as a Medicare auditor for the Blue Cross Blue Shield Plan of Greater New York and has also worked for a small CPA firm in New York City.

Mr. Berger is a Certified Public Accountant (CPA) and a Fellow of the Healthcare Financial Management Association (FHFMA). He is also a Certified Health Executive of the American College of Healthcare Executives (CHE). He has a Bachelor of Science in History and a Master's Degree in Accounting, both from the State University of New York at Binghamton.

Over the last 10 years, Mr. Berger has taught Master's level courses in healthcare financial management at two universities and spoken on a variety of healthcare financial subjects at seminars and educational conferences around the nation. He currently teaches two two-day courses several times a year for the Healthcare Financial Management Association. One of these courses, Fundamentals of Healthcare Financial Management, is the basis for this book. The other course, Turning Data into Useful Information: How to Effectively Collect, Analyze, and Report Financial and Clinical Data to Enhance Decision Making in Healthcare, trains both data users and data crunchers how to understand each other's needs and practical ways in which to meet those needs.

Mr. Berger has also published dozens of articles, columns, and commentary on all aspects of healthcare financial management over the past 12 years in local HFMA chapter magazines. He has also cowritten two articles for the national HFMA magazine, *Healthcare Financial Management,* on healthcare information system issues.

In addition, Mr. Berger is the President-Elect of the First Illinois Chapter of the Healthcare Financial Management Association and currently serves on the national Board of Examiners for the Healthcare Financial Management Association. In each of these capacities, Mr. Berger is part of a team that actively strives to improve the services available to the organization's members.

Mr. Berger is married to the beautiful Barbara. They have four highly active children who provide many fun-filled and fruitful days. When not working, the family enjoys participating in all varieties of sports.

I N D E X